Understanding Biological Psychiatry

Understanding Biological Psychiatry

Robert J. Hedaya, M.D.

W. W. NORTON & COMPANY • NEW YORK • LONDON

The author and publisher wish to acknowledge and thank the following authors and publishers for granting permission to reprint the following illustrations:
Figures 1.1, 1.2, and 1.3, from Hendelman, W.J. (1994) *Student's atlas of neuroanatomy*. Philadelphia: Saunders. Reprinted with permission.
Figure 1.4, from Ashton, H. (1992) *Brain function and psychotropic drugs*. Reprinted by permission of Oxford University Press.
Figure 1.8, from Tamminga, C.A. (1994) Images in neuroscience: Human brain receptors, II *American Journal of Psychiatry, 151*(3):342. Copyright 1994, the American Psychiatric Association. Reprinted by permission.
Figure 1.9, from Shepard, P.D., & Tamminga, C.A. (1994) Images in neuroscience: Human brain receptors, II *American Journal of Psychiatry, 151*(7):956. Copyright 1994, the American Psychiatric Association. Reprinted by permission.
Figure 3.4, from Soutre, E., et al. (1988) Twenty-four-hour profiles of body temperature and plasma TSH in bipolar patients during depression and during remission and in normal control subjects. *American Journal of Psychiatry, 145*(9):1136. Copyright 1988, the American Psychiatric Association. Adapted by permission.

NOTICE
The reader is reminded that times and medical knowledge change, transcription or understanding error is always possible, and crucial details are omitted whenever such a comprehensive distillation as this is attempted in limited space. We cannot, therefore, guarantee that every bit of information is absolutely accurate or complete. The reader should affirm that cited recommendations are still appropriate by reading the original articles and checking other sources including local consultants and recent literature.

DRUG DOSAGE
The author and publisher have exerted every effort to ensure that drug selection and dosage set forth in this text are in accord with current recommendations and practice at the time of publication. However, in view of ongoing research, changes in government regulations, and the constant flow of information relating to drug therapy and drug reactions, the reader is urged to check the package insert for each drug for any change in indications and dosage and for added warnings and precautions.

Manufacturing by Haddon Craftsmen, Inc.

For information about permission to reproduce selections
from this book, write to
Permissions, W.W. Norton Company, Inc., 500 Fifth Avenue,
New York, NY 10110

Library of Congress Cataloging-in-Publication Data

Hedaya, Robert J.
    Understanding biological psychiatry / Robert J. Hedaya.
        p.   cm.
    Includes bibliographical references and index.
    ISBN 0-393-70191-3
    1. Biological psychiatry.   I. Title.
    RC341.H425   1996
    616.89 – dc20   96-2429   CIP

W.W. Norton & Company, Inc., 500 Fifth Avenue, New York, NY 10110
http://web.wwnorton.com
W.W. Norton & Company Ltd., 10 Coptic Street, London WC1A 1PU

2   3   4   5   6   7   8   9   0

I dedicate this book to those, before and after, who pursue and then integrate knowledge, understanding, and wisdom. I hope that my patients and progeny will always be among them.

Contents

Acknowledgments

THIS BOOK HAS GROWN from a seedling thanks to many people. Chief nurseryman among them is Dean Schuyler, my mentor. During my early years at Georgetown University Department of Psychiatry, Dean always challenged my thinking and automatic beliefs and supported my quest for understanding without trying to win me over to his own point of view. I have been luckier than most to have found such a mentor and now friend. In 1991, when I showed Dean a short set of notes from an all-day workshop on biological psychiatry for nonphysicians, he commented that I had the outline of a useful book. Dean encouraged me to contact his friend and editor, Susan Munro, at Norton Professional Books. Susan has helped keep me on track when detours seemed quite attractive and has had the ability to keep my vision clear as to the purpose of this book.

I was fortunate to be trained in the fertile psychiatric environment of the Georgetown University Department of Psychiatry, which, under the wise hand of the late Richard Steinbach, was grounded in tradition yet vibrant and flexible enough to foster my exploration of the various psychiatric domains, including the National Institute of Mental Health, where I trained under William Potter and Matthew Rudorfer.

Following residency training, I was offered a teaching position at Georgetown University. The transition from student to teacher was extremely difficult; were it not for Patricia Meyer, my supervisor in Bowen family theory, I would surely have quit: "Don't quit until you have mastered it, then if you still don't like it, quit." What wisdom! After five years, I liked teaching, and after ten years I loved it. Once again, Georgetown had provided me with fertile soil for growth.

Throughout this process, from college to medical school, residency, and private practice, my wife Mindy has been the consummate partner. Without her, I could not be where I am today. She has always been my supporter, giving me the gifts of time and love that made pursuit of my interests possible. My children, Adam, Josh, and Caroline, have supported me in the writing of this book by dropping into my office and pulling me out for a breath of air, fun, laughter, and a few tears.

Finally, to my mother and father, Caroll and Joe, I can only say thanks for your constant belief in me, without attempts to control (which many parents cannot resist). You gave me a model of the best learning environment of all.

Introduction

THIS BOOK WILL TAKE you on a tour of your brain. I will provide you with a lot of information, in significant detail. At times, you may feel lost. I suggest that you refrain from worrying too much about the detail, that you simply get the flow of the main ideas. I also suggest that you put this book in your office; use it to educate your patients about brain function, how it relates to their symptoms and to their cognitive and emotional life. As you do this on a regular basis, you will find over a period of a month or six weeks that the ideas and concepts become internalized and integrated; you will then have the firm beginning of an exciting new model of human behavior, including cognitive and emotional function. This model will provide you with new ways of conceptualizing clinical problems and new directions for psychotherapy.

Many think that "the biology of mental illness" is a euphemism that refers primarily to medication and psychopharmacology: "To medicate or not to medicate. That is the question!" In reality, biological psychiatry is much broader than psychopharmacology. I hope to help you achieve an appreciation of this broadened perspective. Whether you are treating an individual, a child, a family, or a couple, you have an opportunity, an ability, and an *obligation* to examine and consider the biology of the individual(s) in the system as an integral part of the whole picture. As you develop the skill to think in this way, you will notice that you have found another piece of the puzzle of human behavior.

Paradoxically, the biological perspective will give you more therapeutic leverage. Consider these examples:

- A shift in perspective will occur when you are evaluating a marriage in which one spouse complains, "No matter what I say, he doesn't seem to listen. It just infuriates me so! We can't even have an in-depth discussion without him getting up and doing something else!" When the possibility of an attention-deficit hyperactivity disorder (ADHD) is entertained, and confirmed, it becomes clear that the husband's behavior is not personally directed at his wife. In addition, benefits of this trait (people with ADHD are never boring, like to explore, etc.) can be incorporated into the therapy, reframing a previously negative view of the marital situation.
- You are treating a person with narcissistic personality disorder. Taking a biological perspective, you wonder if the narcissism is the result of an inborn affective instability (an unstable internal emotional environment), a trait that causes the patient to constantly try to maintain internal balance and avoid excessive emotional reactions to stimuli. When you understand this concept, you can explain to the patient that, because she was, in all likelihood, born with this trait (alternatively, it became "wired in" at a very early age as a result of a very unstable external environment), and has had to constantly struggle with her reactivity, she has not learned to look outside of herself, except as a means of keeping the internal overreactivity under control. This internal turmoil has reduced her capacity to truly see another person. This has resulted in people around her feeling diminished and has affected the quality of her relationships. This conceptualization is freeing and often makes sense to patients.

Chapter 1, Foundations, will start with the gross anatomy of the brain (the view of the brain with the unaided eye). Following this, you will explore the microscopic view of the brain, examining the actual functional building blocks of the nervous system, the nerve cells. This will be followed by a discussion of the most important chemicals of the brain, which are used for the communication process between cells in various areas of the central nervous system (the central nervous system [CNS] is made up of the brain and spinal cord, as opposed to the peripheral nervous system [PNS], which is the extension of the nerves from the spinal cord into the muscles, organs, and skin). Finally, you will learn the basics about how nerve cells function (e.g., how we learn).

Chapter 2, Core Concepts in Biological Psychiatry, is the heart of this book. Biological theories of mental disorders are growing more complex as researchers successfully focus in on the core biological functions. This portion of the book will simplify these theories, as they are currently understood. Seven general biological concepts areas are covered: (1) heredity and genetics; (2) reactivity, temperament, and dysregulation; (3) personality; (4) sensitization and kindling; (5) biological rhythms (chronobiology); (6) psychoendocrinology; (7) brain plasticity, learning, and memory. These concepts offer you the potential to approach clinical problems with surprising versatility and will strongly affect your understanding of the development of personality as well as mental health and illness. This will be followed by an exploration of the current state of genetic studies, the role of hormones in psychiatry, and a discussion of current findings in the exciting new area of brain imaging.

In chapter 3, Biological Theories of the Major Psychiatric Disorders, you will apply the concepts you have learned in chapters 1 and 2. Each clinical disorder will be discussed (where relevant information exists) in relation to classification, diagnosis, and associated comorbid disorders; biology (including genetics, animal models, neurology, neurotransmitters, hormones, markers, brain imaging studies); psychosocial theory; and the clinical implications of these theoretical models. The discussion will be interspersed with case presentations and concluded with integration and a summary. This chapter will enable you to develop more effective treatment techniques, avoid common but harmful treatment approaches, and respond to patients from a biological framework, in addition to your usual models.

Chapter 4, Medical Mimics of Mental Disorders, involves actual case presentations, followed by a discussion of some general rules of thumb that can help you to spot medical mimics of mental disorders. The chapter closes with the presentation of three cases involving medical mimics that presented as psychiatric disorders. Screening for medical mimics is something any responsible clinician must do, regardless of how obvious it may seem that psychosocial explanations can account for the presenting problems. In my opinion, there are few errors we can make as clinicians that are worse than treating an individual, couple, or family for months or years only to discover (after much frustration, or worse) that the problem, the focus of our psychosocial therapeutic efforts, has been largely medically caused. Most clients will appreciate the thoroughness and open-mindedness demonstrated by your willingness to consider nonpsychosocial factors in your evaluation.

Chapter 5, Practical Considerations in the Use of Medications, begins with an exploration of the split treatment model, in which a psychiatrist prescribes medication and another mental health provider treats the patient with psychotherapy. (I call this the therapeutic triangle, although with the advent of managed care some would call it a therapeutic rectangle.) The discussion will help you to manage the triangle to maximize the patient's improvement. This is followed by a discussion of how to work with the biological psychiatrist (including how refer patients to the psychiatrist effectively), as well as the therapist's role in facilitating the success of pharmacotherapy. The remainder of the chapter explores the frequent questions about practical issues, such as medications and dependency, long-term side effects, pregnancy, nursing, driving, the elderly, treating recovered addicts, lifestyle issues (e.g., sleep and diet), compliance, drug interactions, length of treatment, polypharmacy, and multiple medication trials.

Chapter 6, The Psychotropic Medications, is devoted to a review of all classes of medication used in biological psychiatry. Each class of medication is reviewed with regard to when it is being used clinically, how and where we believe it works, dosages, side effects, and significant risks.

It is my hope that this book will stimulate your curiosity, generate new ways of thinking about clinical problems, and, of course, result in improved outcome for your clients.

Understanding
Biological
Psychiatry

CHAPTER 1

Foundations

GROSS ANATOMY

OUR BRAIN IS WHAT makes us human. It coordinates all of our internal body functions, as well as our interactions with the external world. It follows, then, that to have a full, well-rounded understanding of mental health and emotional dysfunction we must understand not only the psychological, social, and spiritual aspects of mental health and illness, but also the biological structure and function of the nervous system. Recognizing this need, as well as the rapid progress in the neurosciences, the United States Congress declared the 1990s "The Decade of the Brain."

Of all the organs in the human body, the brain (figure 1.1) is the most difficult to study, due to its protective encasement in the skull. While modern imaging techniques have recently elucidated the structure and function of the living brain, medical science has known its gross anatomy for hundreds, if not thousands, of years. As a result of this history, the language of neuroanatomy is essentially Latin. However, I suggest that you leave the Latin for last; it is more important to learn the concepts, always developing a mental picture of the subject before moving on. This chapter provides the foundation for the rest of the book and, more importantly, for the development of confidence in working with biological psychiatrists and clients.

1

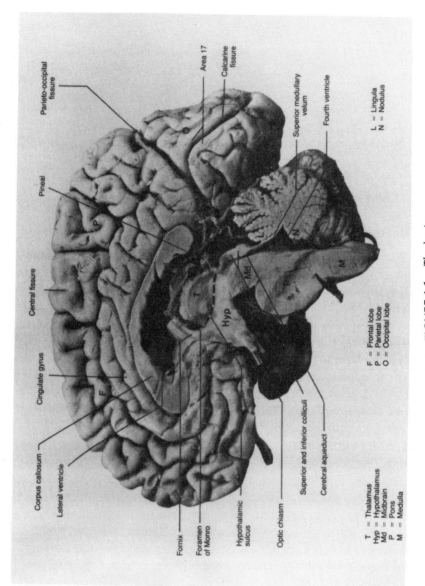

Corpus callosum

Central fissure

Cingulate gyrus

Parieto-occipital
fissure

Pineal

Area 17

Calcarine
fissure

Lateral ventricle

Fornix

Foramen
of Monro

Hypothalamic
sulcus

Optic chiasm

Superior and inferior colliculi

Cerebral aqueduct

Superior medullary
velum

Fourth ventricle

T = Thalamus
Hyp = Hypothalamus
Md = Midbrain
P = Pons
M = Medulla

F = Frontal lobe
P = Parietal lobe
O = Occipital lobe

L = Lingula
N = Nodulus

FIGURE 1.1.   The brain.

2

Section Overview

The brain can be subdivided in three different ways, all of which are useful. Each approach reflects our increasingly sophisticated understanding of nature's most fascinating organ.

First, the brain can be divided by its obvious *structure* into physical units:

- hemispheres (right, left)
- lobes (frontal, temporal, parietal, occipital)
- nerve tracts (groups of nerve fibers carrying signals to and from the same area)
- nuclei (dense collections of nerve cells with common specific functions)

Second, the brain can also be subdivided according to its presumed *time of evolutionary development*. In this scheme, postulated by Paul MacLean (1978), the most recent parts of the brain to evolve are most advanced in function, and have been added on to the earlier, more primitive layers of brain. These deeper structures are presumed to control more primitive, basic functions. This model divides the brain into the thinking brain (late mammalian), the emotional brain (early mammalian), and the primitive brain (reptilian).

Third, the brain can be subdivided according to *functional systems*. In the most sophisticated approach to date, any function of the brain is seen as the product of a very complex interplay of activity in different brain regions, both advanced and primitive, which occurs in a perfectly synchronized, sequential manner.

A more in-depth review of each of these approaches follows; it will serve as your vehicle to the study of gross anatomy of the brain.

The Structure of the Human Brain

This approach to the human brain involves the identification of **hemispheres, lobes, nerve tracts,** and **nuclei.** Abnormal function of the individual nerve cells making up these specific structures is associated with specific clinical syndromes such as depression and panic disorder.

Hemispheres

Visual examination of the human brain reveals that it is divided into two halves, the right and left hemispheres, which are almost identical reflections of each other. The dominant hemisphere (usually the so-called left brain in right-handed people) processes information in an analytic, sequential, linear fashion, while the nondominant hemisphere (usually the right brain in right-handed people) processes information in a visual-spatial, emotional, gestalt, holistic manner.

Lobes

Within each hemisphere one can visually identify four large segments called lobes (figure 1.1): the frontal (in the front), temporal (by the temples), parietal (above the ear), and occipital (the rear) lobes. In a general sense, various functions are known to be associated with, but not limited to, each lobe.

The frontal lobes are generally involved in self-awareness (introspection, physical and emotional sensation) and executive functions (focusing, planning, judgment, decision making, social functioning). Closely associated with brain regions that involve emotion, they regulate the expression of emotion and of motor behavior. Neuropsychological testing and brain imaging studies indicate that the frontal lobes seem to be involved in schizophrenia, disorders of attention such as attention deficit disorder, obsessive compulsive disorder, and mood disorders.

The parietal lobes are generally associated with the coordination of sensation and motor behavior (such as the coordination of language functions), spatial orientation (knowing where your body is, in a physical sense), and recognition of people and objects.

The temporal lobes are intimately involved in memory formation, language, and learning. Clinically, euphoria, auditory hallucinations, and delusions are usually associated with impaired function of the dominant (usually left) temporal lobe, while dysphoria, depression, irritability, and inappropriate affect are associated with abnormalities of the nondominant (usually right) temporal lobe.

The occipital lobes are associated with vision and visual memory.

Nerve Tracts

On examination of the surface of the brain, each lobe appears to be separated from its neighboring lobe by clear and obvious surface folds and cleavage called **fissures**. This apparent separation of the lobes is belied by the extensive submerged connections: the various nerve tracts. Just as tertiary and secondary roads feed into main highways, individual nerve cells carrying signals from one location to another are bundled into nerve tracts. These communication pathways, or information superhighways, may carry signals locally, between hemispheres (corpus callosum and anterior commisure), or between higher and lower brain centers. Much of the brain is made up of these communication tracts, which are often named (in Latin of course) according to their site of origin and destination. (Thus, the mesocortical tract carries information between the mid[meso]-brain and the cortical areas.) Several tracts are of clinical importance in biological psychiatry, and you should develop some visual idea of their location (figures 1.1–1.5).

The Corpus Callosum: Bridge between Hemispheres
As a body (corpus) of nerve fibers of colossal proportions, this tract allows each hemisphere of the brain to receive and send information to the other hemisphere, so that functions can be coordinated between the left and right sides of the brain. It has been implicated as abnormal in schizophrenia and attention deficit hyperactivity disorder.

The Cingulum: Emotional Superhighway
On the same level as the corpus collosum is the main information highway of emotion, the cingulum. This central highway seems to be involved with the summation and integration of emotion and thinking in preparation for final input to the hypothalamus, a central integrating station (discussed below). Thus, in contrast with the corpus collosum, which facilitates an integrative function of the left and right sides of the brain, the cingulum facilitates an integration from higher (thinking and emotion) to lower (the hypothalamic nuclei) brain regions. The cingulum is larger in women, whereas structures controlling aggression seem to be larger in men.

The Median Forebrain Bundle: Reward
The various tracts involved in the processing of pleasurable experience and reward (see mesocortical and mesolimbic tracts below) come together in a pathway called the median forebrain bundle. This bundle of reward fibers interconnects areas of the brain involved in

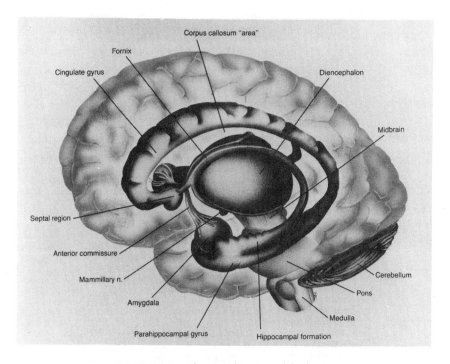

FIGURE 1.2.   The septal region of the brain.

mediation of emotion (the limbic system, discussed below), learning, arousal, memory, and hormonal control. It runs between the hypothalamus (figure 1.1) and the septal region (figure 1.2). This tract has clinical importance in depression, mania, and schizophrenia. In these instances, researchers have postulated that there is a fundamental imbalance of activity between the median forebrain bundle reward system and the inhibitory (punishment) center of the brain. In mania the pleasure centers are hypothesized to be overactive and/or the inhibitory centers, underactive. In depression the reverse would be so.

The Periventricular System: Punishment
This tract follows a path around (peri) the fluid-filled spaces within the interior parts of the brain (the ventricles, figures 1.1 and 1.3),

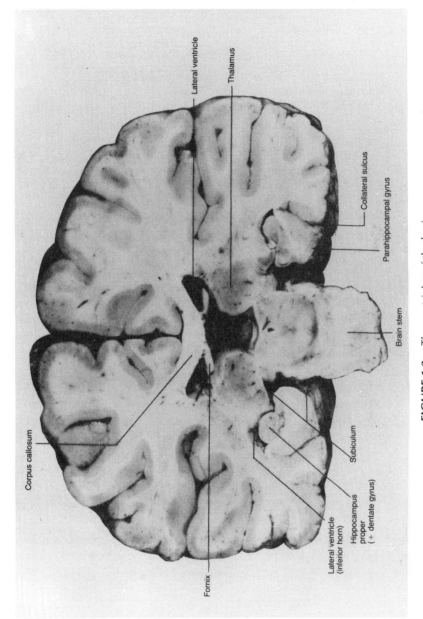

FIGURE 1.3. The ventricles of the brain.

Lateral ventricle

Thalamus

Collateral sulcus

Parahippocampal gyrus

Brain stem

Corpus callosum

Lateral ventricle
(inferior horn)

Hippocampus
proper
(+ dentate gyrus)

Subiculum

Fornix

7

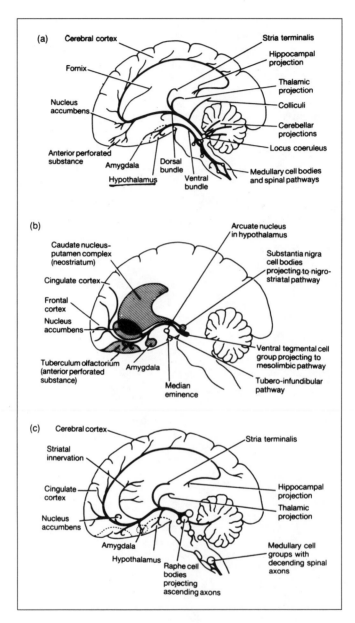

FIGURE 1.4. Monoaminergic pathways in the brain. (a) Noradrenergic pathways. (b) Dopaminergic pathways. (c) Serotonergic pathways. Note wide distribution of noradrenergic and serotonergic pathways and more discrete dopaminergic projections. Diagrams are based on animal data.

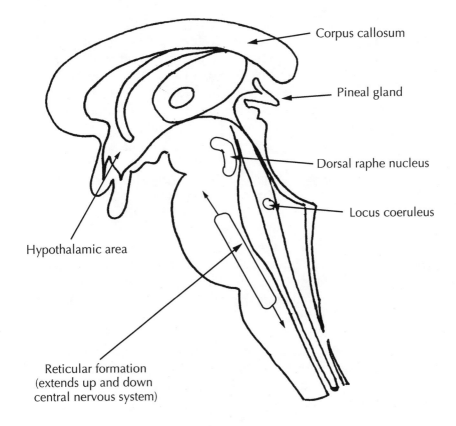

Corpus callosum

Pineal gland

Dorsal raphe nucleus

Locus coeruleus

Hypothalamic area

Reticular formation
(extends up and down
central nervous system)

FIGURE 1.5. The brain stem.

connecting the emotional, thinking, and hormonal functions of the brain. This is the primary inhibitory or punishment pathway in the brain; activation of this pathway seems to initiate avoidance behaviors. This tract is in balance with the reward tract, mentioned above. Together they modulate varying degrees of excitation and inhibition of behavior in various areas of the brain involved in learning, emotion, arousal, and hormonal activation.

Mesolimbic and Mesocortical Tracts: Reinforcement
These two pathways carry information between a part of the brain stem (figure 1.1) called the mid (meso) brain and the limbic system

(figure 1.2) and frontal lobes of the brain, respectively. The pathways that appear most involved in reinforcement are the mesolimbic and mesocortical pathways. These two pathways join to pass through the median forebrain bundle (above). Abnormal function of nerve cells in these two tracts has been implicated in the positive symptoms of schizophrenia, such as hallucinations (mesolimbic tract), and the deficit symptoms, such as flat affect (mesocortical).

Nuclei

Nuclei (figures 1.4 and 1.5) are kernel-like aggregates of nerve cells, which are the hub of specialized functions. One way of understanding a nucleus is to think of the map an airline might use to show all of its routes across the country. The larger cities, such as New York and Boston are the destination or transfer points of many routes; as such they are analogous to the nuclei of the brain. The brain has numerous nuclei, all of which are involved in a complex network of communication. Certain nuclei have been identified as having a clear role in specific clinical states. Knowing both the location of these nuclei, so you can draw a rough schematic diagram for a client, and the functional role they play in the biology of a particular client's problem can quell the anxiety of many clients. Following are some nuclei of current interest, along with their locations and clinical relevance (table 1.1).

Locus Coeruleus

This primitive brain stem nucleus, named for its bluish color on fresh examination, contains all the norepinephrine-producing nerve cell bodies of the brain! Hence, activity of the cells of this locus helps maintain arousal when activated and permits sleep when inactive. Full activation of this nucleus will evoke a clinical state of panic. Moderate activation will facilitate learning and cause anxiety. It is easier to create a memory when one is moderately stimulated and aroused, than when either asleep or overstimulated. Here's an example of arousal facilitating learning:

!!!LOCUS COERULEUS!!!

TABLE 1.1
Brain Nuclei: Clinical Relevance

NUCLEUS	NEURO-TRANSMITTER	MEDICATION	LOCATION	CLINICAL RELEVANCE
Locus coeruleus	NE	Tofranil, Nardil, Xanax, Inderal, Depakote	Brain stem	Panic disorder, posttraumatic stress disorder (full activation), arousal, anxiety, learning (moderate activation)
Amygdala	DA ACH	Anticonvulsants, antipsychotics	Limbic system	Involved in control of emotional tone Implicated in inappropriate rage, fear, sexuality, seizures
Suprachias-matic nucleus	5-HT EAA GABA	SSRIs	Hypothalamus	Internal pacemaker Possibly involved in seasonal and nonseasonal affective disorders
Solitary nucleus	NE 5-HT (?)	Tofranil, Nardil, Inderal, SSRIs	Brain stem	Involved in suffocation alarm theory of panic disorder
Dorsal raphe	5-HT	BuSpar, Klonopin, SSRIs	Brain stem	Involved in decreasing anxiety Site of action of Buspar
Corpus striatum (basal ganglia)	DA	Antipsychotics, L-DOPA	Cerebral hemispheres	Mediates involuntary muscle movement, tone Site of Parkinson's disease, medication side effects Involved in affective disorders and OCD
Hypothalamus	NE DA 5-HT EAA	Almost all psychotropics	Immediately above the brain stem	Directs homeostasis, mind-body link, interface of nerve, hormone, and immune systems Regulates autonomic nervous system
Accumbens	DA	Antipsychotics	Limbic system	Mediates the reinforcing properties of drugs of abuse Involved in deficit schizophrenia

EAA = excitatory amino acid neurotransmitter NE = norepinephrine 5-HT = serotonin DA = dopamine GABA = gamma amino buteric acid ACH = acetylcholine SSRI = selective serotonin reuptake inhibitors (e.g., Prozac, Zoloft)

The Amygdala

The amygdala is a group of nuclei involved in the control of emotional arousal, rage, and fear. Because it is easily stimulated, seizures (spontaneous, uncontrolled, spreading bursts of nerve cell activity) frequently develop in the amygdala. These seizures are accompanied by rage, as well as stereotypic chewing and/or lip smacking. Conversely, in monkeys (Kluver & Bucy, 1937), destruction of parts of the amygdala results in a syndrome of docility, clinging, inappropriate sexual behavior, as well as mouthing of objects (the Kluver-Bucy syndrome). Certainly a clinician must be aware of this diagnostic possibility when working with patients who have a history of rage or violence. Ruling out a seizure disorder is a necessary prelude to any psychological formulation of episodic rage.

Suprachiasmatic Nucleus

This group of cells sits on top (supra) of the nerves that come from the eyes (optic chiasm). As a pacemaker of internal circadian rhythms, this nucleus helps keep the internal physiological rhythms and the day-night cycle in synchrony by monitoring the amount and timing of daylight, and then sending that information to other centers for integration and adjustment of the hourly, daily, and seasonal pulses of hormonal output. This nucleus has been implicated in the biological basis of seasonal affective disorders, as well as the abnormal rhythms of sleep, appetite, and energy in the affective disorders.

Solitary Nucleus

This nucleus receives input from the larynx, pharynx, and thorax (the throat and upper respiratory tract). It is involved in monitoring the amount of CO_2 (carbon dioxide) in the blood. Normally, when breathing decreases, the level of CO_2 increases. When the amount of CO_2 in the blood rises past a certain "set-point," the solitary nucleus is activated and a "suffocation alarm" goes off. One takes a deep breath, and a panic response may ensue, via the locus coeruleus. Klein (1993) believes that a solitary nucleus that is too easily triggered may very likely be the basis of one type of panic disorder.

Dorsal Raphe

This is one of a number of a nuclei that sit in the midline (raphe) and on top of (as in the dorsal fin of a shark) the brain stem. This group of cells is involved in the regulation of anxiety. Apparently, when the locus coeruleus stimulates anxiety, activity is triggered in this nucleus, which then feeds back to dampen the anxiety. Nerve cells in the dorsal raphe are the target sites of action of Buspar (buspirone), a nonaddictive antianxiety medication.

Corpus Striatum

This group of three to five nuclei (depending on who is defining it), sometimes called the basal ganglia, is very intimately involved with motor control, muscle tone, and involuntary movement. Medication activity at these nerve cells is the cause of the movement disorders (called Parkinsonian effects) caused by many antipsychotic medications. Since the newer antipsychotics do not have as much activity here, they are much less likely to cause movement disorders as side effects. Abnormalities of nerve cell function at this site is the cause of Parkinson's disease. The caudate nucleus, part of this group, has been shown to have abnormal levels of activity in obsessive compulsive disorder.

Hypothalamus

The hypothalamus is a neuroendocrine (neurons which produce hormones) group of nuclei that lie under (hypo) the thalamus (a part of the brain with sensory, motor, and integrative functions). The hypothalamus is the interface between the mind (psycho) and the body (somatic) (figure 1.6). It directs the internal regulation (homeostasis) of appetite, thirst, growth and development, immune system function, metabolism, and sexual and reproductive functions in two ways. As an integration and relay point, the hypothalamus converts the summation product of thinking (cortical activity) and feeling (limbic) into hormonal output, causing both a carefully orchestrated adjustment of basic vegetative functions (e.g., sexual desire and activity, hunger, thirst, temperature regulation) and immediate physical changes (e.g., heart, lungs, intestinal, and glandular activity) via the autonomic nervous system. Since the thinking (cortex) and emotional areas of the brain (limbic system) send information to the body via the hypothalamus and autonomic nervous system, it becomes quite understandable that **thinking and emotion influence the heart and blood vessels** (hence the higher rates of heart attacks and hypertension in people with untreated manic depression), **intesti-**

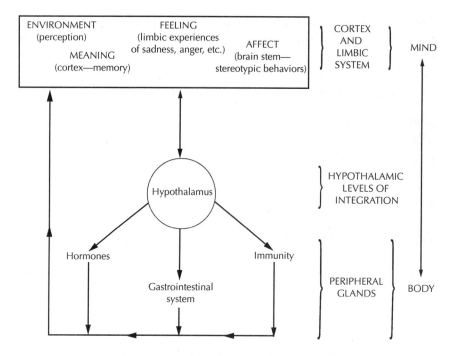

FIGURE 1.6.   The mind-body linkage via the hypothalamus.

nal functions (irritable bowel syndrome is associated with affective disorders), **lungs and breathing** (asthma is associated with affective and anxiety disorders), **urinary and reproductive tract function**, and **skin and gland functions** (the pancreas and the adrenal, salivary, and sweat glands are all affected by emotional state).

It is important, from a clinical perspective, to recognize that this is a two-way street: Neural input from the brain affects hormonal output (e.g., a stressed woman may not conceive a child), and hormones and substances produced by the body affect brain function (e.g., a man with a steroid producing kidney tumor becomes manic, while a woman with an underfunctioning thyroid gland may suffer from depression). Thus psychophysiological dysfunction is bidirectional.

Accumbens Nucleus
This nucleus of cells in the limbic (emotional brain) system is intimately involved in self-reinforcing behavior, pleasure and reward.

This nucleus is a major destination of neurons in the mesolimbic tract discussed above. Abnormalities of function in the dopamine receptors of this nucleus have been implicated as a final common pathway for all forms of drug abuse. In addition, the flat affect, social isolation, and loss of interest that occur in some schizophrenics (deficit type) seem to be related to this nucleus. Interestingly, all effective antipsychotic medications affect the "shell" of this nucleus, which may very well be an essential location for antipsychotic activity.

The Evolutionary View of the Human Brain

A second way of understanding brain structure involves Paul MacLean's (1978) formulation of the triune brain. In this formulation, we actually have three brains, each anatomically layered above the more primitive one. These three brains have, theoretically, evolved over the course of time. A highly simplified view of MacLean's scheme, with some modification, follows. Realize that these divisions are not as clear-cut as presented here; considerable overlap exists. The most recently developed, most evolutionary advanced layer in this scheme is called the **neo(new)cortex**: the thinking, perceiving, remembering, planning, problem solving, talking, and conscious brain, which is present in higher mammals. Below this is the **limbic system**: the emotional brain, which first developed in early mammals. The third layer, the **reptilian brain**, is composed of two parts: a neurohormonal brain (the hypothalamus, discussed above) and the brain stem (figure 1.5). The brain stem controls basic functions such as breathing, blood pressure, pulse, and arousal, and includes three sections, the medulla, pons, and midbrain. These various parts of the brain are interconnected by numerous nerve tracts and function in mutually interacting ways. Let's look at the triune brain in greater detail, paying special attention to areas of importance in biological psychiatry.

The Thinking Brain: Neocortex

The neocortex, sometimes referred to as gray matter because it has a gray color, is made up of six layers of nerve cells. It is primarily involved in integration and modulation of perception, conscious thought processes, memory, planning, and emotion. The bulk of this most evolutionarily advanced part of the brain is primarily made up of interconnections (see tracts above) among various centers of the brain and various parts of the cortex itself. These areas of communication are called the association areas. Other parts of the neocortex are involved in specific functions such as sight, hearing, speech, and voluntary motor behavior such as deciding to move your hand to turn this page. When we dream, we might connect one concept, sensation, or image, with something that seems, in our awake state, to be absolutely unrelated. This probably occurs in the association cortex, which seems to be at least as active in dream sleep as it is during the normal waking state.

The prefrontal cortex is the part of the neocortex in the very front of the brain (behind the forehead). It appears to be involved in planning complex behaviors (foresight), introspection (insight), and execution of novel and complex behavior. Modern brain imaging techniques indicate that abnormalities in networks involving the prefrontal cortex are present in disorders such as schizophrenia, depression, and attention deficit syndromes.

The Emotional Brain: Limbic System

Earlier in the course of evolution came the early mammalian brain. The limbic system (limbus means boundary or edge) is the interface between the newer centers and the oldest centers (figure 1.2) and as such has numerous two-way connections with the neocortex, above, and the lower brain centers (described below). The specific functions of the limbic system relate to the regulation of emotional states such as feeding, fighting, fornicating, family, and forgetting (the five Fs). The limbic system is fashioned from various nuclei (e.g., amygdala, corpus striatum, hypothalamus, discussed above), tracts (e.g., the cingulum, discussed above), and paleo(old)cortex—the hippocampus. The hippocampus is a critical area in biological psychiatry, and thus deserves more attention.

The Hippocampus

The hippocampus, or paleocortex, is much older than the neocortex. While the neocortex covers the surfaces of the brain, the older cortex has actually been folded in over time, so that it no longer is on the surface of the brain. Rather than six layers of cells (as the neocortex has), the hippocampus has only three layers, evidence of its primitive origins. The hippocampus is essential for learning and the consolidation of new memories. Cells of the hippocampus (and its neighbor, the amygdala) are exquisitely sensitive to the environment. As you will discover later, states of extreme stress can actually destroy the cells of the hippocampus; in fact, modern brain imaging techniques have demonstrated reduced hippocampal size in people with posttraumatic stress syndrome.

The Reptilian Brain

Our primitive reptilian brain is composed of the brain stem (like the stem of a wineglass, the rest of the brain sits on top of this structure) and hypothalamus (discussed above). In addition to basic life support functions, the reptilian brain controls stereotyped behaviors, which enable us to deal reflexively with the external environment. Such ritualistic behaviors include grooming, imitation (often seen in infants), and deception (such as simple stalking behaviors). Affective reflexes, such as opening the eyes wide with surprise, showing teeth with rage, withdrawing with fear, and some aspects of courting behavior (such as automatic body language) are additional examples of the reptilian behavioral repertoire. The brain stem contains the **reticular formation** (figure 1.5), a diffuse network of nuclei (including the locus coeruleus, discussed above) that seems to control the general level of arousal. The reticular formation has been implicated in attention deficit disorder and anxiety disorders.

A Functional Systems View of the Brain

This approach to the brain is based on functional networks involving various parts and levels of the brain operating in a sequential, synchronized fashion. Luria (1973, 1980), a neuropsychologist, suggests that the brain is composed of three functional units:

1. The most fundamental unit regulates attention and arousal and is diffusely present throughout the brain. It includes, but is not limited to, the reticular formation of the brain

stem and contains the locus coeruleus and raphe nucleus. This unit receives information from almost all sensory systems and relays that information, after much communication between different receiving stations (nuclei), to almost all the higher brain centers.

2. The second functional unit is a sensory network that receives, integrates, and stores perceptions (hearing, touch, smell, movement). This system includes parts of the brain stem, thalamus (an integrating and relay station), paleocortex (hippocampus), and neocortex.

3. The third functional unit is a motor network that controls the output, or motor behavior. It involves the frontal lobes, the corpus striatum, and other lower centers.

In essence then, Luria's model is made up of three units, which involve structures at all levels of the brain: One turns the machine on, the second takes in information, and the third controls output. All three units operate together in a holistic, synchronized manner.

Section Summary

Our understanding of brain structure and function has emerged after centuries of slow progress. This section has described three approaches to understanding gross anatomy of the brain. In the current functional systems model multiple structures at various levels participate in various processes via a carefully synchronized network of activity and feedback. Higher level structures show progressively greater degrees of response flexibility. The clinical importance of this information lies in:

- recognizing the anatomical basis of psychosomatic disorders: how perception, meaning, and experience are translated into hormonal, immune, cardiovascular, gastrointestinal, and sexual/reproductive symptoms and disease states.
- being able to educate clients regarding the nonpsychological aspects of their difficulties, thereby alleviating guilt without eliminating responsibility.
- understanding that similar cellular and chemical abnormali-

ties (such as "too much serotonin") occur in different brain regions and are associated with a variety of syndromes, yet are often treatable by the same medication!

- understanding the need for continually increased awareness and consideration of possible physical brain disease as a cause of abnormal behavior in individuals, couples, families, and coworkers.

THE STRUCTURE AND FUNCTION OF THE NERVE CELL

Understanding the structure and function of the nerve cell, the basic unit of the nervous system, has become a necessity for all mental health clinicians as a result of the explosion of knowledge over the last 35 years. This section will present the basics of nerve cell structure and function, enabling you to understand current theories of how medications work and how psychotherapy works, and provide a basis for appreciating the clinically important processes discussed in chapters 2 and 3.

Section Overview

After the chemicals (**neurotransmitters**) and essential structures (**membranes, channels, receptors, nucleus, axons**, etc.) of the **neuron** are described, the actual functioning of the nerve cell will be explored. The nerve cell exhibits two types of functional responses: immediate and long-term (**neuromodulation**). These two responses will be described in some detail, since grasping these concepts will take you a long way toward being able to view mental (dys)function in a holistic way.

Neurotransmitters

Nerve cells (neurons) carry information along themselves in the form of electrical currents. However, they transfer information between themselves via chemical signals. So, unlike wires, which must touch each other in order to pass along information or signals, neurons secrete molecules called neurotransmitters, which when released migrate almost instantaneously across the void between neurons. They act, as the word implies, to transmit signals from one **neuron** to another. Neurons in different parts of the brain contain different neurotransmitters. While individual neurons use only one type of neurotransmitter to send signals, most neurons contain numerous different receptor types and subtypes to receive many different signals from different sources that converge on it. The neurotransmitters currently thought to be of most importance in biological psychiatry are listed in table 1.2, along with related information.

Neurotransmitters are separated into three categories: **amino acids, biogenic amines**, and **peptides**.

Amino Acids

Included in this group are L-tryptophan, glutamate, GABA (gamma-aminobutyric acid), glycine, tyrosine, and tyramine. The major excitatory amino acid neurotransmitters are glutamate and aspartate, and the major inhibitory amino acid neurotransmitters are glycine and GABA (which is derived from the excitatory amino acid glutamate!). Most amino acids can be made in the body. Some, called essential amino acids (such as L-tryptophan), can only be obtained through the diet. For this reason serious dietary imbalances, as in severe depression, psychosis, bulimia, anorexia, and carbohydrate addiction, can affect the functioning of the nervous system. Amino acid deficiencies can impair the ability of antidepressants to act effectively.

Biogenic Amines

The biogenic amines are involved in the treatment mechanism and possibly the genesis of the major psychiatric disorders. The activity of these biogenic amines is the target of many psychotropic medications. The biogenic amines are derived from a series of minor changes in two dietary amino acids: tyrosine and L-tryptophan (table 1.3). **Norepinephrine**, also called noradrenalin, is the adrenaline of the brain. **Serotonin**, first discovered as a substance controlling the tone of blood vessels, was later found in various areas of the body, including the intestines, brain (where the effects of serotonin vary depending on the activity level of the norepinephrine nerve cells), and the immune system (where it seems to have an inhibitory effect). Knowing this, one can easily understand why psychiatric syndromes

TABLE 1.2
Neurotransmitters of Known Importance in Biological Psychiatry

NEURO-TRANSMITTER	TYPE	DERIVED FROM	CLINICAL RELEVANCE
GABA	Amino acid	Glutamate	The most ubiquitous Involved in sleep, anxiety reduction, muscle relaxation Involved in relaxing effects of alcohol
L-tryptophan (L-T)	Amino acid	Can only be obtained in the diet	Promotes sleep, especially when taken with a high carbohydrate, low protein meal Dangerous when consumed with MAO antidepressants
Tyramine (Tyr)	Amino acid	Fats and carbohydrates	Dangerous when consumed with MAO antidepressants
Glutamate (Glu)	Amino acid	Fats and carbohydrates	MSG reaction to Chinese food The major excitatory amino acid May be associated with neurotoxic effect in alcoholism
Dopamine (DA)	Biogenic amine	Tyrosine, fats, and carbohydrates	Mania, schizophrenia, Parkinson's disease, attention deficit disorder, substance abuse, tics, blood pressure regulation Antipsychotics (major tranquilizers) inhibit DA action Some antidepressants act here
Norepinephrine (NE)	Biogenic amine	Dopamine	Depression, anxiety, panic, blood pressure regulation Necessary for learning and memory Some antidepressants act in these conditions via this neurotransmitter
Serotonin (5-HT)	Biogenic amine	L-tryptophan	Depression, mania, anxiety, blood pressure and temperature regulation Many antidepressants, new antipsychotics, and nonaddicting antianxiety agents act on these conditions via this neurotransmitter

TABLE 1.3
The Formation of Biogenic Amines from Dietary Amino Acids

AMINO ACID	INTERMEDIATE COMPOUND	BIOGENIC AMINE
Tyrosine ⟶	DOPA ⟶	Dopamine ➤ Norepinephrine
L-tryptophan ⟶	5-hydroxytryptophan ➤	Serotonin (5-hydroxytryptamine)

that involve serotonin dysregulation (depression, mania, obsessive compulsive disorder, eating disorders, impulse disorders, anxiety) are often accompanied by irregularities in cardiovascular disease, abnormal bowel function, and allergy. **Dopamine** is involved in many of the higher brain functions, including attention, reward, and planning, as well as movement and muscle tone. Dopamine is found primarily in the frontal lobes of the brain and in the limbic system.

Peptides

Peptides are short chains of amino acids. This group of neurotransmitters is not as well studied as the previous groups, but it is known to be the largest, encompassing hundreds of neurotransmitter substances. The functional role of peptides is poorly understood, and to date none has been identified as causing any disease state. One example of a clinically important peptide neurotransmitter is CCK (cholecystokinin), a substance that provokes panic attacks in panic disorder patients. CCK was originally discovered in connection with the gall bladder and has been found in high concentrations in the cortex, amygdala, and hippocampus.

Recent Candidates for Neurotransmitter Status

In order for a substance to be classified as a neurotransmitter it must be synthesized and stored in nerve terminals and cell bodies, be released when the neuron is activated, have specific binding sites (receptor sites), affect the firing rate of neurons, and its effects must be capable of being blocked by molecules of similar structure. While these appear to be stringent criteria, new neurotransmitters are being discovered rapidly. Most recently, it seems likely, if not accepted, that nitrous oxide (laughing gas) as well as carbon monoxide (poisonous in large amounts) are produced by neurons. These gases seem to carry signals over short distances.

A CLINICAL ILLUSTRATION   I once gave a workshop to a group of approximately 100 counselors. After a lively first morning session, we paused for coffee and doughnuts. As we reconvened, I advised my audience that they would notice a two-part reaction. First they would experience a rise in mental acuity, and perhaps some jitteriness. Second, in about one hour, most of them would be quite drowsy. As predicted, the majority of my audience appeared dazed within an hour. While this effect might be due to my public speaking style, it was, as I explained to those still awake, at least in part mediated by two neurotransmitter changes.

First, the simple carbohydrate (doughnut) and the release of epinephrine (adrenaline) caused by the caffeine resulted in a rapid rise in blood sugar (the energy source of neurons), which in turn caused the members of the audience to experience increased mental acuity. Besides its direct energizing effect, epinephrine contributed further to the rise in blood sugar by releasing sugar previously stored in the liver. In the next phase of this predictable reaction, the rapid rise in sugar caused the pancreas to release insulin, with a subsequent drop in blood sugar. Finally the carbohydrate (doughnut) helped increase the absorption of L-tryptophan. L-tryptophan was then converted in the brain to serotonin (a biogenic amine neurotransmitter), which caused drowsiness.

Nerve Cell Structure

The individual nerve cell is called a **neuron** (figure 1.7). Neurons come in all different shapes and sizes and vary in length from microscopic to more than one foot. A good sense of the proportions of a neuron can be experienced when one realizes that if the cell body of the neuron were the size of a tennis ball, the dendrites of the cell would fill a room, and the axon would stretch up to a mile, while being only half an inch thick! Inside the central nervous system or CNS (brain and spinal cord), groups of neurons are usually called nerve tracts (discussed above). Outside of the brain in the peripheral nervous system (PNS) these groups of neurons are simply called

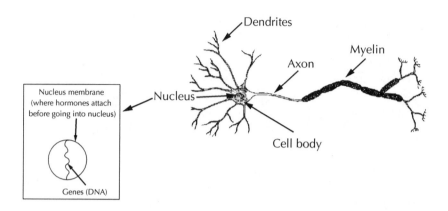

FIGURE 1.7. The neuron.

nerves. The neuron has several basic structures that can be grouped by their location:

- Embedded in the **cell membrane** are the **receptors, ion channels,** and **reuptake pump.**
- The **cell body** contains the **nucleus,** which contains the **DNA (genes).**
- **Extensions** from the cell body include **axons, dendrites, axon terminals, myelin,** and the **synaptic vesicles.**
- The **cell interior** includes **G proteins,** and **second** and **third messenger systems.**

The Cell Membrane, Channels, and Receptors

Neurons (figure 1.7) are visually analogous to a tree with buds. In fact, the visual correspondence is so striking that the terms used by scientists for the growth of neurons include "branching" and "arborization." Using this analogy, the bark of the tree is analogous to the **neuronal cell membrane** (figures 1.8 and 1.9), the "skin" of the cell. However, unlike the bark of a tree, which is hard and static, the cell membrane is a fatty, flexible boundary that keeps the cell as an entity. The cell membrane is made up of two layers of fats (called a phospholipid bilayer). Each layer is made up of individual fat mole-

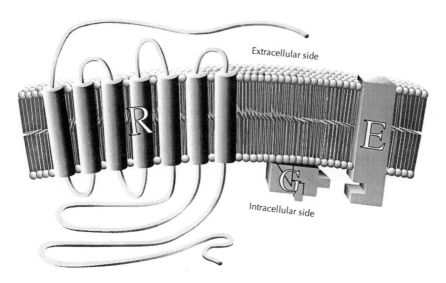

FIGURE 1.8. In the cross section of the cell membrane, note that the receptors (R) have seven sites that span the cell membrane in which it is embedded. The tail of the receptor protein, which is inside the cell, is adjacent to the G protein (G). When a neurotransmitter binds to the receptor, the receptor protein tail changes shape and activates the G protein, which amplifies the original neurotransmitter signal. The G protein in turn activates the effector protein (E), which then activates the second and third messengers, leading to neuromodulation. The site of action of lithium may be at the G protein.

cules shaped like an old-fashioned clothespin. If you imagine a circle made of a double layer of clothespins whose tails face each other, you will have a good mental image of the membrane. The neuronal cell membrane has two primary purposes:

1. The cell membrane keeps the inside environment of the cell stable to the appropriate degree. It functions as the gate-keeper, allowing substances to pass in or out of the cell, via specialized pores called **ion channels** and **neurotransmitter pumps**. The channels are passageways through which a number of positively and negatively charged elements (e.g., potassium, calcium, sodium, chloride) flow into and out of the cell. Pumps, on the other hand, more actively control the intake or secretion of neurotransmitters into and out of the cell interior.

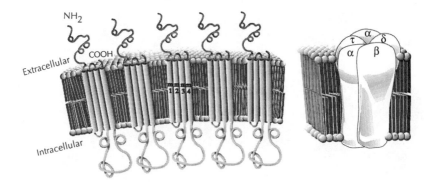

FIGURE 1.9. Ionophore receptor embedded in the cell membrane. Stimulation of the ionophore receptors (which are embedded in the cell membrane) causes rapid but temporary changes in neuronal excitability. On the left of the figure, the receptor is unfolded to illustrate its structure. Note that these receptors have five distinct subunits, and each one itself has four membrane-spanning units (m1–m4). On the right, each of these distinct subunits is labeled with a Greek letter. Note that these five subunits are actually grouped together in the shape of a cylinder with a central channel or pore. Electrically charged particles called ions (such as sodium, chloride, and potassium) can pass through this ion pore, to enter the neuron, rendering it more or less excitable. Many psychoactive drugs act at these receptors (e.g., benzodiazepines such as valium, PCP, and nicotine).

2. The cell membrane also carries electrical signals from one end of the neuron to the other. The difference between the total positive and negative charges inside and outside the cell determines whether a neuron propagates the signal it received on to the next neuron.

Receptors (figures 1.8 and 1.9) are microscopic, folded, protein structures that are transmembranal (they extend across the cell membrane, from the outside of the cell to the cell interior). When they are combined with the neurotransmitters (called **first messengers** because they are the first in a series of carriers of information or messages from one neuron to the next) that bind to them, a cascade of events (via **second and third messengers** inside the cell) occurs to convey information from the outside environment of the cell

*   via ion channels, which then close or open, thereby inducing the cell to be stable to a greater (behavioral inhibition) or

lesser (behavioral excitation) degree. This immediate cellular response affects the transmission of signals, but does not cause long-term neuronal changes (no learning).

* to the innermost sanctum of the cell, the nucleus and genes. Certain receptors initiate long-term changes in the neuron by activating or suppressing certain genes.

There are a number of abnormalities of receptor function in medicine, including a type of diabetes in which the receptors do not recognize insulin and a condition called peripheral resistance to thyroid hormone. This latter condition, although rare, is associated with attention deficit disorder.

Receptors have been the focus of a great deal of research in the neurosciences. There are hundreds of different receptor types and subtypes. As more and more receptors are discovered, their nomenclature is becoming more and more complex. Since the newer medications, such as Buspar (buspirone), Risperdal (risperidone), Prozac (fluoxetine), Paxil (paroxetine), Zoloft (sertraline), Effexor (venlafaxine), Wellbutrin (buproprion), and Serzone (nefazodone) are actually targeted to specific receptor classes and subtypes, some familiarity with how they are named will reduce your confusion.

Broadly speaking, receptors are classified into families, such as the dopamine family, serotonin family, and norepinephrine family. The specific subtypes of receptors (new subtypes are discovered almost weekly) are not relevant to your purposes. Receptors are named after the neurotransmitter that binds to it, for example, serotonin receptors. There are only two types of receptors known at this time:

* Gate or ionophore (think "ion-pore") receptors (figure 1.9) are made up of four or five transmembranal protein subunits. When one of these receptors is activated, the gates or channels of the cell membrane are immediately opened or closed to the flow of potassium (K^+), chloride (Cl^-), sodium (Na^+), calcium (Ca^{++}), and other charged elements (ions). The net result of this ion flow immediately determines whether the neuron is activated to fire (pass a signal to the next neuron) or inhibited (dormant). These receptors

are the site of action of alcohol and the minor tranquilizors, such as valium.

• G protein linked receptors (figures 1.8 and 1.10) also span the cell membrane, and are physically linked to an important protein family, the **G proteins** (over two dozen types have been identified so far). G proteins are the place in the cell where amplification and integration (summation and convergence) of various imputs occur. G proteins are very important in bipolar disorders and may be the site where lithium has its impact. These receptors are made up of seven subunits. Once the neurotransmitter docks in this receptor,

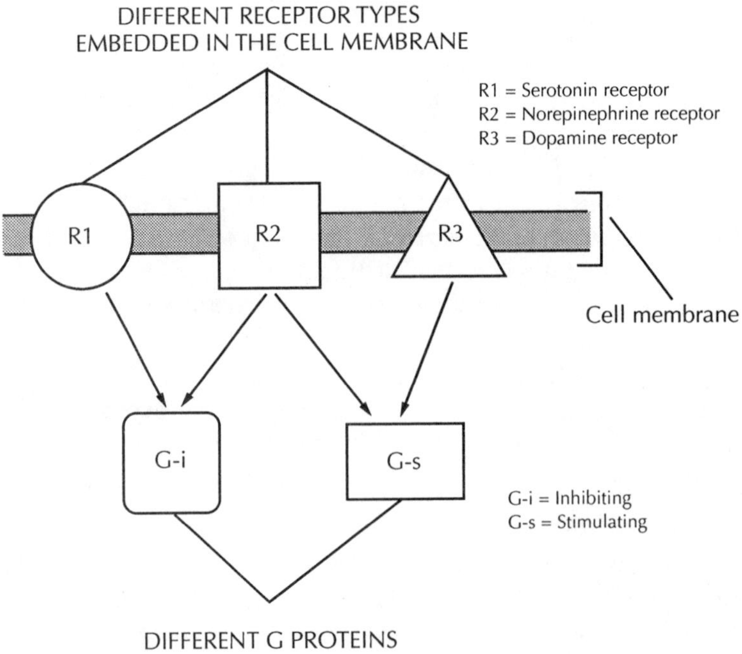

DIFFERENT RECEPTOR TYPES
EMBEDDED IN THE CELL MEMBRANE

R1 = Serotonin receptor
R2 = Norepinephrine receptor
R3 = Dopamine receptor

R1   R2   R3

Cell membrane

G-i   G-s

G-i = Inhibiting
G-s = Stimulating

DIFFERENT G PROTEINS

FIGURE 1.10. G protein linked receptor embedded in the cell membrane. Note that a single type of receptor can be linked to several types of G proteins (both inhibitory and stimulatory). A single G protein can be activated by different receptors. A single neuron may have receptors for a variety of neurotransmitters. This demonstrates the subtlety and complexity with which neural activity can be regulated.

the shape of the G protein is altered. This causes a cascade of internal events, which often leads to long-term changes (neuromodulation) in the types and amounts of proteins produced by the neuron and, therefore, long-term changes in its structure and function. The discovery of this receptor type has been critical in understanding how learning and memory occur, as well as the mechanisms involved in addiction (see nerve cell function below).

The Cell Body and Nucleus

In our analogy of the neuron as a tree, the root ball of the tree is analogous to the **cell body** (figure 1.7). The cell body is a wide area of the neuron that contains the **nucleus**. The nucleus is the command center of the cell, and it is here that the **genes** (DNA) are located. The genes contain almost all of the blueprints, templates, and recipes for cell structure and function. Hormones act at the nucleus to turn certain genes on and off, causing the cell to vary the amounts and types of protein produced for normal development, maintenance, and function of the cell.

Dendrites, Axons, Axon Terminals, and Myelin

Dendrites (figure 1.7) are short processes that receive signals from other neurons. They are relatively close to the cell body, and in our analogy would look like the roots of a tree. Frequently, an axon will have branches that turn back to itself, thereby stimulating receptors (called autoreceptors) on its own cell membrane as a form of feedback control.

Embedded within the dendrite membrane are the receptors, G proteins, and ion channels, discussed above. The **axons**, analogous to the trunk and branches of a tree, are relatively long processes that carry the proteins, chemicals, and electrical signals generated in the nucleus and cell body downstream to the **axon terminals**. In many neurons, fatty white coverings called **myelin** are interspersed along the axon. Since the electrical current can't pass through the myelin it jumps over the myelin, and the electrical current is moved down the axon at an accelerated pace, increasing the response rate. Multiple sclerosis (MS) is a condition in which the myelin sheaths are lost or damaged, causing an irregular and nonuniform slowing of nerve

conduction and a host of symptoms that are often labeled psychosomatic. MS is a great mimic of mental illness, often causing severe
depression or psychosis before it is diagnosed correctly (chapter 4).

Axon terminals are tiny bulging, bud-like structures filled with the
neurotransmitters to be released to the next neuron. Axon terminals
contain tiny sacs or packets called **synaptic vesicles** (figure 1.11),
which are filled with the chemicals that will be released by the activated neuron. These synaptic vesicles lie at the ends of the axon
terminals, ready—when an electrical impulse arrives—to release their
contents into the space between neurons, the **synapse**. The excess
neurotransmitter chemical is taken back into the neuron that released
it by a **reuptake pump**. This pump, which sits in the cell membrane
at the axon terminal, functions to clear the synapse of the neurotransmitter, and thereby end stimulation of receptors on the next
neuron.

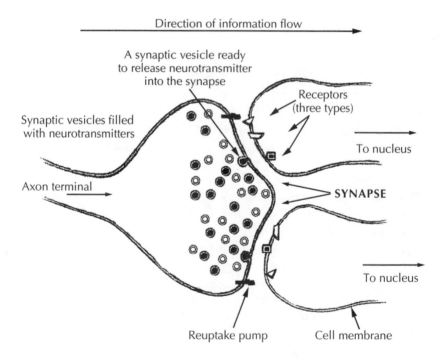

FIGURE 1.11.   The synapse. Left: presynaptic neuron. Right: postsynaptic neurons.

Section Summary

Neurons are the fundamental unit of the nervous system. These cells stretch a variety of distances to reach their communication targets via extensions from the main cell body (axons and dendrites). Neurons receive, monitor, and send information via an intricate cascade of chemical events that can have two possible outcomes (see next section) and a cellular machinery that exists to carry out these functions. This machinery includes a variety of structures for production (dietary amino acids and enzymes), transport (axons), storage (synaptic vesicles), binding (receptors), and removal (reuptake pump) of the neurotransmitters, the first messengers of the cascade. Recent research has determined that the neuron is prepared to receive signals via two different receptor types. One type, the ionophore receptor, controls the "pores" in the neuronal skin (the cell membrane) and thereby raises or lowers the threshold for excitability of the neuron. The second type of receptor — the G protein linked receptor — causes an internal cascade of events (via second and third messengers) that leads to long-term changes in the structures and functions of the nerve cell. Understanding these structures is essential to our conception of how medications work and how the nervous system changes with experience.

NERVE CELL FUNCTION

Section Overview

For our purposes, a discussion of neuronal function is largely a discussion of neurotransmission. Neurotransmission is a multistep process that describes the manner in which neurons communicate via the conversion of electrical signals into chemical signals and vice versa. Neurotransmission may result in either:

- rapid but brief changes in the activation or inhibition of the neuron, via binding of the neurotransmitter with gated ionophore receptors, or
- longer-term modulatory changes in the actual structure and functioning of the cell, via the binding of the neurotransmitter with a G protein linked receptor. The process by which

these long-lasting changes occur is called **neuromodulation**. Learning about neuromodulation will help you understand memory formation and the basic characteristics of how the brain, as a whole entity, functions and changes over time. This information has implications for treatment of the major psychiatric syndromes and is useful in guiding treatment with both psychotherapy and medication.

Neurotransmission

The first step in neurotransmission is the production of neurotransmitters. There are primarily three types of neurotransmitters (table 1.2 and discussion above): amino acids found in the diet (e.g., glutamate), biogenic amines (serotonin, norepinephrine, and dopamine), and peptides. Amino acids in the bloodstream circulate through the body and into the tissues. In the brain, they are taken up by neurons. Once in the neuron, these amino acids may be used as neurotransmitters or they may be transformed, via various enzymes and steps, into the biogenic amine neurotransmitters (dopamine, norepinephrine, and serotonin; see table 1.3). At this point the neurotransmitters are packaged into the synaptic vesicles (figure 1.11) and shipped to the axon terminal. They are ready for release when this neuron (neuron A, or presynaptic neuron) is stimulated, causing the electrical signal (which travels along the cell membrane) to arrive at the axon terminal.

Activation and Inhibition of Neurotransmission

The presynaptic cell (neuron A) may be stimulated or inhibited when neurotransmitters bind to the gated ionophore receptors on its cell membrane. This process of activation or inhibition occurs via an opening or closing (respectively) of the ion channels (pores in the membrane). This, in turn, either facilitates or blocks a rush of charged elements (ions) to enter or exit the cell. If the channel is opened, this temporary change in the balance of electrical charges produces an electrical current that is transmitted along the membrane of the axon of neuron A. Within milliseconds of the initial neurotransmitter-receptor binding, the electrical current reaches the axon terminal (figure 1.11) and the synaptic vesicles, containing the neurotransmitter, empty their contents into the synapse, the space between neuron A (the presynaptic neuron) and neuron B (the post-synaptic neuron). The neurotransmitter released from neuron A almost instantaneously migrates across the synapse to the surface receptors of neuron B. When the neurotransmitter fits into these receptors, the receptor changes shape, causing a cascade of events. At this point, again depending on the particular receptor-neurotransmitter combination (gated ionophore or G protein linked receptor, and inhibition vs. activation), the neurotransmission process may repeat itself, this time from neuron B to neuron C. Excess neurotransmitter that is not bound to the receptors on the synaptic surface of neuron B is then taken back up into neuron A. This is accomplished by the reuptake pump. Once back inside neuron A, an enzyme called monoamine oxidase (MAO) breaks down the neurotransmitter for recycling or waste.

Alternatively, the ion channel may be blocked, decreasing any chance of neuronal activation and putting an end to the neurotransmission. In this event, no signal is generated to neuron B and the process is over.

The path just described is a rapid response that enables the neuron to react quickly to incoming signals. It does not cause any permanent changes in the neuron. This rapid process occurs when an amino acid neurotransmitter binds to a gate type of receptor. Once the neurotransmitter binds to this receptor, the receptor is able to control the flow of ions into and out of the neuron, through the channels or pores in the membrane. The end result is either inhibition or activation of neurotransmission. The determining factor of whether a neuron is activated or inhibited is the type of neurotransmitter that binds to the gate receptor. If the neurotransmitter is inhibitory (such as GABA), the neuron is stabilized and its chances of activation are diminished. If the neurotransmitter is glutamate (an excitatory amino acid found in the popular flavor enhancer MSG and involved in neurotoxic effects of alcohol abuse), the neuron is activated.

Neuromodulation

Another result of neurotransmission is neuromodulation. This process causes more substantive changes (short-term or long-term) in the neuron. Neuromodulation starts with neurotransmission, but only occurs when biogenic amine neurotransmitters bind to the G protein linked receptors. These neurotransmitter-receptor complexes start a cascade of events inside the neuron, cell nucleus, and DNA (as opposed to electrical changes along the membrane in the neurotransmission process). This neuromodulation of neuronal function takes place over minutes, hours, and years, causing changes in the actual structure and function of the nerve cell and the growth of new connections between nerve cells (or conceivably the opposite).

The process of neuromodulation is responsible for short-term and long-term learning, memory, and change. Thus it is very important for the psychotherapist as well as the biological psychiatrist. For the purpose of understanding these two processes, paths A and B (table 1.4), in greater detail, a useful, although highly imperfect analogy can be made: Think of the neuron as a fast food restaurant. Just as a neuron takes in information and raw materials in order to put out a product (neurotransmitter and information), so does a restaurant. This restaurant has front and rear doors, as well as two types of specialized drive-in windows: windows for ordering, and windows for delivery.

TABLE 1.4
Results of Neurotransmission

PATH A	PATH B	
	Neuromodulation	
A transient process	Short-term modulation	Long-term modulation
Activation or inhibition of neuron	Short-term memory	Long-term memory and learning
Ion gated receptors	Adjustment of neurotransmitter (and enzyme) production, and release, receptor sensitivity	Synthesis of structural elements of the cell: receptors, channels, new connections between cells
	G protein linked receptors	G protein linked receptors

Path A: Routine Neurotransmission

Customers (excitatory neurotransmitters) drive up to the ordering window (bind to gate receptors) to place an order. The food, which is already prepared and wrapped (just as neurotransmitters are prepared and wrapped in synaptic vesicles), is released. A transaction then follows at the delivery window (the pores or ion channels in the membrane) in which substances may be exchanged, and the restaurant is active (the neuron is activated).This is the equivalent of path A. The transaction is transient, efficient, and causes no long-term changes.

Path B: Neuromodulation

Imagine the chain of events, the domino effect, that occurs when the restaurant owner finds out from the home office that a new community is being developed in his area, and his business activity will be increasing. He must effectively transmit this message to his restaurant in such a manner that effective, efficient changes will take place, so that he is prepared for the future increase in activity. The restaurant owner (biogenic amine or peptide neurotransmitters) is the first messenger sent from the home office. As the first messenger, he opens the front door lock (the receptor). Putting his key in the lock activates a trigger mechanism (the G protein) that gets the manager's attention. The owner supplies the letter from the home office containing the following information to the manager (second messenger): "Some new recipes must be activated from our master restaurant management book, and added to the menu. Order more meat, potatoes, and rolls; increase the production of hamburgers. If necessary, buy more equipment to get the job done. Also, construct more drive-in windows, both for ordering and delivery."

The manager (the second messenger) relays the information to the assistant manager (the third messenger), who in turn orders the chief cook (a transcription factor) to go to the master restaurant management book (DNA), which is locked in a vault (the cell nucleus) for safekeeping. The chief cook copies (copies or transcribes) the requested recipes and necessary construction orders (specific genetic codes) from the book. He then sends them to the assistant cook (messenger RNA), who transforms all the raw materials (hamburger meat, etc.) into the required products (new proteins). The chief cook is a man of many talents, and so he also builds new drive-in windows of both types (receptors and channels).

Section Summary

In neuromodulation, when the neuron is stimulated by the first messenger (neurotransmitter), the G protein activates the second messenger, which in turn activates the third messenger and transcription factors. These factors then go to the nucleus of the cell, which contains the genes (DNA) of the cell. The genes have billions of recipes and plans for every substance that the human body needs to make, in order that it may function properly, replace parts, and grow. Within seconds to hours after a stress, or even after normal nerve transmission, these transcription factors activate or inhibit the production of a specific recipe, usually a protein (a long chain of amino acids) or a peptide (short chain of amino acids). Much of the cell, including the enzymes, receptors, nerve growth factors, and even neurotransmitters, are made up of proteins or their smaller cousins, peptides. Activation of these transcription factors can have long-lasting, permanent effects on the structure and function of the nerve cell. Neuromodulation can alter the type of neurotransmitter a cell uses, the number and type of receptors in the cell membrane, the amount and types of enzymes available to make the neurotransmitters, and the number and location of new branches and connections (arborization and pruning; see chapter 2 and figure 2.10).

SUMMARY

The base of the human brain controls basic life support functions and seems to be hard-wired at birth. It does not appear to have changed much over the millennia. In the emotional circuits of the brain we begin to see how the processes of neuromodulation enable us to learn from our experiences. At the highest levels of the brain, our problem solving, planning, and social adjustments are taken to new highs.

Only 50 years ago the brain was viewed as a static organ. As a result of advances in cell biology and brain imaging we now know that the brain is constantly changing and developing, even into old age. We used to think of structural brain maps. We now think of functional brain maps in which a network can be visualized as a three-dimensional net extending from higher centers to lower centers and from side to side. These neural networks are plastic. They are continually adjusted by neuromodulation, becoming more efficient with time, needing fewer and fewer branches to accomplish the same task. We used to believe that each area of the brain subserved one function, and that there was little if any duplication of function. We now know that there is a great deal of duplication of function, and it is often possible after cell injury to recruit other neurons to recover function. We used to believe that the folds of the cortex were fixed. We now know that the shape of these folds is influenced by both environment and genes.

Finally, our new knowledge has allowed us to identify structures that prove that the mind and the body are inseparable, that psyche equals soma, and vice versa.

CHAPTER 2

Core Concepts in Biological Psychiatry

INTRODUCTION

THE GOAL OF THIS CHAPTER is to help you understand the biological aspects of mental function. Seven current core concepts in biological psychiatry will be introduced sequentially, from the nearly pure biological level (heredity and genetics) to concepts that reflect greater degrees of interaction between biology and environment. The core concepts are:

1. Heredity and genetics
2. Reactivity, temperament, and dysregulation
3. Personality
4. Sensitization and kindling
5. Chronobiology (biological rhythms)
6. Psychoendocrinology
7. Plasticity, learning and memory.

If this is your first exposure to this material, I suggest once again that you don't sweat the details—instead, get the gestalt (use your right brain)!

HEREDITY AND GENETICS

When an individual is conceived, an **ovum** (egg) unites with a **spermatocyte** (sperm cell) to form the first cell of its being. This first cell contains a full blueprint of instructions for every process necessary for the development and functioning of the human. Contained in 46 volumes, each called a **chromosome**, these blueprints actually exist in duplicate, so that there are 23 pairs of chromosomes, numbered from 1 to 23. Twenty-two of these chromosome pairs are the same in males and females, but the 23rd, called the sex chromosomes, are different in males and females. In females, this 23rd sex chromosome is represented by two large chromosomes called the X chromosomes. In males, the 23rd pair contains one large X chromosome and a smaller chromosome designated the Y chromosome. As the individual grows, cells divide in two, but before they do, they must prepare a new set of chromosomes (so there are actually four copies of each chromosome). Once this is accomplished, the cell divides in half, each cell getting its own full set of chromosomes (23 pairs). Each chromosome pair holds tens of thousands of individual sets of coded instructions, each called a **gene**. Just as a computer stores information by coding everything as a series of zeros and ones, the gene code stores information in a string of codes. The genetic code is made of four molecules called bases, which form pairs. These base pairs form a template upon which specific **amino acids** line up and are linked together, forming the **proteins** (chains of amino acids) that direct all the bodily processes. Although the genes have protective mechanisms, an alteration of just one base can render the output of that gene useless, causing a cascade of related body functions to go awry. Until recently it was commonly believed that the genes were independent of the environment. We now know that genes and environment shape each other. Environmental events can actually turn some genes related to memory and learning, called immediate early genes, on (or off) within seconds.

In 1987 researchers believed that they had finally found a gene responsible for a major psychiatric disorder: Chromosome 11 was identified as the site responsible for manic depression in an Amish family. A new era in psychiatric research was proclaimed by the media, and the psychiatric community took notice. Less publicized was the fact that the findings did not stand up to subsequent analysis. Despite numerous promising leads and the successful identification of specific genes that account for other medical diseases, *no single gene has yet been identified for any psychiatric condition.* However, despite the lack of a smoking gun, a great deal of evidence exists (from twin, adoption, and family studies) for the proposition that *the vulnerability for the major psychiatric disorders is inherited.*

Goodwin and Jamison (1990) point out that monozygotic twins (identical twins with identical genes, because they developed from the one [mono] egg [zygote]) will both have bipolar disorder 62–72% of the time. Dizygotic (two [di] egg [zygote]) twins and siblings both have bipolar disorder 0–8% of the time. Conversely, this means that 28–38% of the time, some factor(s) other than genes themselves must be necessary for the genes to express themselves as a bipolar mood disorder. All in all, the evidence indicates that there are several genes responsible for bipolar disorder, and that the expression of these genes ranges from schizoaffective disorder, in the most severe cases, to bipolar I, bipolar II (depression with hypomania), and unipolar depression.

Similar types of studies (e.g., Kendler, 1983) strongly indicate that genes account for approximately 60–70% of the variance in transmission of schizophrenia. This is based on the study of over 800 monozygotic twin pairs and 1000 dizygotic twin pairs in a variety of study designs. Interestingly, there seems to be a higher rate of paranoid and schizotypal personality disorders in relatives of schizophrenics as well (Kendler, 1995b; Kety et al., 1994).

Studies of panic disorder are much fewer. In fact, only 29 twin pairs have been studied, of which 13 were monozygotic. The monozygotic studies indicate a 31% concordance (e.g., Crowe, 1995), which indicates 69% of the factors causing panic disorder are environmental. Family studies of panic disorder, which are more numerous, support the idea that there is a genetic vulnerability for panic disorder.

There is good evidence that a gene that directs the production of a certain type of dopamine receptor (D2) is associated with substance abuse (Crowe, 1995). This dopamine receptor is of the G protein linked type (see chapter 1) and, as such, is associated with short- and long-term changes in neuron structure and function. This receptor is found in abundance in the mesocortical and mesolimbic tracts, which are associated with reward behavior. Since reward is an important factor in other clinical areas of mental function, it is not surprising that this receptor is associated with other psychiatric disorders as well. This gene does not *cause* substance abuse, but probably acts to increase vulnerability to various types of substance abuse (via the reward system) by modifying the actions of other genes.

In addition to the effect of genes on the individual, a recent large twin study by Kendler and colleagues (1993), which examined recent life events and difficulties, found that personal and social factors that predispose to stressful life events are substantially influenced by an individual's genetic background as well as the commonly assumed effect of family background. He suggests that *stressful life events may also be a result of genes* and that we abandon the "unidirectional idea" that environment influences the individual and not vice versa.

Integrating Genetic and Environmental Influences

As our knowledge has become more sophisticated, we have gradually moved away from the extreme positions that any disorder is caused by purely biological or psychosocial factors (figure 2.1). In the same way, genetic researchers have moved away from extreme positions regarding the genetics of psychiatric disorders. Until recently, researchers have tended to fall into two opposing and extreme perspec-

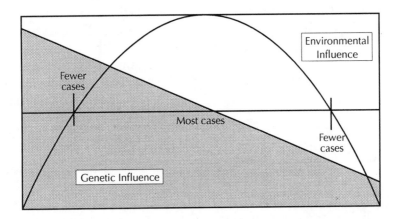

FIGURE 2.1. Estimating the genetic influence. The bell curve indicates that for most people with a psychiatric disorder, both the environment and genes are important. For a smaller number of people, genes or environment are primary. In extreme cases (much less common), the genes or environment are the only factors involved.

tives. One perspective was that there was a general genetic tendency (either high or low) toward psychiatric illness. The type of illness one developed would depend on environmental influences. The other perspective was that each psychiatric disorder was distinct and was related to a specific genetic vulnerability to that particular disorder. It now seems clear that neither position is accurate.

Kendler and colleagues (1995b) studied the relationships between six common psychiatric disorders in women (phobia, generalized anxiety, panic, bulimia, major depression, and alcoholism). In this study, Kendler also determined what model best explained his data on 1,030 female twin pairs so that he could tease out the relative contribution of genetic factors (GF), family environment factors (FEF), and environmental factors specific to the individual (ESI), such as personal illness and trauma.

There seem to be two major genetic liabilities to the disorders studied. The first factor seemed most closely related to phobia, panic, and bulimia, disorders that manifest brief paroxysms of symptoms. The second factor seemed very closely related to major depression and generalized anxiety disorder and is thought to be related to a general vulnerability to recurrent episodes of dysphoria. Except for bulimia, where the family effect was substantial, family environment played little or no etiologic role. Instead, contrary to common belief but supported by numerous studies Kendler has conducted, environmental experiences that are not shared by a twin and her cotwin seem to be the strongest environmental contributors to the risk of developing these disorders. Finally, alcoholism was significantly more heritable than any of the other disorders he studied and was most closely related to major depression in these women.

Clinical Application

Genetic studies generally support the notion that the psychiatric disorders are, to varying degrees, the result of multigenetic predispositions: The more genes there are predisposing one to a certain disorder, the earlier the onset, the more severe the symptoms, and the less important the environmental influence. **Genetic loading** can be assessed in a general sense by taking a careful and thorough history of the individual and three generations of the extended family. In order for this to be effective, the patient and other historians must be questioned about each individual in the system ("Did Joe ever experience depression, alcohol use, etc.?" not "Did anyone in your immediate or extended family ever abuse alcohol or suffer from depression, etc.?"). Questions regarding substance abuse, depression, suicide, panic, psychosis, psychiatric hospitalizations (nervous breakdowns), and temperament are important in assessing an individual's genetic loading.

The more genetic loading one has, the more easily the environment can tip him or her over the edge, the more likely (if Kendler is correct) and the earlier in life that disease is likely to manifest itself. This does not mean that psychotherapy is without benefit, only that the therapist must help the patient to understand that degree to which he/she/environment (family, etc.) is or is not responsible for the problem. This, of course, can alleviate guilt and anger, but it can also increase hopelessness unless the therapist holds out hope for assistance in managing the problem, while helping the patient understand that this is his or her area of personal responsibility.

REACTIVITY, TEMPERAMENT, AND DYSREGULATION

Reactivity is a term that refers to the duration, type, and degree of **response** that any entity exhibits in response to a **stimulus,** as well as the threshold of stimulation required to elicit such a response. The essential questions concerning the measurement of reactivity in any system are: What is the range of fluctuation of the system at rest (background noise) and under stress, and how long does it take to recover? The response measured may be physiological, behavioral, or psychological. Reactivity is a term that is used in a broad sense, as well as in a more specific one. In the specific sense, reactivity refers to one particular temperamental quality (e.g., the degree of inhibition/harm avoidance in response to a noxious stimulus) as a response style. As a general term, we can talk about the reactivity of the heart rate, the reactivity of the immune system, the hormonal system, or even the reactivity of a shock absorber on a car!

The analogy of the shock absorber is quite useful clinically: To determine if a shock absorber is functioning adequately, one can measure it with a ruler. If it measures below a certain measurement, it is defective. This is a **static** measurement, which will detect only the most defective shock absorbers. A **dynamic**, and more sensitive test of the reactivity of the shock absorber is to apply a stress (push down on the car) and observe the up and down motion of the car (the degree of reactivity). If the motion of the car fluctuates too widely and for too long, or too stiffly for too little time, the shock absorber, which measured a normal length on the static test, is deemed defective, or approaching that point. Biological systems function in the same way. In clinical practice patients may exhibit extremes of reactivity in numerous areas of function (table 2.1).

It is quite remarkable that leading researchers in various branches of the brain and behavioral sciences have independently come to recognize the importance of the concept of reactivity, each in his own area of study, be it biological, psychological, behavioral, or social.

Bowen, the father of family systems theory and therapy, observed a direct relationship between the increasing degrees of emotional reactivity of an individual and the failure to develop a sense of self separate from one's family of origin (Kerr & Bowen, 1988). He called this concept, central to his theory of family systems, the *differentiation of self*. He considered the basic level of differentiation of an individual to be fixed, although structured effort or unusual life experiences could boost an individual to a higher level of differentiation.

Jerome Kagan (1994) is one of the primary researchers in the area of temperament. His work is focused on the ease and extent of arousal (reactivity) in infants and young children to various stimuli. Neurotransmitter systems normally operate within a limited range of activity. In abnormal states of depression these systems are highly variable, unstable, and inappropriately responsive to incoming information; they may even become disconnected from normal biological rhythms (Parry, 1995)!

In essence, these pioneers are saying the same thing: If your emotional "shock absorber" system works well, your emotions stay in a reasonable, consistent range, the boundary between self and non-self is relatively clear, and a sense of self can develop. Your nervous system and the nervous systems of those around you will not be shaken by every bump in the road of life. Explaining the concept of

TABLE 2.1
Some Systems Relevant to Mental Health that Exhibit Extremes of Reactivity

SYSTEM	CLINICAL MANIFESTATION OF HYPER(OVER) REACTIVITY	CLINICAL MANIFESTATIONS OF HYPO(UNDER) REACTIVITY
Motor	Impulsivity (present in mania, ADHD, borderline, antisocial, and histrionic personality disorders, Tourette's syndrome, self-mutilation, violent suicides)	Inhibition of behavior (present in depression [as decreased initiative and psychomotor retardation], Parkinson's disease, autism, catatonia, thyroid disease)
Affect	Affective instability or hyperthymia (present in bipolar disorder, rapid cycling, and borderline, antisocial, and histrionic personality disorders)	Alexithymia, difficulty experiencing and expressing emotion (present in schizoid, schizotypal, and paranoid personality disorders, syndromes of apathy)
Attention	Distractibility (present in ADHD, schizophrenia)	Obsessive and stereotypic behavior (present in obsessive compulsive disorders, excessive doses of amphetamines)
Immune	Allergy (eczema, hay fever)	Immune deficiency, lack of immune system reaction (present in cancers, AIDS)
Hormones	Excessive hormonal reactions (present in hypoglycemia [excess insulin], Cushings disease [excess corticosteroids])	Inadequate hormonal response (present in menopause, a type of diabetes [inadequate insulin production], Addison's disease [inadequate production of corticosteroids])
Gastrointestinal	Increased motility (present in diarrhea, colic)	Decreased motility (present in constipation)

reactivity to clients, along with a drawing of figure 2.2, has uni-
formly allowed clients to feel relief. The discussion would go something like this:

"Joan, If I were to measure the level of norepinephrine (NE) in
the brain of a depressed person, the graph would look like this
(point to the left side of the upper graph in figure 2.2, preceding
the stress). Notice the variation in the baseline? Now if I were
to put that person's hand in ice water (labeled stress in figure
2.2) and measure the NE level, it would rise to some degree,
and then take some time to return to the earlier noisy background. Now, if I were to measure NE in a nondepressed person, it would look like this (point to left side of bottom graph).
Notice how stable the baseline is? If I then put *that* person's
hand in ice water, the NE response would be much greater, and
then it would return to the stable baseline more quickly. This is
a more efficient response. Joan, translated into your life, this
means that internally you are always working with an emotional
baseline of being somewhat upset. When a stress comes, you
cannot react efficiently or effectively, and then it takes you a
long while to recover. This is hard work. When you have this

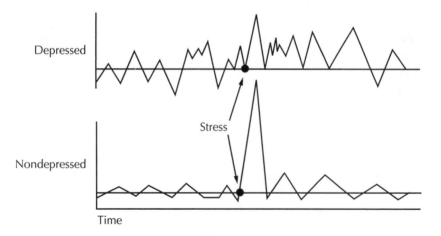

FIGURE 2.2. Reactivity in depressed patients: norepinephrine (NE) in depressed
and non-depressed patients, with and without stress.

constant level of excess reactivity to deal with, it's hard to deal with the world, and your self-esteem suffers. What's wrong with me, you wonder. Why does everything bother me? Why am I so sensitive? Then you deal with this in any number of ways. You might stay away from people, try to control people and events, use drugs to calm yourself. But the bottom line is you become self-absorbed trying to deal with this internal reactivity. Everything around you bothers you, and you are so busy with this internal state that you can't focus on others and learn about the world. Most of your strategies are aimed at trying to calm this internal reactivity. The nondepressed person responds efficiently, and then recovers quickly. Medication can help move your reactivity from here (upper graph) to here (lower graph)."

Temperament can be defined as emotional or behavioral qualities that appear early in life and are substantially determined by genetics. Temperament may be modified to a greater or lesser degree by environmental influences over time. Since temperamental characteristics are emotional traits, it is not surprising that they originate in large measure within the limbic system (the emotional brain, discussed in chapter 1). Under the umbrella of temperament, a small number of core traits has been identified and studied. As you read this section be aware that researchers are in some disagreement about these core traits and often use different language to describe the same trait. These traits are probably independently inherited and can be thought of as four axes or dimensions that reflect an individual's propensity toward:

1. **inhibition** of behavior in response to a stimulus (also called **harm avoidance,** this limbic response involves intense *reactivity* to aversive stimuli),
2. **impulsivity,***

---

*Impulsivity is not always considered to be a separate temperamental quality. Impulsivity seems to be mediated by serotonin neurons, as is harm avoidance. This common chemistry suggests that impulsivity is merely the opposite extreme of harm avoidance. Thus often only three temperamental qualities are identified. Because of its clinical importance, however, I will treat it as a separate temperamental quality.

3. **maintenance** of behavior that has already been established as pleasurable (**reward dependence**), and
4. **activation** of behavior in response to potentially pleasurable stimuli (**novelty seeking**).

Recently, studies have been published indicating that identification of temperament may have predictive value. One controversial study (Bell et al., 1995) indicates that shyness, possibly in combination with depression, may help predict one's risk of developing Parkinson's disease! Thus, serotonin and dopamine dysregulation may manifest themselves differently over time: early in life as shyness and late in life as Parkinson's disease.

Researchers have been struggling for years to identify some factor(s) that could be used to predict which medications will work, thereby decreasing the need for multiple drug trials by biological psychiatrists. Recently, a few studies (Ansseau et al., 1991; Joyce, Mudler, & Cloninger, 1994; Peselow, Fieve, & DiFiglia, 1992) have actually been able to do this. These researchers have found that different temperaments predicted which type of antidepressant would work (e.g., serotonergic vs. noradrenergic). Joyce found that severely depressed women high in fear (harm avoidance) with low need for approval (reward dependence) responded to desipramine (a noradrenergic antidepressant). High need for social approval (reward dependence) predicted clomipramine response (a serotonergic antidepressant). Depressed patients with an antisocial temperament (high novelty seeking, low reward dependence, low harm avoidance) did poorly with either drug. Patients with high levels of fear (harm avoidance) and need for approval (reward dependence) did well on either drug. If these findings are replicated, they will be quite valuable as clinical tools. Because of the potential pharmacologic value, as well as the clear psychotherapeutic value, let's review these temperamental traits in detail.

Inhibition of Behavior (Harm Avoidance)

The more easily and intensely emotionally upset one is by noxious stimuli, the more one is likely to avoid new stimuli, simply because the experience is so uncomfortable. This inborn emotional response is translated into a behavioral response style called **inhibition** (Kagan, 1994) or **harm avoidance** (Cloninger, 1987). It is closely related to shyness; moreover, there is an association between this temperament and certain physical characteristics and disorders (table 2.2). Let's examine the views of these two premier researchers in the field of temperament, in order to develop a sense of where this research is heading and, more importantly, its clinical value.

Studying three sites of reactivity (frontal, limbic, and behavioral) in four-month-old infants, Kagan (1987) was able to identify two extreme temperamental types (inhibited and uninhibited) and two middle-of-the-road types (aroused and distressed). These four groups were defined by: (1) their ease of arousal (highly reactive vs. minimally reactive) to stimulation and (2) the type of behavioral state that resulted from the stimulation (calm and smiling or distressed and fearful).

The highly reactive group, characterized in table 2.2, tends to be behaviorally inhibited. Kagan found that the behavioral measures in the high reactors at four months of age (e.g., extreme crying and muscular movement) were significantly correlated with inhibited behavior at 3½ years of age, although the correlation was not perfect.

TABLE 2.2
Characteristics of Behaviorally Inhibited Children

- Reluctance to initiate spontaneous comments with unfamiliar children or adults
- Absence of spontaneous smiles with unfamiliar people
- Relatively long time needed to relax in unfamiliar situations
- Impaired recall memory following stress
- Reluctance to take risks; cautious behavior in situations requiring decisions
- Unusual fears and phobias
- Large heart rate accelerations to stress and to a standing posture
- Large pupillary dilation to stress
- High muscle tension
- Greater cortical activation in the right frontal area
- Allergies
- Light blue eyes
- Narrow face
- Higher frequency of Parkinson's disease in relatives
- Gastrointestinal problems (colic, irritable bowel)

From Kagan, 1994. Copyright© 1994 by Basic Books, Inc. Adapted by permission of BasicBooks, a division of HarperCollins Publishers, Inc.

Similarly (but not identically), the stability of the calm, uninhibited group can be predicted over the same time period.

Cloninger's concept of harm avoidance, measured in adults, is identical to Kagan's concept of inhibited and uninhibited temperaments in infants and young children. Cloninger defines harm avoidance (the tendency toward inhibition of behavior) as a heritable tendency to respond intensely (high reactivity) to aversive stimuli. This causes inhibition of behavior in order to avoid the "punishment" of subjective discomfort brought on by novelty and frustration. Cloninger developed the Tridimensional Personality Questionnaire (1991) to measure three of the dimensions of temperament above (he does not include impulsivity as a separate entity): the inhibition of behavior due to over (emotionally uncomfortable) reactivity, novelty seeking, and reward dependence. His scale of harm avoidance ranges from +3 (severely high harm avoidance, manifested by a consistent state of fearfulness that is nonresponsive to support, pessimism, inhibition in unfamiliar and uncertain situations, and high levels of fatigue) to −3 (severely low harm avoidance, manifested by highly uninhibited calm responses to unfamiliar situations, confidence and optimism, minimal reluctance to risk personal injury, and high levels of energy with rapid recovery after exertion). The correlations of certain personality disorders with temperamental and character traits are summarized in table 2.3.

The Mechanism of Inhibition

The threshold of response of the limbic neurons to various stimuli (how easily the neurons are triggered) determines the degree of emotional reactivity of a person, and the consequent inhibition or lack of inhibition of behavior. The limbic neurons, which are the seat of temperament, are at the limbus (border) of the higher and lower brain centers, and thus connect with higher and lower centers. The higher centers include the frontal lobes (which help regulate emotion) and the hippocampus (which facilitates learning by making associations between emotional states and stored memories). The lower centers include the hypothalamus and brain stem, which control the physiological and behavioral outputs of emotion, such as hormone changes, muscle tension, facial expression, heart rate, etc.

TABLE 2.3
Correlations Between Personality Disorders, Temperament, and Character

PERSONAL-ITY DISORDERS (LISTED IN CLUSTERS)	TEMPERAMENT			CHARACTER	
	NOVELTY SEEKING	HARM AVOIDANCE	REWARD DEPEN-DENCE	SELF-DIRECTED-NESS	COOPERA-TIVENESS
Schizoid	n/s	n/s	Very low	Low	Low
Schizotypal	n/s	High	Low	Low	Low
Paranoid	Low	n/s	Low	Very low	Very Low
Antisocial	Very high	n/s	Very low	Low	Very low
Histrionic	Very high	n/s	n/s	Low	Low
Borderline	High	High	n/s	Very low	Low
Narcissistic	n/s	n/s	n/s	Low	Low
Passive-Aggressive	High	n/s	n/s	Low	Low
Avoidant	Low	Very high	n/s	Very low	n/s
Obsessive-Compulsive	n/s	High	n/s	Low	Low
Dependent	n/s	Very high	High	Very low	n/s

n/s = no significant correlation found. *Very high* = positive correlation, significant at the p = <.0001 confidence level. *High* = positive correlation, significant at the p = <.05 to .001 confidence levels. *Low* = negative correlation, significant at the p = .05 to .001 confidence levels. *Very low* = significant negative correlation at p = .0001 confidence level. From Cloninger, Svrakic, & Przybek (1993). Copyright 1993, American Medical Association. Adapted with permission.

A variety of evidence suggests that harm avoidance is primarily mediated by neurons that involve serotonin.

The Clinical Relevance of Inhibition

This temperamental subtype has relevance in various clinical situations. First, when a nonphysician takes a personal and family history, he should make certain to take an in-depth history of allergy, shyness, Parkinson's disease, chronic pain, phobias, irritable bowel, etc. (table 2.2). The presence of these syndromes is a clue to the possible temperament of the client, the degree of fearfulness the nonphysician will be dealing with, as well as the possible benefit of pharmacological intervention.

Second, when considering pharmacotherapy for a particular person, one should be aware that this temperamental type seems to be quite responsive to the selective serotonin reuptake inhibitors Prozac, Zoloft, Paxil, Luvox, BuSpar, and Serzone, as well as the MAO inhibitor Nardil.

Third, a therapist should realize that patients with high harm avoidance will be less likely to try out new behaviors, and so, all other factors being equal (which they never are!), the therapy will progress more slowly.

Finally, a therapist who understands the biological basis of such a temperament can educate the patient, thereby alleviating the sense of inadequacy he or she feels.

A CLINICAL ILLUSTRATION   Mr. Kay was a 52-year-old married professional, who came from a large family. His father was an aggressive, unstable alcoholic, who was so impulsive with money that he was declared bankrupt on two occasions. Mr. Kay had always felt inadequate next to his father and four older and one younger brothers because they seemed stronger and more masculine (translate: more aggressive and more impulsive = serotonergic activity dysregulated). They were always willing to fight, whereas the patient saw no purpose in this. Not surprisingly, despite his aggressiveness in athletics, Mr. Kay considered himself to be more feminine in nature. His brothers, he felt, had their father's respect, whereas he didn't. Yet Mr. Kay was the most stable and well-adjusted of all the male siblings. His stronger brothers had drug and alcohol problems, as well as numerous incarcerations for illegal activities. When the biological nature of his brothers' and father's aggression was explained and contrasted with his normal degree of harm avoidance, Mr. Kay felt quite relieved. The discussion included the following points: Impulsivity, aggression, and harm avoidance are probably all part of the same chemical brain systems (serotonin). The way our brains react to the possibility of risk, harm, and uncertainty is partially an inborn trait, and this trait is modified, for better or worse, as a result of the early environment we grow up in, the things that happen to us, and the strengths and weaknesses we are endowed with. Unfortunately, Mr. Kay's brothers and father probably inherited a temperament that was unusually low on the inhibition scale. As a young child he could not have known this, and being different (the only one with a normal degree of impulsivity), he assumed that he was bad or inadequate compared to the models immediately around him. In fact, he was probably the only serotonergically well-balanced one! This reframed his thinking, and with further repetition and explanation, became integrated as part of his self-concept.

Impulsivity

Impulsivity may be defined as a decreased threshold for motor (physical) activity in response to internal or external stimuli. As mentioned above, impulsivity may be related to inhibition of behavior (harm avoidance), maintenance of behavior (reward dependence), and/or faulty activation of behavior (novelty seeking). Thus, some researchers do not accord impulsivity its own separate status as a temperamental quality. We will discuss it as a separate entity due to its clinical importance in borderline, antisocial personality disorders (cluster B personality disorders), as well as mania, violent suicide, attention-deficit/hyperactivity disorder, and substance abuse. Nevertheless, the reader should be aware that very often the same pharmacologic agents that are useful in treating the inhibited or harm avoidant individual can be useful in the impulsive individual. (The most likely reason for this is discussed in the section on dysregulation, below.)

Numerous studies have documented a clear association between violent suicide, increased aggressiveness, and impulsivity (Goodwin & Jamison, 1990). It is significant that these three behavioral characteristics are mediated by serotonergic neurotransmission. In fact, one of the most consistent findings in biological psychiatry is that the brain and spinal fluid levels of both serotonin and its breakdown product, 5-HIAA (5-hydroxyindoleacetic acid), are much lower in violent and impulsive suicides. This means that the activity level of serotonin neurons is quite low. These findings are supported by other studies, which show that the higher the levels of aggression and impulsivity as measured by psychometric testing, the lower the spinal fluid levels of 5-HIAA (e.g., Depue & Spoont, 1986). Also, not surprisingly, low 5-HIAA levels are found in recovered alcoholics (Rosenthal et al., 1980). Alcoholics are by nature more impulsive than the general population. These findings have particular clinical relevance due to the frequent presence of impulsivity in the clinical population.

The Mechanism of Impulsivity

Damage to the part of the frontal cortex that lies above the eyes (orbitofrontal cortex) is associated with signs and symptoms of disinhibition of behavior: impulsivity, social inappropriateness, irritability, euphoria, hyperactivity, and emotional lability. This neurological syndrome so closely matches that seen in mania and hyperactivity (ADHD), that researchers strongly suspect abnormal function of the neurons in this area may be involved in impulsivity (Mega & Cummings, 1994). These signs and symptoms are thought to be a result of reduced activity of the serotonergic neurons in this area of the brain, along with a relative increase in the activating neurotransmitters (dopamine and/or norepinephrine).

The Clinical Relevance of Impulsivity

Increasing activity of serotonergic neurons generally, but not always, tends to result in reduced anxiety, calming, and even sedation. This is the basis of folk medicine's recommended warm glass of milk before bed (milk is loaded with L-tryptophan, the building block for serotonin). Since moderate amounts of serotonin lead to a calming effect, it makes sense that reduced serotonin activity leads to aggression, agitation, and anxiety. Therefore, a therapist must respect the biology of the depressed suicidal patient. Knowing that serotonin activity is probably low in your patient (even if it cannot be measured at the time), you can begin to understand that your patient is attempting to control the behavioral output of a powerful biological process. Despite the patient's and therapist's exchange of reassurances, a good therapeutic relationship, 24-hour availability of the therapist, and an antisuicide contract, the final decision to commit suicide is very often an impulsive act, one not counterbalanced by an adequate physiological braking mechanism.

The suicidal patient knows that he or she cannot reliably contract against the impulse. As a 29-year-old manic depressive attorney recently said, "When the impulse is really there, the contract does not even exist in my mind. I really don't know that I can keep the contract, although I'd like to say I could. At those moments, I am consumed by the desire to die." A man heading down a steep hill in a car with failed brakes could no more promise not to crash than a severe depressive could promise not to attempt suicide. Until the brakes have been repaired, and the patient has been treated pharmacologically to normalize the impulsivity in an appropriately safe environment, the therapist cannot confidently rely on other factors to control the suicidal impulse. Lithium, selective serotonin reuptake inhibitors (SSRIs) such as Zoloft, Paxil, and Prozac, as well as the serotonin precursor L-tryptophan, have all been associated with decreased impulsivity and aggression, along with decreased craving for alcohol.

By understanding the inborn nature of the tendency toward impulsivity, the therapist will be able to approach the client with substance abuse problems and cluster B personality disorders (impulsive, novelty seeking) in a nonjudgmental manner. In part, the psychotherapeutic goal is to teach the client how to cope with the impulsivity via strengthening of the character (e.g., increasing self-direction by developing and pursuing long-term goals, increasing cooperativeness and self-transcendence).

Maintenance of Behavior (Reward Dependence)

Reward dependence refers to how easy or difficult it is for a person to become "hooked" on a pleasurable, rewarding behavior, and to what degree his or her behavior remains controlled by it. Reward dependence is defined by Cloninger (1987, p. 575) as "a heritable tendency to respond intensely to signals of reward" (or relief of punishment) and to maintain behaviors previously associated with rewards. Cloninger described a scale of reward dependence which ranges from +3 (severely high reward dependence manifested by high dependency on social support, industriousness to the point of exhaustion, extreme sensitivity to rejection, and persistence of craving for gratification) to −3 (severely low reward dependence manifested by social detachment, independent and nonconforming behavior, minimal desire to please others, and reliance on immediate gratification).

The Mechanism of Reward and Reward Dependence

The brain seems to contain numerous locations which, when stimulated, will bring either pleasure or relief of distress. Most of these "pleasure centers" are located in the limbic (emotional) brain, and come together in the median forebrain bundle (MFB), a bundle of nerve tracts near the hypothalamus (see chapter 1). Similarly, most of the brain locations that generate aversive sensations are also in the limbic brain. These come together in a group of nerve fibers called the periventricular system (PVS), which mediates the experience of punishment. These two systems are closely connected with the systems involving learning (conditioning) and memory. They are in balance in the healthy state, but seem to be out of balance in the disorders discussed above, and are thought to be central to the abnormal biology of depression.

Just as there are multiple reward and punishment centers, there are also multiple neurotransmitters that mediate pleasure and reward. Dopamine, norepinephrine, and the body's own opioids (morphine-like substances) are probable neurotransmitters involved in mediation of pleasure systems. Dopamine neurons must function normally for the individual to experience reward, and rapidly rising levels of dopamine receptor activity seem to be associated with excessive pleasure (see The Mechanism of Impulsivity, above), as when amphetamines and cocaine are used. Norepinephrine (the adrenaline of the brain) neurons, on the other hand, must be activated to a sufficient degree in order to consolidate and store memories of which behaviors brought on the pleasure (or the relief of an aversive sensation). The opioids, such as enkephalin and endorphins, are present in many of the same areas of the brain as norepinephrine, and are very likely involved in the sense of satisfaction as a goal is attained.

The ability to be self-directed and independent from environmental contingencies is mediated by a nerve circuit in the brain that runs from two parts of the frontal lobe to deeper structures (the thalamus and closely related structures). Excess reward dependency, the inability to be self-directed and break the stimulus-pleasure response connection, can be due to abnormal function of these neurons.

The Clinical Relevance of Reward Dependence

It seems quite likely that the nature of what one finds rewarding is related to early experiences and abilities, but is later modified by maturing experiences and thoughtful reflection. Thus, some people may be extremely dependent on social approval, which they find so very rewarding, while others may find pleasure in a sense of control or power or in an ability to be loving.

Clinically, we all too often see individuals whose conditioned response of pleasure to social approval can be so powerful and so ingrained that they have difficulty developing a sense of self. Often these individuals find themselves acting like chameleons, changing behavior and beliefs automatically to suit the needs of those around them. In severe cases, the people-pleasing behavior is maintained despite objective evidence that it is not presently rewarding. Being in a group setting is intolerable for these individuals, since each individual in the group may have different expectations of them. Thus, they are in a situation of confusion and anxiety, as their need for reward is frustrated.

If the biological substrate of approval-seeking behavior is explained thoroughly to the client, the shame which these individuals experience can be reduced, they can begin to understand the basis for their difficulty in giving up the rewarding behavior, thoughtfully resist the reward, and develop a more positive self-concept. The explanation should include the following points:

1.   The persistence with which a person maintains previously rewarded behavior is an inborn temperamental trait.
2.   This trait is mediated by overly sensitive neurons in specific parts of the brain, which are geared toward maintaining pleasure.
3.   This occurs via the easy and persistent formation of memory of the situation and the behaviors that produced the pleasure, and/or inadequate levels of activity in the nerve pathways that extend from the (lateral/orbital/prefrontal) cortex to the emotional brain.
4.   This trait can be modified with persistent effort.

For the psychotherapist who is working with personality disorders, table 2.3 shows the significant correlations between the various personality disorders and temperament and character (as defined by Cloninger, Svrakic, & Przybeck, 1993). Moderately high reward dependency along with high cooperativeness seems to be incongruent with having a personality disorder. Interestingly, excessively high levels of reward dependence seem to be present only in hysterical and dependent personality disorders, while excessively low levels of reward dependence are present in most other personality disorders!

Those in the aloof cluster A (schizoid, schizotypal, and paranoid) are lowest in reward dependence; antisocial personality disorder runs a close second. It may be significant that these personality disorders are among the most refractory to treatment. Some significant level of reward dependence (perhaps specifically social reward) seems to be important in successful psychotherapy as well as drug responsiveness (Joyce et al., 1994). Borderline personality disorder, although difficult, is amenable to treatment and seems to exhibit normal reward dependence.

The anhedonia (lack of ability to anticipate and/or experience pleasure) of depression and the apathy and some of the negative symptoms of schizophrenia are also related to impaired reward dependence. Depressed patients do not seem to maintain the behaviors that normally were rewarding to them, probably due to the experience(s) of helplessness in achieving the reward. Their reward centers are underactive relative to their punishment centers. When trying to identify the psychosocial factors that lead to an individual's depression, it is important to realize that lack of expected reward (disappointment) as well as punishment will be aversive, and that in the treatment of such individuals a lack of expected punishment (relief) as well as reward will be pleasurable (Ashton, 1992).

A CLINICAL ILLUSTRATION   This morning Mr. Zand and his wife of 42 years were in my office for couples therapy. Two years ago, Mrs. Zand was ready to terminate the marriage out of a sense of complete frustration. I persuaded her that a trial of couples work was indicated, and she agreed. Over the past two years it has become apparent that there is a deep bond between these two people, and they have made significant progress as a couple. One recurring theme is Mr. Zand's overfocusing on projects to the exclusion of other aspects of life — including his wife. For example, when Mr. Zand began to explore underwater photography, he became obsessed with it, purchasing the best equipment, etc. This hyperfocusing was fine to some degree, and in fact contributed to his material success; it was not fine, however, in regard to his inability to stop drinking and driving, which he acknowledged was irrational and dangerous. With discussion about the common theme of his overfocusing, we began to explore times in his life when he wanted to change his focus but could only do so after a prolonged period of great struggle. I explained to Mr. Zand the neurochemical basis for the ability to be self-determined, as opposed to reward-dependent, as well as the influence of nature and nurture. I invited him to think about this theme in his life, and to put the drinking behavior in that context. He found this to be intriguing, and was more open to the idea that his resistance to change was not so much a choice as a result of a trait with a neurochemical basis. In order to overcome this trait (which had enriched his life in a variety of ways), understanding what he was up against was an important first step. This morning he had started the session with an announcement that, despite the logic of discontinuing the drinking and driving, he felt "something inside" that rebels at the thought of giving it up. This is the language of reward dependence in Mr. Zand.

Ms. Duffy, my second patient of the day, was also a highly successful, persistent, overfocused person who used her talents well in her career. However, after meeting her "soul mate" five years earlier she was hopelessly hooked! Despite the rapid deterioration of the relationship over several months, and the destruction which ensued in both lives as a result of this "match made in heaven," Ms. Duffy could not let go. She followed her soul mate to three different states, persistently trying to reunite with him. His refusals had no effect. When he would finally give in to her plea for intimacy, this would rapidly be followed by sexual liaison, a deep sense of connection, and relief of loneliness (the rewards). Intense conflict would inevitably follow, with the entire cycle repeating within 24 hours or less. Ms. Duffy gave up an exciting high-level executive position (to which she had aspired), family relationships, friendships, and financial security to pursue a reward that no longer existed. Ms. Duffy loathed herself for her inability to disconnect her behavior from the need for reward.

Activation of Behavior (Novelty Seeking)

Novelty seeking may be defined as a heritable tendency toward intense exhilaration or excitement in response to novel stimuli or cues of previously established behaviors associated with pleasure or relief of discomfort. Novelty seeking can also be called behavioral activation (similar to Freud's pleasure principle). Behavioral activation can be caused by anticipated pleasure or anticipated relief of an unpleasant state (e.g., hunger or monotony). One may or may not become dependent on these rewards, depending on the tendency toward reward dependency (maintenance of the behavior).

Cloninger (1987) again defines a scale ranging from +3 to −3 to quantify the novelty seeking component of temperament. Very high novelty seeking behavior is characterized by consistent thrill seeking and exploration, intolerance of structure and monotony regardless of consequences, unpredictability, and disorganization in relationships and work. Very low behavioral activation (−3 on Cloninger's scale) is reflected in people who like being in a rut; they demonstrate serious resistance to all attempts to modify routines, lack of exploration regardless of benefits, extreme predictability and organization, fondness for structure, and rigid consistency in work and relationships.

The Mechanism of Novelty Seeking

Novelty seeking seems to be mediated in large measure by dopamine neurons in the limbic system. These neurons receive input from the arousal centers in the brain stem ("Wake up, stay alert!"), from the hypothalamus ("Get the muscles, heart, stress glands, etc. ready for action!"), and from the cortex, or thinking brain ("Let's see, what's going on here?"). Once the information is integrated, the dopamine pathways send the information back to the forebrain (frontal lobe), which initiates the execution of the goal directed behavior ("Do it!"). When the frontal lobe structure or function is impaired (as it seems to be in various brain diseases [Parkinson's, Alzheimer's], attention deficit disorders, depression, and schizophrenia) patients exhibit difficulty planning and executing goal-directed tasks.

The Clinical Relevance of Novelty Seeking

Novelty seeking behavioral activation is excessive in certain personality disorders (table 2.3), attention deficit hyperactivity syndrome, mania, and substance abuse. It is inhibited in depression, Parkinson's disease, and often in chronic schizophrenics.

Behavioral therapy of depression can be defined as a collaborative effort between therapist and patient directed at behavioral activation (e.g., forced novelty seeking) via homework assignments broken into small achievable steps. I often use the concept of behavioral activation with depressed patients who have little initiative. I give a thorough explanation that the graded task assignment very likely works by reactivating the reward centers of the brain, and that doing the task will actually change the chemistry of the brain, helping to bring it back into balance. This explanation enables the patient to reframe the homework. It is no longer a chore and a burden, but a mechanism of control over a chemistry that has gone haywire. It is quite effective!

Dysregulation refers to the failure of one or more components of the nervous system to maintain itself in a relatively narrow range. In the early years of biological psychiatry the monoamine hypotheses of affective disorders and schizophrenia postulated, quite simply, that these disorders were the result of too little or too much norepinephrine or dopamine. These hypotheses generated much valuable research, which eventually laid the monoamine hypotheses to rest. We know that there is no simple one-to-one correlation between an neurotransmitter and any psychiatric disease state. Once again, humankind outgrew the cause and effect model, and we were forced to look at brain function in a less rigid, static, and categorical manner. We now know that the action of a particular neurotransmitter may vary depending on the state of the other systems. For example, serotonin, in the face of high levels of norepinephrine activity (as in panic disorder) will calm anxiety and reduce norepinephrine levels, but in the setting of reduced norepinephrine activity serotonin will raise norepinephrine levels, perhaps even causing anxiety! This information helps to explain the different responses to Prozac. Anergic patients may get agitated, while patients with panic may actually be calmed. Thus serotonin is best described as a modulator, keeping the activity of norepinephrine circuits in a well-regulated range. This discovery, among others, helped researchers to come to the concept of dysregulation. By definition a dysregulated system may:

1. vary widely from too much activity to too little activity, resulting in instability, failure to react adequately, efficiently, and selectively to incoming information,

2. show excessive baseline (unstimulated) activity,
3. exhibit a slow return to baseline conditions after a stress, and
4. become disengaged from normal biological rhythms (daily, monthly, and seasonal).

An Analogy for Patients

Patients often can relate to the thermostat analogy of dysregulation, which can easily be applied to depression and dysthymia (figure 2.2). When a thermostat is functioning well, it keeps the temperature of a home between 68 and 72 degrees, despite extreme variation in outside temperatures (stress on the system). Cold temperatures below 68 degrees will trigger the heating system, and warm temperatures above 72 degrees will trigger the air conditioner, thus the temperature within the internal environment remains in a relatively narrowly pre-defined range. When the system is dysregulated, the temperature in the home may rise to 78 degrees before the air conditioner kicks in, and it may then overcool the house to 62 degrees before shutting off. This wide fluctuation keeps the temperature in the home unstable; if it is extreme enough, it may cause other systems to break down (e.g., the pipes freeze).

In the same way, when a person has a temperamental tendency toward emotional overreactivity (which looks very much like figure 2.2) and affective instability (which leads to a reluctance to be active called inhibition of behavior or harm avoidance), minor changes are experienced as stressful, provoking relatively strong emotional/physical feelings. This makes it quite difficult to cope, since almost everything affects the person's sense of emotional stability.

In situations such as this, biological psychiatrists aim to normalize the dysregulation of the emotional system (the lower part of figure 2.2) via a healthy life style, elimination or treatment of medical problems, and the use of antidepressants or mood stabilizers. Having done this, the client can be free to develop him- or herself, without the extra burden of being buffeted by minor events and thoughts. The client's personal ability to develop his or her life is thereby enabled by biological psychiatry, but assured by psychotherapy. Many patients are relieved to hear this explanation, since it mirrors their experience. Even more impressive to patients is the counterintuitive but clearly established fact that people whose limbic systems are dysregulated actually respond less strongly to stressful stimuli. In other words, people who are overreacting internally are often under-reacting in their behavior!

A CLINICAL ILLUSTRATION   The following case illustrates how an understanding of the concept of dysregulation can be essential to successful pharmacological treatment.

Mr. Jordon, a 41-year-old male public relations officer, was referred to me for evaluation by his therapist. The evaluation revealed a number of possible diagnostic possibilities, including attention deficit disorder, bipolar disorder, sleep apnea, and hypothyroidism. Sorting out these possibilities was quite difficult due to the patient's low level of self-awareness, trouble communicating clearly, and general difficulty responding directly to questions. After a thorough evaluation ruled out the possibilities of sleep apnea and hypothyroidism, I initiated treatment with lithium. After three weeks, Mr. Jordon concluded, "It's no help." He reported no benefits and few side effects. While it was premature to give up on lithium (the benefits can take as long as one year to appear), I was not optimistic. Several days later, however, I received a call from the therapist, who reported that the patient casually reported that he was able to speak up to his coworker for the first time. Mr. Jordon had reported, "In the past I would have said nothing [inefficient, inadequate response to a stressful stimulus], and stewed over it for days [slow return to baseline]." Understanding the concept of dysregulation, it became clear to both his therapist and me that perhaps the lithium was beginning to work after all. Eventually, we determined that Mr. Jordon was suffering with attention deficit disorder as well. Ritalin calmed his thinking and distractibility, and his communication skills improved very significantly. The effective medication response resulted in decreased background noise and an increase in Mr. Jordon's ability to respond to specific stimuli in an efficient manner.

PERSONALITY

There is a clear and continuous interaction over the entire life span between the genetically determined temperament (T) and environmental (E) factors. Temperamental qualities (e.g., harm avoidance) are modified by environmental influences to form **personality (P)**. Environmental influences include environmental quality (e.g., lead contamination, air quality, allergens), culture, spirituality, parenting, birth order, trauma, and degree and quality of exposure to values. While this is not a mathematical formulation, this relationship can be represented as:

$$P = T \leftrightarrow E$$

Personality and Environment

Despite the fact that temperament is inherited, most research indicates that the environment and genes have roughly equal effects on a person's personality.

These interactions were recognized over 1700 years ago in Galen's treatise: *On the Passions of the Soul* (Ellenberger, 1970). There he described his method for mastering the passions, which is really akin to modern psychotherapy of the narcissistic, borderline, and antisocial personality disorders. Galen's first step was abstaining from the crudest kind of emotional outburst (kicking and biting in his day, acting out behaviors in ours). Next was to find a wise, older mentor who would point out one's defects and give advice. This was difficult to find in his time, by his account, but perhaps more easily found in our time under "psychotherapists" in the yellow pages. Galen's final step was to "engage, with the help of one's mentor, in an unceasing effort to control one's passions" (long-term therapy). Ultimately, the genetic temperament would no longer define the behavioral response style or personality.

The interaction between genes and environment, which Galen sought to control, was more recently explored by Jerome Kagan. In keeping with our culture's research-oriented, quantitative approach to problems, Kagan was not merely content to be descriptive, as Galen was. Rather, he attempted to quantify. Kagan's (1994) study of 600 infants aged 4 months to 3½ years shows that there is an interdependence between nature and nurture. In fact, it appears that infants who are moderately inhibited or uninhibited at 4 months of age will very often drift to the opposite physiological response style by 3½ years of age! Even infants in the extreme ranges of inhibition or disinhibition at 4 months may drift to the opposite response style by 3½ years of age, depending on the presence of stressors (which would cause the disinhibited to become inhibited) and the quality of the maternal approach. Highly inhibited infants show less fear at 3½ years when raised by mothers who extinguish the fear response by limit setting, demanding obedience, and providing lesser amounts of holding. Highly reactive, inhibited, or harm avoidant infants at 4 months of age who are raised by "laissez-faire" mothers (who are less firm and more protective) remain in the high fear state at 3½ years of age. This may be due to excessive comforting and protectiveness which could lead to a failure to learn to cope with uncertainty and novelty—a failure to become desensitized. Infants will move from the uninhibited to the inhibited response style with greater frequency than vice versa, suggesting that it is easier to create fear via trauma than it is to remove innate fear responses via desensitization.

Character

Two of the environmental contributors to personality are the socialization process (social cooperativeness) and the mirroring process via which the perceived environmental responses to one's presence and actions promotes the development of a self-concept about one's place and purpose in life (self-concept and self-directedness). The amalgam of self-concept and degree of socialization results in what is often thought of as the characterological component of personality.

Psychotherapy of the character disorders leads to improvement in character, i.e., development of a sense of self-direction and a nonjudgmental and cooperative attitude toward others.

The Clinical Relevance of Personality

The findings that are being generated in the area of temperament, development, and character have numerous implications for individuals and society. Morality, in its extreme forms (completely absent or excessively rigid) may be born of excessively high or low thresholds for arousal in the frontal cortex-limbic tracts, rendering one person impervious to emotion (hence lacking empathy) and another extremely susceptible to anxiety and shame. The development of morality therefore may be automatic in some overly sensitive individuals and environmentally induced in others, but only when there is a sufficient neurological mechanism (i.e., the frontal-limbic tracts must be in good working order). As clinicians we will be less judgmental if we remember that extreme temperamental characteristics, such as extreme fear, reward dependency, and novelty seeking, are difficult, additional burdens for people to carry. These traits require strong mentoring and character building, yet all too often individuals with these inherited or acquired temperaments attempt to cope with drugs, sex, religion, or crime.

A CLINICAL ILLUSTRATION   Karen was a highly anxious, depressed 28-year-old college graduate, who was drifting (poor self-direction) through her personal life and her career as an editor. She was extremely sensitive to rejection (reward dependent), self-mutilating at times, demanding, frequently suicidal, impulsive in her spending and alcohol use, and intensely tearful. Karen was referred for medication of her depression while her therapist of three years continued to work on her personality disorder, with the main success being the fact that she was still alive. Eventually Karen was treated with a serotonergic antidepressant (Prozac) and a therapeutic level of nortriptyline (Pamelor), a tricyclic antidepressant. Her chronic suicidal ideation cleared, as did her depression. She began to make good progress in her therapy, identifying "who she was" (this was easier to see now that her mood was stable) and becoming more self-directed; individual differences no longer signified rejection. Karen eventually found a job that suited her quite well and established a number of satisfying relationships. By the end of the therapy interaction, Karen was very different: She would smile, be appreciative, feel free to disagree. She felt optimistic about her life. Her reward dependence and harm avoidance had decreased, and her tolerance of novelty and uncertainty increased along with her cooperativeness and self-direction.

SENSITIZATION AND KINDLING

Sensitization and kindling are types of learning characteristic of certain parts of the nervous system. In sensitization, a **stimulus (S)** that initially causes little or no observable **response (R)**, eventually, with repetition, produces a full response. Given further exposure to the same stimulus, the full response will soon occur even with lower stimulus levels than the original stimulus. Eventually, with further repetition, the response occurs spontaneously, in the absence of any stimulus. Once the response begins to occur automatically, without external stimuli, kindling has occurred.

It seems that kindling, as a property of different functional systems of the central and peripheral nervous system, is involved in hypertension, seizure disorders, and, according to most evidence (Post, 1992), in the unipolar (depression only) and bipolar (mania and depression) affective disorders. The concepts of sensitization and kindling have great significance for the treatment of affective disorders.

In the following paragraphs I will present two nonpsychiatric models of sensitization and kindling: an animal model (seizures), and a real world medical model (high blood pressure). The analogy to the affective disorders is not perfect, but it remains clinically important. First, let's look at the animal model of sensitization and kindling.

Sensitization and Kindling of Seizures: An Animal Model

In this model (figure 2.3), an animal is taken from its home cage to an experimental cage where a low level electrical current is episodically applied to the brain (phase 1). Initially, the low level of electrical current does not produce any response, but with some repetition the brain becomes **sensitized** and the low level current causes a seizure (an escalating electrical activation of wider and wider areas of brain tissue, eventually leading to unconsciousness and involuntary muscle movements, depending on the area of brain tissue involved). At this point the animal has been sensitized: It is having seizures in response to a stimulus that was previously incapable of causing any seizures. Given further stimulus repetitions, less and less current is required to induce a seizure (phase 2), and soon seizures begin to occur spontaneously (phase 3) and we can say that kindling has occurred. Without further external stimulation the kindled (i.e., spontaneous or unprovoked) seizures gradually increase in frequency (phase 4). Thus, there has been progression from nonresponse to

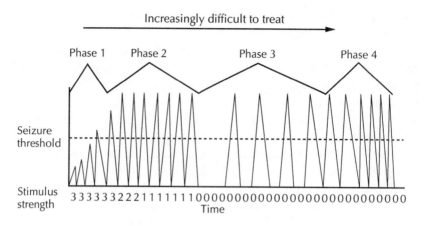

FIGURE 2.3. Sensitization and kindling.

a stimulus, to sensitization and response, followed ultimately by spontaneous seizures without external stimulation.

In experimental animals the kindled response is context dependent. That is, the sensitization or kindling is strongly associated with the environment (e.g., the experimental cage) in which kindling was accomplished. Removal of the animal from the context in which the event was kindled may lead to an absence of further seizures, as long as the animal is not returned to the original experimental cage. Even applying the electrical current to the animal (remember that it was sensitized and seizures were kindled) in its home cage will not produce a seizure! This has strategic clinical implications for psychotherapists, as will be illustrated in the clinical vignettes below.

Sensitization and Kindling of High Blood Pressure: A Human Model

Rick, a 48-year-old executive, commutes 45 minutes to work each day from his new home. "It's a bit far from the office," he initially reasoned, "but it's worth the commute." Over the next few years, traffic jams (the stimulus) gradually become more frequent, and Rick becomes increasingly frustrated (phase 1, figure 2.3). One day Rick has a crucial meeting to attend, but is delayed by another traffic jam. He becomes agitated, and his blood pressure (the response) rises for the first time (he has been sensitized), but eventually returns to normal during the day (end of phase 1/beginning of phase 2). The next day, unbeknownst to Rick, while sitting in another traffic jam, his blood pressure rises again, and soon his blood pressure begins to rise every day that he encounters a traffic jam. In fact, Rick's blood pressure rises even with the slightest increases in traffic (phase 2)! Soon, Rick's blood pressure may become elevated even when there is no traffic at all. The hypertension now occurs without stimulus and is therefore considered to be a kindled phenomenon (phase 3). Finally, Rick's blood pressure begins to rise on a regular basis, increasing in frequency, and eventually remaining elevated (phase 4).

The Mechanism of Sensitization and Kindling

Sensitization and kindling seem to occur via the process of neuromodulation (see chapter 1). In this process, psychosocial events (which, via the meaning assigned to them, may be stressful), and/or the affective episodes themselves, change the long-term activity or expression of the genes. The altered amounts and types of gene products can change the actual structure and function of the neuron. The alteration of reactivity of the individual neurons can occur via changed amounts and types of receptor protein, as well as alterations in the number of connections the cell has with other cells (by the sprouting of new dendrites or, conversely, withdrawal of dendrites and even actual cell death). The areas of the human brain most likely to be sensitized and to kindle are the hippocampus (the seat of much of our memory and learning) and the limbic system (emotional brain). Only valproic acid and possibly Valium-type drugs seem to inhibit kindling. Both of these medications affect the same neurotransmitter, GABA.

The Clinical Relevance of Sensitization and Kindling

There is an old saying in medicine: Hypertension begets hypertension. Research now seems to indicate that affective episodes beget affective episodes. It seems that some people with affective disorders clearly become sensitized and experience kindled episodes, while others do not. In the majority of patients, it seems that later episodes are significantly less likely to be associated with identifiable psychosocial stressors (figure 2.4).

A recent study by Kendler (1995b) indicates that people with high genetic loading (close relatives with affective disorders) are 2.4 times more likely to respond to stressful life events with an affective episode than those with minimal genetic predisposition. Thus, while we cannot separate out or predict for whom this model will apply, we can look at the family history of affective disorders to assess an individual's sensitivity to stressful stimuli and the likelihood of future depression, and thereby assess the risk for sensitization and kindling.

Thus, the sensitization/kindling model implies several considerations:

1. It is imperative to identify and treat early episodes of affective disorders aggressively, with psychotherapy (cognitive, couples, family, or interpersonal therapies), structural life changes (to decrease the frequency whenever possible of negative, depressogenic, and helplessness-inducing environments), skills training (for the workplace), and pharmacology to prevent further episodes. It is no longer acceptable

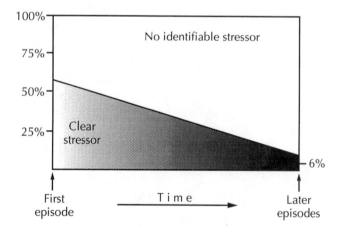

FIGURE 2.4. The percent of episodes with identifiable stressors precipitating an affective episode (based on a literature review).

for any therapist to fail to screen carefully for affective disorders and genetic vulnerability or to continue treatment (for a first episode) more than a few weeks without evidence of response to psychotherapy. Patients with multiple episodes of affective disorders require multimodal treatment, including intervention in the biological arena, in order to maximize prevention of sensitization and kindling.

2. Affective disorders beget affective disorders. Inadequate treatment places the patient at substantial risk of spontaneous episodes and increasing episode frequency (e.g., rapid cycling), and may be more difficult to treat with medication (table 2.4). This risk may be significantly greater in patients with genetic loading.

3. Maintenance medication with therapy is the most beneficial course for prevention of episodes (Kupfer, 1992).

TABLE 2.4
The Progressive Phases of Kindling

DISORDER	PHASE 1 INTERVENTION	PHASE 2 INTERVENTION	PHASE 3 INTERVENTION	PHASE 4 (MALIGNANT PHASE) INTERVENTION
Unipolar depression	Psychotherapy/ environmental change	1 + antidepressant	1 + 2 + lithium (augmentation strategies)	1 + 2 + additional antidepressant or ECT
Bipolar disorder	Lithium/improve sleep, diet, lifestyle habits	1 +/− Valproate	1 + 2 + Tegretol	1 + 2 + 3 + thyroid ECT
Hypertension	Diuretic/dietary, lifestyle changes	1 + Inderal (beta receptor blocker)	1 + 2 + calcium channel blocker (e.g., Procardia)	1 + 2 + 3 + +
Seizures	Valium type medication/lifestyle changes	1 + anticonvulsant	1 + 2 + additional anticonvulsant	1 + 2 + 3 + + psychosurgery

Effective treatment of a kindled event (be it seizures, hypertension, affective disorders, panic, or anticipatory anxiety) is more difficult, requiring progressively more medication and environmental intervention, as one progresses from phase 1 to phase 4. Therefore it is critical that the clinician identify the disorder as soon as possible. This requires a careful longitudinal and family history to determine the frequency of the event, what triggers it, and whether those triggers are still necessary or can somehow be removed. (Numbers in column text refer to previous phase interventions.)

4. Changes in context may be of benefit even in late stages of
    affective disorders, particularly when they have developed
    in a particular context. In such cases, direct recommenda-
    tions for structural life changes (e.g., leave a job, a spouse)
    may be indicated, despite the traditional therapeutic stance
    of allowing the patient to come to his or her own conclu-
    sions, as in the following case.

A CLINICAL ILLUSTRATION   Every health care provider has had experiences that were so powerful that they have forever transformed
his or her thinking and approach to patients. The following was such
a case. It demonstrated a number of things to me, including the
importance of context, the limitations of medication, and the failure
of psychiatrists—myself included—to educate their nonmedically
trained therapist colleagues in the rapidly progressing biological
realm. At a time when the secrets of the brain are being unraveled,
and research in the brain sciences is burgeoning like few other medical fields, we as psychiatrists are not spreading the news to our
colleagues.

Some time ago, when the concepts of sensitization and kindling
were first being published in the psychiatric literature, I began to
look at clinical cases from an additional, broader perspective. What
I saw—and what I knew I needed to do—went against all of my
psychotherapeutic training.

Jenny was a 40-year-old attorney and a divorced and remarried
mother. She was referred by her therapist of two years, Ms. Troy,
for psychiatric evaluation and consideration of medication to treat
her worsening depression. At the initial interview, Jenny's husband,
Frank, an accountant, was present in order to provide some history.
He was quite cooperative yet strangely detached. He answered all
queries in a genuine manner—as he worked on his paperwork! After
ruling out any medical causes of Jenny's depression, I prescribed
medication and encouraged her to continue her therapy with Ms.
Troy. Jenny responded nicely to the medication but soon relapsed.
Over the course of one year she relapsed four times, each time requiring a change in medication.

It gradually became clear that the source of Jenny's unrelenting
depression was her husband's lack of accountability and responsibil-

ity regarding the marriage. While Frank said all the right things, he would frequently and unpredictably be late for couples sessions, not follow through on promises, etc. Jenny was helpless to achieve her dream of a satisfying marriage. This context (an uncooperative spouse, combined with a desire to make the marriage work) was powerful enough that Jenny's depressions were recurring repeatedly, but, as may occur in a poorly managed split-treatment setting, I as her psychopharmacologist had only peripheral awareness of these dynamics. This changed, however, when I was paged to a long distance number at 11:30 p.m. on a Saturday night.

Jenny was in a hotel 2000 miles from home, threatening suicide. After arranging for her safety, I made sure that she was escorted to a friend's home the next morning. When Jenny came in my office she looked haggard. As she filled me in on the details of the episode, I realized that the episode was again triggered by the ongoing helplessness within the marriage. Her husband, it turned out, had discontinued couples therapy several weeks earlier and was clearly not engaged in her attempt to improve the marriage. Jenny felt trapped between failure in a second marriage and helplessness about improving the relationship. That Saturday night she saw suicide as the only way out.

Now, at the crucial moment, she wanted me to tell her whether she should stay out of the house or go back to her husband. Based on the sensitization and kindling models, as well as the learned helplessness and other models of depression, I (gulp!) advised Jenny that a change in her context was medically indicated, and that was my firm recommendation. Her husband was creating a depressogenic context that attitude change and/or medication could not counterbalance. Continued depression caused by this context — a context in which her level of control over the outcome was negligible, a context that was in conflict with her deep need to love and be loved — led to more severe, frequent depression (sensitization, which could lead to kindling), and of course, suicidal ideation. I advised her to stay out of the home; if she and her husband chose to, they could continue in couples psychotherapy. Jenny followed my advice, and one- and two-year follow-ups revealed that she did not relapse into depression. Jenny's therapist was surprised by the advice I had given Jenny; she, too, had been taught that therapy was not about giving advice.

CHRONOBIOLOGY

Investors have always known it. Now psychiatrists know it too: Timing is everything.

Chronobiology is the study of rhythmic or periodic changes in biological functions over particular time periods. In the mental health arena, we must be concerned with daily, monthly, and seasonal rhythms. Hormones (messenger molecules released from various glands closely associated with the nervous system, which travel through the blood to reach their target organs) seem to be essential pieces of the chronobiological mechanisms, and will be reviewed in more detail in the next section. In this section your awareness of the rhythms most important for mental health professionals will be raised. It is my hope that whenever you see a patient with worsening emotional symptoms, you will wonder: Is this tied to a rhythmic pattern? Is this client worse because of the time of year, the time of month, or even the particular time of the day?

Circadian Rhythms

Circadian rhythms are fluctuations that occur within and around the daily 24-hour cycle. Temperature, energy, sleep, arousal, motor activity, appetite, hormones (e.g., thyroid, cortisol, sex hormones, melatonin), and mood all demonstrate circadian rhythms. Abnormalities in these rhythms are apparent in and relevant to the study and treatment of depression, hypomania, mania, and, to a lesser degree, some anxiety disorders (panic, obsessive compulsive disorders, dissociative disorders).

The Mechanism of Circadian Rhythms

There are two parts to the proposed regulation of circadian rhythms: external cues and internal pacemakers (figure 2.5). As a piano player might adjust or entrain his internal rhythm to the beat of a metronome, so the body adjusts its natural internal rhythm to the beat of the external world. When it works well, we have a masterpiece, but when it doesn't, life loses its rhythm. The external metronome or cues (chronobiologists call them zeitgebers) include light, temperature, mealtimes, social interactions, posture, and activity levels. The

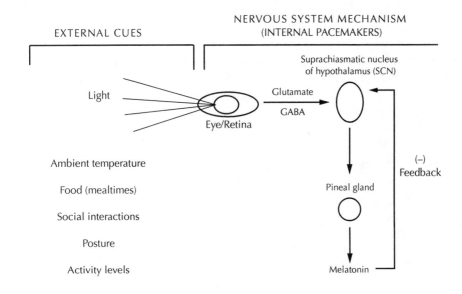

FIGURE 2.5. The link between the environment (external cues) and the nervous system mechanism (internal pacemakers) of circadian and seasonal rhythms.

internal pacemaker in the brain that regulates the daily rhythms is called the suprachiasmatic nucleus (SCN) (see chapter 1, Nuclei). As the name implies, this nucleus sits above (supra) the nerves that emanate from the retina of the eye. The SCN is one of the many nuclei of the hypothalamus, the central integrating station that controls hormonal and autonomic nervous system output. The neurons in the SCN are stimulated by glutamate, an excitatory neurotransmitter, and GABA, an inhibitory neurotransmitter. Dopamine is also involved in this neural circuit. The external environmental cues lead to activation or inhibition of the SCN, which then causes the pineal gland of the brain to increase or decrease the release of the hormone, melatonin. Melatonin is thought to play a role in the sleep-wake cycle, adjusting the body clock (SCN) via a negative feedback loop, according to the external light cues.

The Clinical Relevance of Circadian Rhythms

Chronobiology offers a new way of conceptualizing mood and anxiety disorders. From the chronobiologist's perspective, the affective disorders and possibly the anxiety disorders reflect a desynchronization between the external cues and internal pacemaker. The desynchronization may originate internally or externally. Affectively disordered patients exhibit a variety of abnormalities in the external-internal linkage. There is some evidence of instability of the internal pacemaker (SCN), difficulty entraining to external cues, as well as over and undersensitivity to external cues. It appears that different individuals are likely to have abnormalities in different phases of this external-internal linkage.

Hormones are released from the various organs of the body in predictable, internally paced pulses that are generally entrained to the external cues, with the light-dark cycle and social cues probably being most relevant. In mood disorders, severe depression is often marked by a high frequency of variation from the norm in mood and energy. Normally, one's energy begins to pick up early in the day, with a mid-afternoon peak. In severe depression, mood and energy are shifted, so that the depressed person will only begin to feel some improved mood and energy by late afternoon. This type of disturbance, commonly refered to as **diurnal variation**, has traditionally been thought to be strongly indicative of a biological dysregulation requiring pharmacologic intervention. **Reverse diurnal variation**, that is, a worsening of mood and/or energy as the day progresses, is sometimes thought to be more common in anxious, rejection sensitive, seasonal, and bipolar (those with a history of either hypomania or mania) depressives.

As a result of the research that has been conducted in this area, it also seems clear that sleep deprivation (partial—asleep at 8 p.m., up at 2 a.m.—or complete—up for 40 hours continuously), and rapid eye movement (REM) sleep suppression (accomplished via antidepressants, research methods, or partial sleep deprivation) are both effective in treating depression. REM sleep suppression, which takes 2–3 weeks to work, seems to last longest and be most effective. Sleep deprivation, on the other hand, provokes an antidepressant response within one day, but lasts only one or two days.

Do the psychosocial stresses act, at least in part, by disrupting the normal routines and their entrained internal rhythms? If your energy and mood rise in the morning with the sound of the birds, breakfast, your husband's smile, and taking out the garbage (!), and, like Pavlov's dog, your biological clock is entrained to this daily rhythm, what happens if your husband travels frequently or, worse yet, leaves you? Does the loss of the normal routine throw off your internal hormonal rhythm, as the loss of the metronome throws off the rhythm of the amateur (read: vulnerable) piano player? The tendency toward dysregulation of this internal clock is probably inherited, but it is also influenced over the course of the life cycle by stresses, lifestyle (e.g., shift work), sex hormones (depression is twice as common, and rapid cycling three times more common, in women than men), and normal aging. Does psychiatric hospitalization and/or regular psychotherapy, with their regularizing schedule, promote stabilization of internal rhythms around a new set of cues? Are the sleep-wake cycle, temperature cycle (5 a.m. is the low for the day), hormonal rhythms, etc., of depressed or manic people overly sensitive to disruption of social cues such as loss of an established social role? One study indicates that widowed subjects who had highly disrupted social patterns were more likely to experience depression than those who maintained their routines (Ehlers, Frank, & Kupfer, 1988). Are infants who have difficulty establishing a regular routine of sleep and waking more prone to depression? While the answers are not in, you as the clinician now know the questions to ask. You can listen for these factors and begin to form your own impressions and hypotheses.

A PERSONAL VIGNETTE   Last week I had a personal experience that supported the importance of maintaining rhythms in my own life. My mother-in-law, who has been in a nursing home for five years, had a sudden setback and became semicomatose. My wife and I suddenly were torn from our daily routines, and I noted how anxious I felt about my mother-in-law's possible death, as well as the disruption in my own life (less sleep, cancelled patients, no writing, etc.). I thought that was a fairly selfish thought on my part until I recalled the study by Ehlers and colleagues (1988), which I referred to in the previous paragraph. I realized that both my wife and I needed to maintain our usual activities as much as possible, and we supported each other in that. The reduction in anxiety and stress was impressive and was experienced by me on a physiological level. This experience has deepened my appreciation of the importance of maintaining one's rhythm.

As a result of my own experience, I reiterated the need for daily structure to a 39-year-old recently unemployed female with a rapidly cycling bipolar disorder. This time around, however, I related my own experience. She then offered me a piece of history that I had previously overlooked. She told me that the events that led up to her job problems and subsequent hospitalization actually began with the illness of her grandmother, to whom she was particularly close. During her grandmother's illness, my patient was often up late at night and experienced numerous disruptions in her rhythm, which actually precipitated her decline! Reviewing further, I found that at least 50% of her previous episodes were precipitated by events that disrupted her daily rhythms (e.g., a move to a different school).

Monthly Cycles

Aside from the sleep-wake cycle, the most commonly recognized chronobiological cycle is the female reproductive (menstrual) cycle, beginning at puberty and tapering off at menopause. Given the large number of hormonal fluctuations that occur on a monthly basis, it would not be very surprising if the internal pacemakers of most women in the reproductive years were desynchronized on a regular basis, leading to a mood or anxiety disorder and all of their consequences. Yet this is not the case, and most women do not suffer from significant premenstrual dysphoric disorder (PDD is the more narrow mood-related disorder, formerly called PMS, which encompasses the exacerbation of any premenstrual problems), although some researchers believe it is underreported. Nevertheless, it seems highly likely that these hormonal swings are partially responsible for the increased incidence of unipolar depression and rapid cycling bipolar disorder (four or more episodes per year) in women.

Dalton (1984) has studied PMS extensively in her clinical population and views premenstrual dysphoria as one of a number of premenstrual "syndromes" that exhibit a cyclical worsening of symptoms, much like seasonal worsening of a number of disorders. Thus, the rate of change and the degree of change during the seasonal and monthly cycles will unmask or worsen any underlying infirmity. Premenstrual dysphoric disorder, in DSM-IV, is therefore restricted to a mood disturbance occurring during the 15th–28th days (second half) of the cycle. Dalton, however, takes a broader view and notes that there is a statistically significant increase in tension, depression, irritability, lethargy, migraine, epilepsy, fainting, acne, herpes eruption, itching, asthma, allergy, joint pain, arthritis, glaucoma, styes, sinusitis, sore throats, violent acts, suicide attempts, criminal acts, alcoholic binges, panic attacks, psychotic episodes, and hospitalizations (medical and psychiatric) in the premenstrual period!

The Mechanism of PDD/PMS

In view of the complexity of the hormonal and subsequent physical changes that occur each month, and the increased difficulty women have with depression, it is clear that only minor entries into the maze of PDD/PMS have been made. Various theories regarding its mechanism have been proposed, as researchers reason backward from what seems to work. (This pharmacologic dissection of PDD/PMS is consistent with the approach that has brought biological psychiatry so far since the 1950s.) A leading theory suggests that the relative rates of change in progesterone and estrogen are the source of the problem. Another proposed mechanism for PMS/PDD is that of opioid withdrawal, following the mid-cycle peak in a naturally occurring morphine-like substance called beta endorphin. This is based on the observation that naltrexone, a drug that stops opiate withdrawal syndrome, was found to be significantly more effective in PMS/PDD than placebo (Chuong, 1988). Additional theories include abnormalities in melatonin regulation (sometimes bright lights are effective in PMS/PDD — even without a seasonal pattern), elevations in prolactin levels (the hormone that *pro*motes *lact*ation), abnormal thyroid function, abnormalities of B6, magnesium, water balance, etc. Finally, there is the fact that the sex hormones strongly influence the internal pacemakers, slowing them down (progesterone) or speeding them up (estrogen), and enhancing synchronization between different pacemakers (estrogen). Thus, it seems clear that alterations in the sex hormones affect the biological clock, other hormonal systems, and neurotransmitters (progesterone increases activity of the inhibitory neurotransmitter GABA, causing a calming

effect). There is ample opportunity for dysregulation of neurotransmission, desynchronization of internal and external pacemakers, and
exacerbation of other preexisting problems.

A CLINICAL ILLUSTRATION   Nancy is a 39-year-old married, employed mother of one very precocious three-year-old girl. She had
been in psychotherapy for seven years when she was referred for
evaluation of her mood disturbances. As it turns out, Nancy had had
a severe postpartum depression (almost to the point of psychosis),
which was never evaluated (postpartum thyroid disturbances or severe abnormalities of the hypothalamus can look like depression or
psychosis, but can also be medical emergencies). Evaluation at the
time of early meetings with Joan revealed that her thyroid function
was indeed low, and treating this cleared a number of symptoms (dry
skin, hair loss, bloating in the ankles, low energy), but did not alleviate her depression. Nancy was very patient as we proceeded through
a number of medication trials. Often, Nancy would show a good
response to a medication, and then: "Whamo!! I get close to my
period and the depression is back! How can I beat this thing, when
my period keeps setting it off? I think it's hopeless!"

Nancy was correct about the process, but not about the outcome.
Eventually Nancy did quite well on Nardil (a monoamine oxidase
inhibitor type of antidepressant) with Ritalin (methylphenidate, to
help with the side effects of the Nardil). She broke through the
medication during her premenstrual phase twice, but an increase in
dosage finally stabilized her.

At the time of this writing, Nancy is tapering off the Nardil,
getting ready to have her next child. Given her history of postpartum
depression, she has a 50% increase in the risk of recurrence in the
postpartum phase; if she had been psychotic after her first child, that
risk would increase from 1 in 500 to 1 in 3 for this pregnancy! I have
advised her of these risks and will follow her closely in the months
following her delivery. Nancy has elected not to breast-feed, so that
she can restart her medication quickly.

Seasonal Rhythms

Given the above discussion of entrainment of internal pacemakers to
external circadian rhythms, it is not surprising that researchers have

recently turned their attention to the more subtle and gradual seasonal rhythms, as Hippocrates did 2000 years earlier (Jackson, 1986). It may seem, therefore, that there's really nothing new under the sun; however, that is decidedly not the case! In fact, as we shall see, highly effective treatment is now available.

Seasonal variations in numerous illnesses occur, including but not limited to the psychiatric disorders of depression, mania, panic, obsessive compulsive disorder, and bulimia. In addition to this list, I have treated four cases of dissociative disorders, including multiple personality disorder, which demonstrated clear seasonal exacerbation (Clark, Hedaya, & Rosenthal, 1995) of the dissociative disorder.

About 10% of all affective disorders are seasonal, of which there seem to be two types. Type A is the classic fall–low, spring–high pattern; type B is the reverse: spring–low, fall–high. A large number of seasonal affective disorder (SAD) patients are known to be bipolar type I or II, and this seems to be more common if the patient falls into a type A pattern. The frequency with which SAD patients are bipolar ranges from 49 to 93% (Faedda, 1993). Eighty percent of all SAD patients are female. Given the entrainment of internal rhythms to environmental cues, it is not surprising that the highest frequency of onset of mania or depression comes at the times of greatest change in the seasons: April and September. Seasonal depression (type A) seems to be primarily associated with low energy, hypersomnia (excessive need for sleep), hyperphagia (excessive appetite, carbohydrate craving, possibly related to abnormalities in serotonin neurons of the brain's feeding center), and depressed mood. In clear-cut SAD, the depressed mood may be secondary to the frustration and helplessness these patients experience around a profound lack of energy and inability to carry on with their lives. Very little research has been done on type B SAD, although some researchers speculate that temperature may be the primary factor in these cases.

Treatment of type A SAD involves phototherapy, which requires that the patient be exposed to full spectrum lights (10,000 lux, no ultraviolet) for a specific amount of time, and at a certain distance from the light source (usually a light box). The timing of the exposure to the light seems to have little impact on efficacy, as opposed to the importance of duration of exposure. Treatment frequently works within 5 days, and the only side effects seem to be possible eye strain and irritability (too much light). Recent research seems to indicate that certain drugs that suppress melatonin secretion, such as Inderal (propranolol), are also effective in SAD. Type B SAD is currently treated as other affective disorders are, although further research will undoubtedly change this approach.

The Mechanism of Seasonal Rhythms

No consensus has been reached about the mechanism of light therapy, and there are at least eight hypotheses according to Wirz-Justice (1995). SAD may be related to the length of the photoperiod, the total number of photons taken in per day, melatonin secretion, instability of the circadian rhythms in conditions of extreme daylight or darkness, retinal deficiencies, abnormalities of alpha-2 and/or serotonin receptors in the paraventricular nucleus (PVN), which controls food selection, etc. It seems certain that the simplified circuit diagrammed in figure 2.5, as well as its branches, are involved in the abnormalities of diminished arousal and excessive carbohydrate intake, and that serotonin dysregulation is involved as well.

A CLINICAL ILLUSTRATION   Bill is a 27-year-old physicist with bipolar SAD, type A. He agreed to take lithium, which eliminated his spring-time hypomania, but only partially alleviated his winter depression. Light therapy was added with good results. After three years, Bill married, and two years later he and his wife decided to move to a farm, which is at the same latitude, essentially, as his home of origin (the frequency of SAD goes down as one moves toward the equator and sunlight increases, and vice versa). I will never forget the conversation Bill and I had after his second year on the farm, because the transformation was so remarkable.

"Doc, I gotta tell you, I finally felt like I was ready for this fall!"

"What do you mean?" I inquired.

"Well, I worked all spring and summer. From dawn till after dark in the fields. It was really hard, but I was out there all day. When fall came, I was really ready for it! I'm really in synch with the seasons now! I'm looking foward to the winter for the first time in my life. I need the rest and relaxation, the short days and long nights. I'm looking foward to it!"

I have followed Bill over four years since that phone conversation, and he has not had one depressive episode since, despite the death of his mother two years ago.

PSYCHOENDOCRINOLOGY

Psychoendocrinology is the study of the interaction between psychiatry/psychology and hormones (endocrinology). **Psychoneuroendocrinology** includes the study of the neural systems that mediate the interaction between psychiatry/psychology and hormones, and thus is the most complete approach to this aspect of biological psychiatry (figure 2.6). Remember that while psychological, social, and neural factors mediate the release of hormones, the brain is itself a target organ of these hormones.

While research over the past 25 years indicates that there are clear

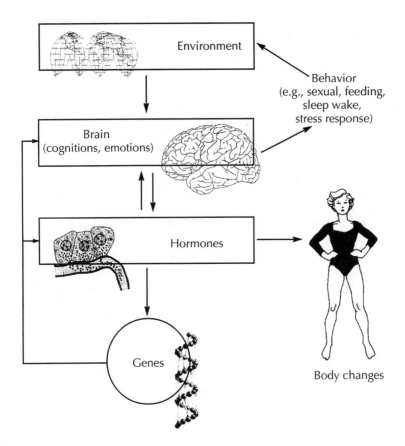

FIGURE 2.6. How hormones interface between the environment, brain, and gene expression.

abnormalities of hormonal regulation accompanying many psychiatric syndromes (e.g., affective disorders, seasonal disorders, postpartum disorders, late onset psychotic disorders), this knowledge has not yet been applied in any generally accepted manner to the practice of biological psychiatry. There has been minimal research on the effects of the sex hormones on affective disorders, despite the increased incidence of affective disorders in women (unipolar depression is twice as frequent in women as in men), rapid cycling (three times more likely in women than men), frequent onset of the affective disorders around puberty (men and women), the menses, the postpartum phase, and postmenopause. As psychoneuroendocrinological research progresses, it is virtually certain that hormonal assessment and manipulation will play a widely accepted role in the standard care of the major psychiatric syndromes, particularly in those patients who respond poorly to the currently available interventions.

Hormones

Hormones (from the Greek word *hormaein*, meaning "to set in motion") are chemical substances produced by individual cells within an organ or gland. Hormones are manufactured and then stored in the individual cells of the gland. When the cells receive the appropriate signal, usually from the nervous system, they release an appropriate portion of the stored hormone into the blood (circulation), which carries them to their target(s). While traveling in the bloodstream, hormones are often bound to "carrier" proteins; they are inactive until released from these carrier proteins. The levels of carrier proteins are affected by factors such as birth control pills, certain medications, and nutritional status, and therefore changes in these proteins will affect the amount of active hormone in the blood.

Hormonal Axes

The triad of hypothalamic, pituitary, and peripheral (i.e., outside of the central nervous system) hormones and glands constitutes what biological psychiatrists refer to as an axis. Just as one would think of an axis as a line "spearing" the earth from the north pole to the south pole, so one can imagine various axes connecting the hypothalamus, pituitary, and peripheral glands. Thus we talk about the HPA axis (hypothalamic-pituitary-adrenal), the thyroid axis (hypothalamus-pituitary-thyroid), or the reproductive axis (hypothalamus-pituitary-ovaries/testes).

Hormonal Controls

A cascade of several different glands and their respective hormones, along the axis, may be involved in the regulation of one peripheral target organ. In general, a particular cascade follows four steps (figure 2.7):

1. The hypothalamus releases a **releasing hormone**. The amount of releasing hormone secreted is determined by input to the hypothalamus from at least three sources: (a) the internal pacemakers (whose own activity is modified by the external cues to which they are entrained) — these cause predictable pulsatile stimulation of the releasing hormone, which may occur hourly, daily, monthly or annually (see Chronobiology, above), (b) the actual amount of the endproduct of the cascade that is already present in the blood, and (c) the higher cortical and limbic centers, via the cingulate tract.
2. The releasing hormone stimulates the pituitary gland to release a **stimulating hormone**, which will then
3. activate a particular target gland outside of the central nervous system, such as the thyroid or adrenal gland, which will then
4. secrete a hormone into the blood, which will act on a large number of the body functions and cell types.

The amount of this "final" hormone will feed back to the hypothalamus and pituitary glands which produced the releasing and stimulating hormones: Higher levels will turn off the cascade; lower levels will turn it on.

How Do Hormones Work?

Once released and attatched to their targets, hormones may generate two types of responses (figure 2.7):

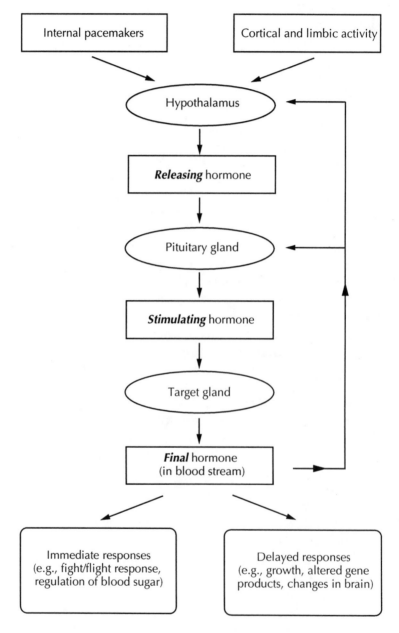

FIGURE 2.7. The hormonal axis: cascade and response.

1. An **immediate response**, for example, the fight/flight response of epinephrine (also called adrenaline), which is released from the innermost part of the glands situated on top of the kidneys—the ad(above)renal(kidney) medulla (innermost part). The immediate response is involved in rapid adjustments of bodily function such as the fight/flight response to a threat or the adjustment of blood sugar levels to accommodate suddenly changing conditions.

2. A **delayed response**, for example, the stress response of the adrenal cortex (outer "shell" of the adrenal gland). This response is involved with the bigger picture confronting the individual and the production of long-term changes in the structure and function of the body (e.g., growth). This delayed response changes the structure and function of the brain via tailoring of gene expression. This characteristic ability of the brain to constantly change its structure and function in response to the environment is sometimes referred to as **plasticity** and is mediated in part by hormones. In the brain, these changes caused by hormones can result in nerve cell growth or death over various periods of the life span, as well as maturational changes (e.g., pubertal changes, menopausal changes) during the life cycle. Interestingly, it has been shown that hormones influence neurons in the female rat brain to rhythmically sprout and wither with each reproductive cycle—just as the leaves of a tree bloom and whither in their annual cycle! These findings challenge our view of the brain as a static organ and highlight mechanisms by which stress, as well as psychotherapy, can cause brain changes.

The Stress Response

Aside from mediating conservation of the organism and development of maturational and reproductive changes in the body, hormones also play a major role as the "shock absorbers" of the body. When stressed by physical or psychological trauma, such as rape, military combat, divorce, etc., the hormonal system secretes adrenal hormones (epinephrine and corticosteroids) that counterregulate each other. The stress response also activates brain neurotransmitters and the immune system. As a result, the victim of trauma will respond in a balanced manner, neither overreacting or underreacting. In the case of repeated uncontrollable stress (figure 2.8), as in the learned helplessness model of depression (see chapter 3), there is poor or absent feedback by the stress hormones (corticosteroids such as cortisol) to the hypothalamus and hippocampus (Young et al., 1991). This often results in higher than normal levels of corticosteroids, which can destroy the cells involved in memory integration (the hip-

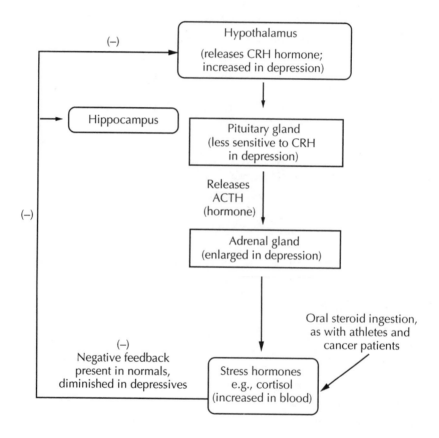

FIGURE 2.8.   The stress response system and its dysregulation in response to uncontrollable stress.

pocampal cells). Depression can thus be regarded as a case of dysregulation of the normal feedback mechanisms in response to stress. This statement is supported by numerous studies of the HPA axis in affective disorders, eating disorders, and late onset psychotic disorders (but not schizophrenia) over the past 15 years. This is important to remember in the treatment of depression and dissociative disorders, as well as PTSD.

A CLINICAL ILLUSTRATION   Five years ago, Lois, a very pleasant, highly intelligent woman in her late thirties, was referred to me for evaluation and treatment of her depression, presumably (according to the referring therapist) for medication and cognitive therapy. In the course of the evaluation, she related a long history of intermittent low grade depression since the onset of her menstruation. This was not unusual. What was unusual, and remained a mystery to me until one month ago, was her recounting of a sudden onset of severe, "almost psychotic" depression and "incredible panic" at the age of 26, shortly after she stopped smoking cigarettes. During the early months of her treatment with me, Lois struggled in vain to communicate the uniqueness, intensity, and mystery of her experience at that "turning point" in her life. She had had depressions and anxiety before, but never like this. Somehow, she insisted, this was different. She felt her confidence was "never the same" afterward, despite building a successful law career and becoming an excellent and devoted mother.

Frankly, I was skeptical of the association between her near psychosis and panic with discontinuation of smoking, but respecting her intelligence and hearing the earnestness in her voice I always wondered what I wasn't understanding. Somehow the pieces of the puzzle didn't fit together. In July of 1995 I received my weekly *Journal of the American Medical Association*, which contained the formerly private internal documents of the tobacco industry called the "Brown and Williamson Documents" (Glantz et al., 1995). The answer to the mystery was in the documents:

Chronic intake of nicotine tends to restore the normal physiological functioning of the endocrine [hormonal] system, so that ever increasing dose levels of nicotine are necessary to maintain the desired action.

Nicotine . . . is an addictive drug effective in the release of stress mechanisms.

Apparently, after years of smoking, when Lois quit smoking her hormonal "shock absorber" system (endocrine system) quit working too, since her stress response was conditioned over years to respond to the cigarette/nicotine! Lois was essentially without a stress response for a number of weeks, the equivalent to having your hormones turned off abruptly, a very dangerous state. This patient's mood disorder was ultimately treated successfully with thyroid hormone replacement and progesterone. No psychotropic medications were needed.

The Clinical Relevance of Hormones

Hormones act inside the nucleus of the cell to tailor the expression of certain genes. As a result, hormones play a very major role in controlling the production levels of proteins, which are necessary for proper function of innumerable bodily processes. For the biological psychiatrist, consideration of hormonal dysregulation as a cause of or contributor to psychiatric problems should be routine. It is well-known that androgens (testosterone), estrogens, progesterone, thyroid hormone, parathyroid hormone, and adrenal-steroid hormones can cause mood or anxiety disorders when dysregulated. These abnormalities—when detected and treated—usually result in enhanced response to antidepressant or mood stabilizing therapies and, on occasion, to complete remission of the "psychiatric" problem. Unfortunately, these hormonal abnormalities are often missed.

A PERSONAL VIGNETTE   Because of my awareness of these facts, I am facinated by psychoendocrinology and convinced that it is an important piece of the diagnostic and therapeutic puzzle. I have been fortunate to know a prominent endocrinologist, Helena Rodbard, M.D., who has assisted me in my continuing education in this field. After working with Dr. Rodbard for several years, my knowledge of the thyroid (a gland in the neck that is primarily involved in growth, neural maturation, and energy and metabolism in the body) began to develop to the point that I was discovering a fair number of thyroid disorders in the process of my evaluation of new patients. As a result, numerous internists and even some endocrinologists became upset with my assumptions, conclusions, and territory violations ("What is a psychiatrist doing, mucking around with the thyroid anyway?"). My improved detection rate was, I thought, a result of a high index of suspicion, careful history and physical examination, and the use of a dynamic test of thyroid function called the TRH (thyroid releasing hormone) stimulation test (figure 2.9). Let me take a brief detour to explain thyroid testing and the TRH test in particular, before returning to my story.

Thyroid tests are some of the most frequently ordered tests in medicine. However, the usual thyroid function tests employed as screening tools are often indirect tests such as the T3RU (similar to calculating the volume of a balloon by measuring the amount of water it displaces when immersed in a tub), calculated indexes (the free thyroxine index), or momentary static measures of the hormone levels (free T4 or thyroid stimulating hormone [TSH]) at one particular moment in time, which may not be reflective of more subtle dysregulations. Often these tests are done as screening measures on a routine basis by primary care physicians. Specific questions relating to possible dysfunction of the thyroid gland are usually not even asked, since it is assumed that the tests will be abnormal if anything

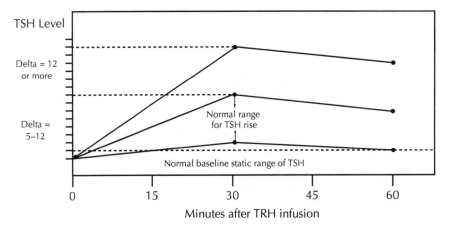

FIGURE 2.9. The thyroid releasing hormone (TRH) stimulation test.

significant is wrong. If the tests come back in the normal range the thyroid is assumed to be fine, and the physician looks elsewhere to account for the symptoms, with many patients being sent to their local mental health professionals since "nothing physical" is identified. These routine static tests will not pick up a mild dysregulation, which would become manifest under stress, unless it is present at the time of the test. Here patients find my shock absorber analogy useful.

As previously described, it is best to use dynamic, rather than static, tests to measure the shock absorber system. One dynamic test of thyroid function is the TRH stimulation test (figure 2.9). In this test the hypothalamic hormone TRH (thyroid releasing hormone) is injected intravenously, and the response of the pituitary gland (TSH, thyroid stimulating hormone) is measured over about one hour (baseline, 15 minutes, 30 minutes, and 60 minutes). The difference between baseline TSH (the amount before any TRH is injected) and maximal TSH at 30 and 60 minutes is called the **delta**, or absolute, change. If the delta is excessively great, the patient is thought to have a low functioning thyroid axis (subclinical hypothyroidism). The problem, however, is that the normal delta is not firmly established and may range from 12 to at least 30 depending on whom you ask!

Unfortunately, clear standards for normal responses for dynamic tests in endocrinology have not been adequately defined, but in principle they are judged useful as the "best test of subtle endocrine dysfunction" (Griffin, 1985). The use of these tests and their interpretation thus remains part of the art of medicine. With this backround let's move on.

I performed a TRH stimulation test on 35 patients whom I thought might have subclinical hypothyroidism (based on signs and symptoms). All of these patients had normal, routine static tests of thyroid function (free T4 and TSH). The TRH stimulation test is not in common use in the primary care arena. It is rare for a psychiatrist to perform it, so over the course of time I had to deal with numerous internists, family physicians, and even one or two endocrinologists who thought I was out of line. It was very difficult, and finally I thought I had better take a look at my assumptions. Perhaps I *was* way out of line.

I hired an independent statistician to review the records. I stopped performing the test for over 18 months while the charts were reviewed. What I was told astounded me. Fifty percent of those tested turned out to be subclinically hypothyroid! "I must be wrong!" I thought. "I'm probably using an overly sensitive delta. How could 50% of the patients with normal thyroid function tests (albeit they had signs and symptoms) have an abnormal result on this test?" I checked with Dr. Helena Rodbard, who was at the time helping to formulate national standards for thyroid evaluation and treatment. She assured me. "Bob, unfortunately you know more about the thyroid than most internists and some endocrinologists!"

That was, of course, music to my ears. But soon I began to wonder if perhaps Dr. Rodbard could be wrong. I went back over the data and saw that the vast majority (nearly 100%) who were treated with synthetic thyroid hormone responded with improvement in the signs and symptoms that had aroused my suspicion (dry skin, hair loss, brittle nails, cold sensitivity, constipation, weight gain, bloating, irregular period, low energy, mental sluggishness, difficulty with concentration, frequent hoarseness, elevated cholesterol, low B12, sluggish reflexes, increased difficulty getting out of a chair, climbing stairs, or getting out of a car, depression, rapid cycling, and partial response to antidepressants).

I started doing the TRH stimulation test again, this time observing the response to synthetic hormone replacement more carefully. To date, rather than finding results which support the status quo, I am finding that the test is quite useful. I conclude that *the type of routine testing of thyroid function in patients with symptoms suggestive of low thyroid function is inadequate.* These results must be replicated (in a formal study) and published (which I will do when this manuscript is completed) to stand up to scientific scrutiny, but on a personal level I have become convinced that a dynamic test is far more sensitive in this setting and must be employed more frequently when suspicious signs and symptoms exist, despite normal routine thyroid function tests.

In addition to thyroid hormone, estrogens and testosterone can affect mood and libido and should be assessed in appropriate cases. Progesterone (Dalton, 1984) therapy can aid in treatment of premenstrual dysphoria since it has a calming effect. Melatonin can be useful in the disturbed sleep of the elderly, whose pineal glands often are no longer capable of producing the hormone, and in avoiding jet lag.

PLASTICITY, LEARNING, AND MEMORY

One's self-concept and identity are constructed by and dependent on one's memory of past experience, preferences, assumptions, etc. **Plasticity** refers to the fact that the shape of who we are — our identity — at the levels of cell (neuron), organ (brain), and organism (human) can constantly be adjusted based on new experience, changes in our recollection of previous experiences, and forgetting.

The analogy of a tree, with its growth, sprouting of new branches (formation of new connections), and loss of branches (loss of connections) from its earlier stages of development is apt (figure 2.10). The tree changes in time as a reflection of the conditions around it

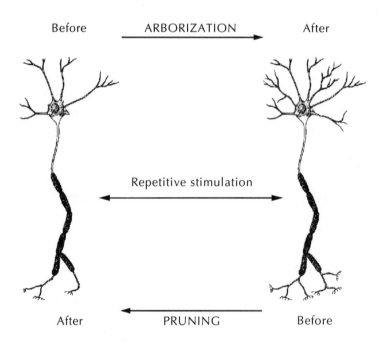

FIGURE 2.10. Plasticity of neurons: arborization and pruning.

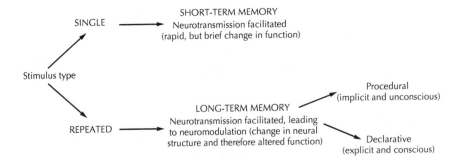

FIGURE 2.11. Short- and long-term memory.

and its own developmental unfolding. It constantly changes shape and appearance — within a limited range. If it started out as an oak, an oak it remains. We as individuals, our brains as organs, and indeed the individual neurons that mediate memory change in the same way. So, in contrast to the view of nerve cells and the brain as static entities that unfold along a predetermined developmental path independent of outside influence, research now strongly supports the view that the brain and its neurons are constantly changing with time and experience, in function and shape, just as our identities and self-concepts change. How these changes occur is interesting and relevant to the psychotherapist. That it occurs at all offers patients hope of change and recovery.

The Mechanism of Learning and Memory

Learning is the acquisition of new knowledge, and memory is the retention of that knowledge for future use. Memory is not a single, fixed entity; it is malleable, changes over time, and involves a variety of distinct brain systems, depending on the type of learning involved. Researchers have found that two relatively independent but interacting memory processes exist (figure 2.11): short-term memory (STM) and long-term memory (LTM). Long-term memory is further subdivided into two types: **declarative** (i.e., explicit) memory, and **procedural** (i.e., implicit) memory.

Long-Term Memory

Procedural memory does not require conscious awareness; it involves the shaping of automatic skills, reflexes, and procedures over time, such as occurs when riding a bike. It involves the parts of the brain that receive the sensation (input) and control motor responses (output). There is no stopover or connection with parts of the brain that mediate consciousness.

Declarative memory involves conscious learning and involves a memory system with three components. First, when an event occurs, information is registered in the various sensory parts of the brain. Thus, as you read this sentence, the parts of the brain involved with vision, language, and speech are activated and short-term memory is activated (via the neurotransmission process, see chapter 1). Second, if the level, duration, and repetition of stimulation are sufficient (i.e., if you read this section over and over, and if you are sufficiently interested and excited about it), the cells of the hippocampus are activated. Like camera film, which changes when exposed to small amounts light, cells of the hippocampus are exquisitely sensitive and are therefore quite capable of being imprinted with new information, as well as being easily overwhelmed by excessive information. The hippocampal cells are involved in the consolidation of the memory information into a whole interconnected memory via the process of neuromodulation (see chapter 1). Theoretically, if the consolidation phase does not occur in a satisfactory manner, appropriate connections between different sensory parts of the experienced event are not established and a "partial memory" or fragmented **neural network** is formed. Third, the memory is stored, in association with the parts of the brain that registered the information in the first place, as a neural network. Activation of one part of the network very likely activates other parts of the network, generating a whole memory.

A PERSONAL VIGNETTE: MY OWN NEURAL NETWORK   As I was writing this, I recalled a striking but common experience that occurred during a visit to my grandmother several years ago. I hadn't been to my grandmother's home for about 15 years, since I had left my hometown for college and medical school, then married and lived in another city. When I returned after 15 years, I was immediately greeted by the smell of kibbeh (a Middle Eastern food she'd prepare on holidays) and the sight of her kitchen. Suddenly, I was transported through time to a memory of a holiday dinner, when I was no more than 10 years old. I was standing by the glossy-white enamel oven, I could smell the familiar spices and was asking for more kibbeh, looking up at my grandmother. I felt that old strange emotion of uncertainty and discomfort: "I want her to give me the kibbeh and then I want to get out of this kitchen before she asks me to help her!"

Aside from being fodder for an undetermined number of psychoanalytic sessions, this is an example of the activation of a neural network by a stimulus. The stimulus — my grandmother's kitchen — evoked activation of the other components of the neural network, including images, feelings, thoughts, etc. This is similar to what happens during a flashback. In the flashbacks of posttraumatic stress disorder, however, the stimulus is generalized so that any number of stimuli activate the memory, the response causes emotional distress, and there is no sense of control over the reliving of the event and its attendant emotional distress — a neural network run amok!

Short-Term Memory

Short-term memory causes temporary changes in the function of neurons. When stimulated *once*, the neurons in areas of the brain involving sensation and motor functions demonstrate an increased sensitivity to (i.e., lower threshold) neurotransmission. This increased sensitivity is affected by how much neurotransmitter (e.g., serotonin) is present, and is the result of an enhanced opening of channels in the nerve cell membrane, which allows the flow of calcium, potassium, and chloride ions to be increased from normal (see Neurotransmission, chapter 1). This sustained flow of ions facilitates the excitation of the neuron, should another stimulus of the same or lower intensity arrive. (Valium-type drugs actually inhibit this and thereby can inhibit short-term memory formation.) This increased sensitivity is only temporary, and if the neuron is only stimulated once, the increased sensitivity decays quickly.

If the stimulation is strong and repetitive, the long-term memory process is activated (see Neuromodulation, chapter 1). This process involves increases or decreases in the number of dendrites connecting two neurons (figure 2.10). Since growth of terminal neuron branches (arborization) is the basis for long-term memory, it makes sense that new genes must be turned on to make new proteins, which result in the new structures. It is likely that pruning, or elimination of dendrites, is associated with loss of memory.

As discussed in the previous section, hormones interface here, in that they either inhibit or facilitate the turning on of different genes. Thus, hormone deficiencies (e.g., thyroid deficiency, corticosteroid excess in PTSD or depression) can affect long-term memory function, as you will see in the next section.

The Clinical Relevance of Learning and Memory

The importance of the above information to the psychotherapist and the biological psychiatrist cannot be overstated. Whether you are trying to explain the basis for your psychotherapeutic recommendations, treating a patient with PTSD or multiple personality disorder, or assessing the possible effects of Valium on your patient's memory, the above information forms the basis of so much that we do as therapists that it cannot be ignored.

A CLINICAL ILLUSTRATION   John, a 29-year-old elevator repair man, was traumatized when he found out that 18 people were killed after a construction cable snapped. He had been the last inspector to certify the cable one month earlier. At first, he recalled nothing unusual in his examination of the equipment and, although upset, was able to continue his work. However, over the subsequent days, John began to "remember" details of the inspection. He thought that he recalled being distracted during his inspection, although he had no way of proving it. This "memory" activated his historically over-developed sense of guilt and fear of social humiliation—which he was sure would occur as soon as his error was discovered. Soon, depressed and obsessed over the accident, he quit his job. John then spent hours each day talking about it, reviewing documents about the development of the cable system, its maintenance record, and similar industry accidents. He began to believe the company was covering up some error he had made, to avoid a lawsuit. As he ruminated over the incident, John gradually "recalled" additional events and built up a "personal history" of his causal role in the accident. *He believed that his memory was accurate.*

Because John was now unemployed, I asked him to make up a

daily schedule. I explained the need for maintaining daily rhythms, and he thought it was a great idea. However, when home, John became distracted by things he "wanted" to do ("paperwork" related to the accident). He didn't understand the importance of the schedule. I then explained to him that, each time he engaged in thinking and behavior about the accident, he was strengthening the neural connections. Distraction and activity, over time, would allow the neural connections to atrophy. Obsession, repetition, and rumination would strengthen them, and he would continue to create a personal history, which would become his identity. He could slowly change the structure of his brain by the activity he chose. This explanation was much more helpful and hopeful to him, and motivated him to throw out his "paperwork" and become active in his own healing process.

In addition, I measured the degree to which his system was overproducing steroids (via a dexamethasone suppression test) and found that he was overproducing steroids in response to the stress. Untreated, his stress was leading to excessive levels of steroids, and steroids can be toxic to memory cells of the hippocampus. This gave further impetus to treat his depression and anxiety with medication, since it would reduce his perceived stress level. The clear recommendation for John's psychotherapist was that uncontrolled emotional catharsis would be damaging and was contraindicated since it would place his hippocampal cells at risk. Medication was important to prevent such damage.

SUMMARY

The recent advances made in understanding brain function have revealed certain fundamental concepts. These concepts range from the almost purely biological (e.g., heredity and genetics), to those which begin to decipher the short-term and long-term interactions between the environment and our brain (e.g., learning and memory). The clinical relevance of these concepts has been addressed in a general manner in this chapter. In the next chapter, these concepts will be applied, along with other cutting edge research, to the major psychiatric disorders.

CHAPTER 3

Biological Theories of the Major Psychiatric Disorders

INTRODUCTION

NOW THAT YOU HAVE a deeper sense of the structure and functioning of the nervous system, it's time to learn to apply this knowledge in the clinical world. The purpose of this chapter is to foster the habit of looking at each client and asking yourself:

- What is the biological component here?
- How does it fit with the psychosocial?

A summary of primary aspects of current biological theory of major psychiatric disorders will be presented, including affective disorders, schizophrenia, disorders of attention, eating disorders, substance abuse, panic disorders, and posttraumatic stress disorder. Each disorder will be discussed from the following perspectives where applicable: diagnosis, prevalence, comorbidity, biological theory and specific biological markers, brain imaging studies, animal models, psychosocial theory, and long-term course of illness. This will be followed by a clinical case, with discussion from the perspective of integration of the biological with the psychotherapeutic.

It is important to avoid the question: Which came first, the biology or the psychosocial stresses? This is a "chicken and egg" question that cannot be answered with certainty in an individual case and can only be guessed at or estimated. The statement "You have a biological depression" can never be truthfully made. It must always be qualified. "Your depression has a strong/moderate/mild biological component" is more truthful. It is from this perspective that I suggest you approach both your clients and this chapter.

Remember, like the three blind men describing an elephant (an elephant is a creature that is smooth [tusks], rough [body], or fuzzy and thin [ears]), each school of thought looks at the elephant from one limited perspective. All perspectives must be integrated to know what an elephant is, and even then you just might have to live with one to truly understand.

The categorization of disorders that I will use generally conforms to that of the DSM-IV (1994), with the exception of the anxiety disorders. In the DSM-IV the anxiety disorders include those associated with generalized anxiety, panic, obsessive compulsive disorder, and posttraumatic stress disorder. However, based on a variety of analyses, including twin (Kendler, 1995b), biologic (Cowley & Arana, 1990), family (Breslau, Davis, & Prabucki, 1987), and developmental (Torgersen, 1986) studies, it appears that *generalized anxiety disorder is more closely related to major depressive disorder than to panic disorder,* and thus panic disorder, and the associated disorders (specific, social, and agoraphobic disorders, as well as posttraumatic stress disorder), are discussed separately from generalized anxiety disorder. For the sake of the discussion, generalized anxiety disorder is considered a mood disorder. It is a state of chronic dysphoria, treatable by antidepressant medications: tricyclics (e.g., imipramine) or MAO inhibitors (e.g., phenelzine). Obsessive compulsive disorder will be discussed as an attention disorder, based on a variety of observations, including the fact that both attention deficit disorder and obsessive compulsive disorder are thought to involve frontal-striatal pathways in the brain, and can be thought of as lying on a continuum of dysregulation of attention processes. Posttraumatic stress disorder seems to involve a large variety of neural circuits involving memory, excessive arousal, and perhaps attentional dysregulation, and will therefore be discussed separately.

MOOD DISORDERS

Overview of Biological Theory

The mood disorders, both depressive and bipolar, reflect disturbed regulation (Siever & Davis, 1985) of specific brain subsystems which normally maintain a good balance in the areas of:

- mood (euphoria/elevation vs. irritability/depression)
- reward/pleasure vs. inhibition/punishment
- vegetative functions (appetite, wakefulness/sleep)
- reproduction (libido, hormones)
- motor function (motor activity vs. motor retardation)
- cognitive function (memory, concentration, judgment)
- social function (isolation vs. interaction)

The dysregulation in these systems is mediated — not caused by — the neurotransmitters (e.g., norepinephrine, dopamine, serotonin) which normally counterbalance each other, while subserving the specific functions (listed above) in specific parts of the the neurocircuitry of the brain. Current research seems to indicate that abnormalities of the G proteins (figure 3.1) may be a vulnerable point in the neural function of patients with mood disorders. G proteins link the first messenger (neurotransmitter) to the second messenger (enzyme within the cell that initiates a cascade of chemical reactions) within the receiving neuron. When, due to either genetics and/or experience, these systems are dysregulated and cannot absorb and adapt to stress effectively, the symptoms experienced by the person will be a reflection of disturbed function in the circuits that are primarily affected. The choice of which medication might be effective is to some degree determined by which subsystems seem most affected, and which neurotransmitters seem to be the main mediators of neurotransmission in that brain subsystem (tables 1.1, 1.3).

Depression, then, is a result of the dysregulated interaction of feedback mechanisms at the experiential, neurochemical, and behavioral levels. The limbic system and its neurons are the final field of action, and are the final neural path (figure 3.2) for depression, regardless of the initiating factors.

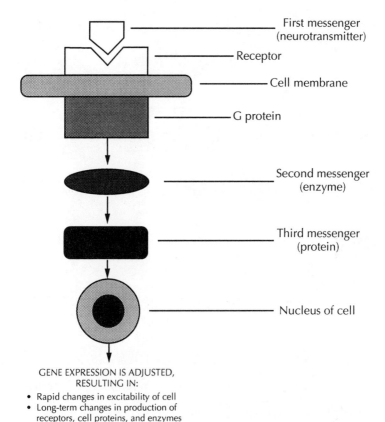

First messenger
(neurotransmitter)

Receptor

Cell membrane

G protein

Second messenger
(enzyme)

Third messenger
(protein)

Nucleus of cell

GENE EXPRESSION IS ADJUSTED,
RESULTING IN:
• Rapid changes in excitability of cell
• Long-term changes in production of
  receptors, cell proteins, and enzymes
  involved in learning and memory

FIGURE 3.1.   Links in the neurotransmission process that may be involved
in the mood disorders.

Classification of Mood Disorders

Most professionals in the mental health field understand the constantly shifting nature of psychiatric diagnostic criteria to be the
result of a number of factors, including new research, changing culture, changing patterns of illness, changes in treatment, and changes
in economic conditions. Thus the search for clear boundaries between different disorders is never-ending, since all these parameters
are shifting at one time or another and since the different mood
disorders probably lie on a continuum with indistinct boundaries.

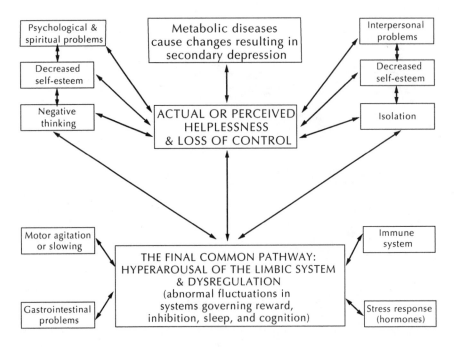

FIGURE 3.2. Depression: the common neural path. The two-way arrows represent the idea that biology can also be a result of developmental, environmental, and interpersonal events. In practical terms, this means "everything" is upsetting and the individual is overly sensitive or reactive in the particular system involved. The emotional brain, no matter how depression starts, is always mediated by the part of the brain controlling the emotional systems of initiative (reward, pleasure, inhibition), sleep rhythms, appetite, etc.

Because of this you must understand that the subtypes defined here are not firm and unchanging, but rather represent the general consensus at the current time.

Mood disorders are usually divided into **depressive** (formerly called unipolar depression) and **bipolar** types. Both may appear with or without the specifiers of psychosis, delusions, or seasonality, but only bipolar disorders may be specified as rapid cycling (more than 4 episodes per year).

Depressive disorders are further subdivided into two primary subtypes. One individual may have more than one subtype, such as the common case of so-called "double depression" in which an episodic major depressive disorder is superimposed on a more continuously evident dysthymic disorder. (It is important to note that the diagnosis applied to an individual patient is always dependent on the longitudinal course of the disorder, not on the characteristics of the present episode. Thus, a patient may present with symptoms of depression, but a thorough history may reveal a spontaneous manic episode 20 years ago. This would classify the patient as bipolar with a current *episode* of depression, not as a major depressive *disorder*.)

1. **Major depressive disorder** (classical unipolar depressive disorder) is primarily characterized by recurrent episodes of continuously depressed mood and affect, middle and terminal insomnia, psychomotor slowing or agitation, appetite loss, and complete anhedonia.
2. **Dysthymic disorder** is characterized by longstanding low-grade depressed mood with some milder symptoms over the course of years. If you are a newcommer to the field, you should consult the DSM-IV for full criteria.

The DSM-IV includes a number of specifiers of both episodes and longitudinal course (the disorder as a whole). The **atypical** specifier (Asnis, Mcginn, & Sanderson, 1995) of a depressive episode is characterized by an unusually excessive need for sleep, overeating (with carbohydrate, sweets, and chocholate cravings), inability to anticipate pleasure (anticipatory anhedonia) but no loss of actual ability to experience pleasure once involved in an activity (no consumatory anhedonia), anxiety, rejection sensitivity, and fluctuating course in response to events (the point here is that the "classic" depressive looks very different from the very common but so-called "atypical" depressive, whose boundaries merge with dysthymic disorder).

Bipolar disorders are subdivided into two essential subtypes:

1. **Bipolar I** patients are those who have had a full-fledged manic episode of such severity that there is a significant degree of loss of contact with reality which often requires hospitalization or causes debilitating dysfunction. Criteria include euphoric/irritable mood, decreased need for sleep, psychomotor activity (increased rate of speech, thoughts,

and goal-oriented activity) or agitation, excessive involvement in pleasurable activities, impairment of judgment, and unusually active and inappropriate social activity.

2. **Bipolar II** disorder is on the less severe end of the bipolar continuum and is characterized by hypomanic episodes (decreased need for sleep, increased energy, impaired judgment, etc.) alternating with depressive episodes. Bipolar II patients seem to share a common boundary with the "atypical" depressives, in that the depressions of bipolar II patients are often (not always) hypersomnic, hyperphagic, and sensitive to rejection.

There does not seem to be as much drift from the bipolar II to the bipolar I category as there is between subcategories within the depressive class. Table 3.1 outlines the clinical and biological differences that exist between the depressive and bipolar disorders, the general clinical course of bipolar disorder vs. depressive disorder, and some biological differences between the two.

Depressive Spectrum Disorders

When the neurotransmitters that are dysregulated involve other areas of physical function that are not usually related to mood disorders, we see what are sometimes thought of as the **depressive** (also called affective) **spectrum disorders** (Hudson & Pope, 1990; see tables 1.1, 2.1), a concept *not* included in the DSM-IV. Often these disorders are treatable by the same medications used in the mood disorders because they share a common physiological abnormality: disturbed regulation of the neurotransmitter function and/or disturbed transduction of the neurotransmitter information signal to the second and third messenger molecules of the receiving cells, which of course then fail to regulate the gene expression in accordance with the demands on the particular organ system. These disorders seem to reflect dysregulations of:

- bowel function (irritable bowel)
- pain regulation in the peripheral nerves and spinal cord (chronic pain syndromes)

TABLE 3.1
Differences between Bipolar and Depressive Mood Disorders

CRITERIA	DEPRESSIVE DISORDER	BIPOLAR DISORDER
Age at onset	Older	Younger, often in adolescence
Sleep pattern (depressed phase)	Middle (1–2 a.m.) and terminal (4–5 a.m.) insomnia	Hypersomnia (>8–10 hours of sleep)
Appetite	Decreased (classic) or increased, craving sweets, chocolate (atypical)	Bipolar I: decreased, craving salts; Bipolar II: often increased as in atypical depression, but may be decreased in more severe classic depressive episodes
Female : Male ratio	2 : 1	1 : 1
Lifetime risk of developing the disorder	5–15% of population will experience at some time; different frequency across cultures	1% of population will experience; stable frequency across cultures
Frequency of substance abuse	More than general population but less than in bipolar	Greater than depressive mood disorder
Impulsivity	Low	High
Novelty seeking	Low	High
Frequency of personality disorders when assessed in normal mood state	High	Low
Extroversion in well state	Low	High
Genetic component	Less	More
Risk of kindling	Yes	Yes
Frequency of episodes	Lower	Greater
Duration of episodes	Longer	Shorter
Divorce rate	Lower	Higher

- feeding centers of the brain (bulimia)
- vascular function (migraine headaches, hyper/hypotension, and possibly chronic fatigue syndrome)
- immune function (allergy)
- attention (obsessive compulsive disorder and attention deficit disorder).
- respiratory function (asthma)

As an example of an affective spectrum disorder, consider allergy (figure 3.3). It is clear that the nervous system has receptors on its neurons for products of the immune system (hence some people feel down with allergies), and it is equally clear that the immune system has receptors on its cells for the products of the nervous system (e.g., serotonin). With such mutual interaction, it is not surprising to find that dysregulation of the nervous system could cause dysregulation of the immune system. An overreactivity of the CNS could certainly be paralleled by allergy. In fact, often patients with anxiety and reactive depressions have allergies that lessen significantly with pharmacological intervention.

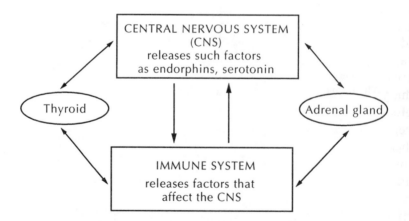

FIGURE 3.3. Mood disorders and allergy: the connection between the central nervous system (CNS), the immune system, and the hormonal system.

Specific Markers of Mood Disorders

Since psychiatric diagnosis is not an exact science, researchers have been searching for objective markers that would make diagnosis easier and more reliable (just as high blood sugar is a marker of diabetes) and that could be used to screen for the disorder, separate it from other similar disorders, and assess treatment. The search for a simple blood test or urine test in psychiatry has not born fruit, and no single simple marker can be used for diagnosis, confirmation of the end of a mood episode, or the prediction of treatment outcomes. Nevertheless, certain markers that are more complex have been found, and can be used both in the research arena and in certain clinical situations.

Sleep Markers

The sleep laboratory provides what are probably the best, most reliable markers for classifying mood disorders. Numerous studies support the usefulness of sleep studies in differentiating between diagnostic categories and response to treatment (Lauer, 1995).

Broadly speaking, there are two types of sleep, defined by the presence or absence of spontaneous eye movements: **REM** (rapid eye movement) sleep, and **non-REM** sleep. REM sleep is when we do most of our dreaming, tends to occur later in the night, and is accompanied by a physical state of paralysis. REM sleep may be involved in the consolidation of long-term memory. Non-REM sleep is divided into stages 1–4, which are defined by EEG (electroencephalographic) recordings of electrical activity of the brain. This electrical activity occurs in a fluctuating, but synchronized, wave-like fashion, which shows progressively greater amounts of slow wave (called **delta wave**) brain activity as one moves from light sleep (stage 1) to deep sleep (stage 4). Stages 3 and 4 are the deepest stages of sleep, when arousal is most difficult. **Delta sleep**, or deep sleep, tends to be most prevalent in the first half of the night, diminishing in frequency with each sleep cycle, while the amount of REM sleep increases with each sleep cycle. Normally, we cycle in sequence through these different sleep stages several times per night, with each cycle being composed of progressively different and predictable percentages of the different stages of sleep.

It is well accepted that the mood disorders are marked by abnormalities of sleep, whether it be **diminished** (the difficulty staying asleep and early morning awakenings in depressive or hypomanic episode), **excessive** (the excessive sleep of atypical, bipolar II, and seasonal subtypes), or **absent sleep** (mania).

One of the most reliable, clinically powerful, but expensive markers of a depressive episode (depressive and bipolar disorder) is the observation that depressed patients go into REM sleep more quickly (sooner than 50–65 minutes) than normal subjects (called **decreased REM latency**), have a deficit of slow wave (non-REM, stage 3 and 4) sleep, and have an abnormality in the distribution of dream sleep through the night, with increased REMs in the first half of the night **(phase shift)**. Successful antidepressant treatments normalize these sleep patterns. Thus, the sleep laboratory, in which the timing and onset of the different stages of sleep are recorded, can be very useful as a diagnostic and treatment marker in biological psychiatry.

In addition, David Kupfer (1988) has suggested that patients who experience decreased REM latency will require medication for effective treatment of their depression, and that if the decreased REM latency persists during treatment, they are more vulnerable to early relapse.

In another study, Kupfer (1990) showed that the degree of phase shift of deep slow wave sleep in depression, as measured by the delta sleep ratio (a measure of the normal decrease in slow wave delta sleep from the first sleep cycle to the second), predicts how long a person will remain free of depression following drug discontinuation, after clinical elimination of the depression.

$$\text{delta ratio} = \frac{\text{slow wave (delta wave count) sleep in the first non-REM sleep cycle}}{\text{slow wave sleep in second non-REM sleep cycle}}$$

In this interesting study all patients were judged to be responders to treatment on the basis of the improvement in symptoms. The ratio accurately predicted who would benefit from maintenance of psychotherapy: If after clinical improvement to normal, the delta sleep ratio was greater than 1 : 1 (i.e., there was enough deep sleep in the first sleep cycle to approach normal), patients stayed well five times longer (101 weeks) than when the ratio was less than 1 : 1 (i.e., despite a clinical appearance of looking like they were better their sleep pattern had not normalized sufficiently), if they are engaged in psychotherapy. These patients stayed depression-free for almost two years on average, after medication discontinuation, if they had once monthly interpersonal psychotherapy. If they didn't engage in psychotherapy, they relapsed almost as quickly (23 weeks) as those whose sleep did not normalize on medication (median time of relapse: 12 weeks or less). *This means that if the medication makes the patient better, including a normalization of his or her sleep pattern, psychotherapy is necessary to maintain the gains.* Those whose delta ratio was less than 1 : 1 (indicating a failure to correct the abnormal deep sleep pattern of depression, despite apparent clinical improvement) relapsed into depression after medication discontinuation whether they had psychotherapy or not! While this study is not the final word, and does need to be replicated, it demonstrates the potential power of sleep studies as markers in affective disorders.

Hormonal Markers

Reference has already been made (figure 2.7) to the function of the various hormonal axes (hypothalamic-pituitary-glandular [adrenal, thyroid, ovarian, testicular]) as the emotional shock absorber systems, which translate emotionally significant information into hormonal responses designed to maintain the equilibrium of an individual. It should be no surprise then that biological researchers have been looking intensely at the response of these hormonal axes to stress in normal states and states of affective dysregulation. Following are some consistent findings.

Dysregulation (Hyperactivity) of the Hypothalamic-Pituitary-Adrenal (HPA) Axis

This has been documented with increased brain fluid levels of the **corticotropin releasing factor (CRF)** in depressives and normalization with clinical recovery. CRF, released from the hypothalamus, is the major regulator of the HPA axis, and results in increased activity of the adrenal glands. A variety of studies has found increased adrenal weight and/or size in victims of violent suicide and depressives indicating overactivity of the adrenal glands. The degree of dysregulation of this axis is measured indirectly by the **dexamethasone suppression test (DST)**. The DST is probably the most widely studied biological marker in psychiatry. In this test, the patient is given 1 mg of dexamethasone (a steroid medication) at 11 p.m. In healthy individuals this will cause the body's steroid production to decrease via an effect on CRF, so that when tested the next day, the level of cortisol in the blood will be suppressed. In 50–70% of patients with a depressive episode, the cortisol level is not suppressed. Recent research indicates that this may be due to an actual switching of the hormones that regulate the HPA axis under stress! The hormone that regulates the HPA axis under normal conditions (CRF) is different from the hormone that regulates the HPA output under stress (vasopressin). This stress hormone is not sensitive to dexamethasone, and thus the dexamethasone doesn't suppress the system. It's as if, under stress, the system changes the control mechanism so that the old "key" doesn't work!

The DST was initially hailed as the first marker of depression, but soon it was shown to be abnormal in a variety of situations, including eating disorders, starvation, and the presence of certain drugs. It is therefore not very specific as a diagnostic tool. However, a great deal of study has found that the DST *is* a sensitive measure of persistent depression. After the depressed patient has responded to treatment, nonsuppression of cortisol on the DST strongly predicts poor outcome (rehospitalization, suicide, or recurrence of severe symptoms), in spite of apparent clinical improvement (Ribeiro, 1993). The DST can also be useful in differentiating dementia from depression.

Blunted Activity of the Hypothalamic-Pituitary-Thyroid Axis
This finding has been documented in a variety of studies, including that of Souetre et al. (1988), which demonstrated a correlation between abnormal body temperature regulation in bipolar depressive patients and an abnormal pattern of thyroid stimulating hormone secretion from the pituitary gland (figure 3.4). In this situation (see chapter 2, Hormones) the normal daily wave pattern of thyroid stimulating hormone (which is itself controlled by the hypothalamic release of thyroid releasing hormone) is flattened and as a result the normal wave pattern of body temperature is also flattened. Clinically, it is often helpful when assessing sleep hygiene (chapter 5) to inquire about the temperature of the bedroom. Sleeping in a cooler environment can actually improve sleep in depressive patients, while a warmer environment can worsen sleep. Temperature dysregulation

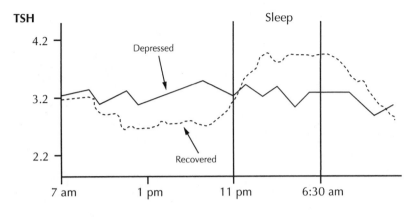

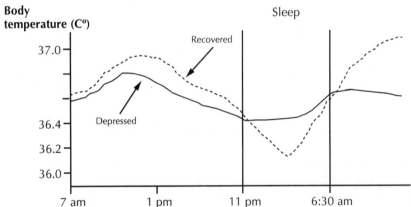

FIGURE 3.4. Temperature and thyroid stimulating hormone (TSH) in depression and recovery.

may also play a role in type B seasonal mood disorder (see chapter 2, Seasonal Rhythms).

Higher Blood Sugars, Resistance to Insulin, and Higher Insulin Levels
Depressive disorder patients who are currently in a depressive episode (Winokur et al., 1988; figure 3.5) tend to have higher levels of sugar in the blood at rest and take longer to return to baseline after a sugar meal. Symptoms of diabetes and depression can be confused (e.g., fatigue, overeating and weight gain, difficulty thinking clearly), and thus the clinician should be aware of this hormonal dysregulation. Therefore, a depressed patient who has not been pre-

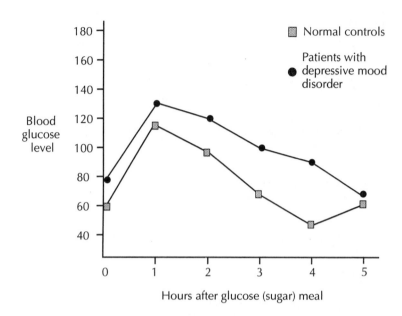

FIGURE 3.5. Insulin resistance after oral glucose tolerance testing in patients with major depression (data from Winokur, 1988).

viously diagnosed as diabetic may lapse into the early phases of diabetes during a depressive episode. Also, diabetics, who generally have more difficulty controlling their blood sugar when depressed, should always have their depression treated.

Neurotransmitter Markers

The neurotransmitters most studied in the mood disorders are serotonin, norepinephrine, and dopamine. Meaningful clinical measurement of these chemicals on an individual basis—which might reflect what is going on in the brain tissue—is difficult. Thus "levels" of neurotransmitters do not provide any clear marker of mood disorders in the individual case. Nevertheless, when *groups* of mood disordered patients are compared with controls, some important and consistent findings about the individual neurotransmitter levels and how they interact with each other in a functional and balanced manner become clearer.

Various measures of serotonergic functions clearly fluctuate on a seasonal basis, being lower in the winter and higher in the summer; this, of course, has implications for the biology of seasonal affective disorders. Dopamine activity, which is associated with motor behavior and initiative, tends to be lower than normal in depression and higher than normal in mania, while norepinephrine activity may be high in mania and depression, although the studies are not consistent on this latter point.

Markers of Suicide

Breakdown products of **serotonin** (5-HIAA) are exceptionally low in those who have attempted violent suicide. Depressed patients with alcoholic relatives are likely to have lower serotonin activity; thus, clinicians must be sure to evaluate suicide risk in depressive patients with family members who are alcoholic. Young male alcoholics with antisocial traits as well also demonstrate low 5-HIAA activity, and must be evaluated for suicide risk.

A recent study (Pandy et al., 1995) indicates that there are a significantly higher number of serotonin receptors on the surface of blood platelets of suicidal patients, independent of primary diagnosis. If replicated, this could be a biological marker for identifying suicide-prone individuals. These two findings, low serotonin function and high levels of receptors, could be linked, in the sense that it is well-known that when there is a scarcity of a neurotransmitter, cells actually increase the number of receptors on their surface (called "up regulation") to "soak up" or become more sensitive to the presence of even small amounts of the neurotransmitter. Another strong marker of suicide is indicated by numerous very large-scale studies (e.g., Golier, 1995) indicating that males (and possibly women) with low cholesterol levels (below about 160 mg/dl) have a significantly greater risk of suicide. Thus, a new male patient who is very depressed should have his cholesterol level checked. If it is low, this should increase your concerns about his suicide risk.

Brain Imaging Studies in Mood Disorders

Most studies that measure either blood flow through various areas of the brain or the activity level (rate of metabolism measured by use of substances such as sugar) of cells in those areas indicate a decreased blood flow and decreased activity in the frontal areas in depressed patients. This seems to be intuitive, as many depressed patients complain of fogginess and trouble thinking clearly, and seem to experience this in the frontal areas of the head. It seems that the greater the depression, the greater the abnormality, and some studies indicate that successful treatment seems to return the brain image pattern to normal.

Other findings indicate that the fluid filled spaces in the brain, called **ventricles,** are larger in patients whose mood disorders have a later onset and are manifested by delusions and hallucinations. This implies that the amount of brain tissue is less in these patients. It may very well be that those patients with late onset mood disorders are suffering from a degeneration of brain tissue, and the depression may be a secondary consequence of impaired ability to cope under stress. Patients with enlarged ventricles are more likely to have abnormalities in their thyroid and adrenal axis as well.

All of the above findings, however, do not tell us about causes of mood disorders, only about the changes associated with the illness, which parts of the brain may be overfunctioning, and which parts are underfunctioning. It is not clear whether the changes seen are trait markers or only associated with the particular state of depression or mania. I must stress that anyone who is treating mood disorders must understand these models thoroughly, be able to apply them to individual cases, and be able to teach them to patients and their families as part of the initial treatment phase.

Animal Model of Depression: Learned Helplessness

In the 1960s Martin Seligman developed the first animal model of depression, which he called "learned helplessness," a concept I consider THERAPEUTIC GOLD. He later published a full account of these experiments (1975), the implications of which are enormous for the psychotherapy of depressed patients. An understanding of this model, along with the biological and social models, liberates patients from guilt and confusion and offers hope.

In this time-honored animal model of depression, three dogs are each placed in a test cage. Dog A is shocked, but can control the shock by turning it off. As a result of this paradigm, dog A experiences mastery over shock. Dog B is also shocked, but cannot do anything to turn it off. Dog B becomes frustrated and soon appears depressed, manifested by immobility, decreased initiative, whimpering, etc. Dog C does not receive any shock and experiences no distress. Each dog is then placed into a "shuttle box" — so-called because if shocked the dog could shuttle or move over a low barrier to escape the shock. As predicted, only dog B, which had received inescapable shock in the first phase of the experiment, never learned to jump over the barrier to escape the shock. When shocked, it just lay there, helpless, depressed, with no initiative, lack of appetite, and abnormal sleep and hormonal patterns. The other two dogs learned to jump over the barrier to escape the shock in a matter of seconds. Seligman concluded that dog B had learned that it was helpless in preventing shock; it had begun to generalize its response to all situations that involved shock. After shocking the helpless dog and pairing that with carrying it over the low barrier (150–200 times), the dog began to initiate normal shuttle behavior on its own, but was always more vulnerable to a helpless response. It had learned that futility or helplessness was possible and, having had the experience, its brain circuitry was most likely altered to encompass the new learning. The result of this experiment is the concept of learned helplessness: Inescapable, painful, uncontrollable events lead to a state of giving up, futility, a belief that one cannot help oneself or do anything to alter outcome. Seligman later went on to show that he could actually inoculate dogs to this learned helplessness by giving them mastery experiences before the experiment (as was the case with dog A).

To cut to the heart of the matter, the core of psychotherapeutic treatment of depressed patients is to identify the current source(s) of their helplessness and direct them in initiating action to solve the problem. The source can be either a situation or erroneous beliefs (top of figure 3.2).

Psychosocial Theories of Depression

Over the years there have been numerous nonbiological attempts at explaining the causes and nature of depression. These attempts go back to biblical times. In the modern era, Freud (1917) postulated that depression is the result of anger turned inward against the part of the self that reminds one of the conflicted part of a lost relationship. While there are anecdotal reports in the literature that support this view, there are no controlled studies indicating that this is a correct or useful way of approaching depressed clients. In fact, encouraging expression of anger can cause a depressed person to feel more guilty, and thereby worsen depression. Following Freud, Bibring (1953) postulated that depression occurs when a person comes to the conclusion that it would be impossible for him to obtain whatever was vital to his or her self-esteem. According to Bibring, one's self-esteem is based on a fixation at one of the three Freudian stages. If this fixation occurs at the oral phase, the patient's self-esteem is dependent on the ability to fulfill the vital goal of being loved. As long as that possibility exists, the patient will not lapse into depression. If, on the other hand, the patient comes to believe that it is impossible for him or her to be loved, then depression will ensue. A therapist using this model will probably aim at correcting that belief, attempting to improve the possibility of achieving the goal of being loved, or changing the goal itself. The other stages of fixation in this model are the anal phase, in which the self-esteem is dependent on the need for control and power, and the oedipal phase, in which the self-esteem is based on the need to perceive one's ability to love as adequate. Bibring's model can be seen as a bridge between Freud's drive model and the later self-oriented models. Bibring's stages are analytically based, and focus not on repressed drives of anger and libido, but rather on conscious values as developed during these stages.

With Seligman's ground-breaking studies, a nearly simultaneous and complementary advance in the understanding of depression was developed: cognitive theory. In cognitive theory, the presumption is made that one's cognitive set, or automatic assumptions, determines one's feeling state. Aaron Beck's (1967) cognitive theory of depression proposed that the depressed person has distortions in his thinking that make him susceptible to depression. In the course of therapy, these distortions are identified, tested, and modified as appropriate in the structured and collaborative therapy setting. Cognitive therapy has been shown to be an effective treatment in mild and moderate depression in at least eight controlled studies of depression (e.g., Beck, Ward, & Mendelson, 1961; Carrington, 1979; Covi & Lipman, 1987; Shaw, 1977; Steuer, Mintz, & Hammen, 1984).

While these studies were being done, Gerald Klerman and Myrna Weissman were developing and formulating social theories of depression into a treatment model that was eventually outlined in a book called *Interpersonal Psychotherapy [IPT] of Depression* (1984). IPT is based on the concept that depression can be conceptualized as a disturbance in interpersonal relationships, and that the therapy should be focused on establishing good quality relationships, dealing with role changes and conflicts, and developing interpersonal skills. IPT was also tested in large-scale clinical trials and shown to be more effective than placebo or "on-demand" supportive therapy (DiMascio, Weissman, & Prusoff, 1979; Weissman, Prusoff, & DiMascio, 1979). IPT was compared with medication, and was shown to be as effective in mild and moderate depression (DiMascio et al., 1979). When IPT was combined with tricyclic antidepressants, the therapeutic benefit of both treatments together was superior to either treatment alone (Herceg-Baron, Prusoff, & Weissman, 1979; Rounsaville, Klerman, & Weissman, 1981; Weissman et al., 1979).

Thus, in summary, there are only three proven types of treatment for depression, each one intervening at a different level of functioning: the biological (e.g., ingested substances such as medication and hormone replacement; rhythm changes by sleep deprivation or phototherapy; electroconvulsive therapy), psychological (cognitive therapy), and social (IPT). At this time there is no statistically proven value to psychodynamic, group, hypnosis, or any other type of therapy in the treatment of depression. The conceptual framework the therapist uses will determine his or her intervention and thus influence the outcome.

A CLINICAL ILLUSTRATION   Carol was a 49-year-old, intelligent designer who was referred for evaluation and treatment of a suspected depression. Upon evaluation she was found to have a history of recurring depressive episodes, most of which were followed by periods of strong hypomania (bipolar II). During her early episodes of depression, a causative stressor could be clearly determined — the loss of a boyfriend, the breakup of an engagement, the loss of a child, a separation, and a job loss. These depressions, which began in adolescence, were followed by periods of increased energy, decreased need for sleep (3–5 hours was plenty), "getting involved," starting projects, elevated mood (although in her later episodes her energy was often elevated, but her mood was irritable—a so-called "**mixed state**") and increased socializing. Carol had been in psychotherapy of one sort or another over the years, and it was often at the point of early hypomania that she would experience an undeniable sense of well-being, declare herself well, thank her therapist for a job well done, and terminate or drop out of treatment. This was followed by overextension at work, impulsive spending that would ultimately be beyond her means, and sexual advances and behavior that she later felt were inappropriate. Her need for sleep, which during her depressed periods was often greater than 10 hours per day, would drop to 3–5 hours per night. After some time Carol would settle down and dig herself out from under "the mess I made." Sometimes she would immediately cycle into depression again.

After taking a careful life history, which involved getting information from both the patient and family members, and charting the episodes on graph paper, I noticed that these cycles of depression and hypomania initially occurred 4–7 years apart, and that frequency of episodes was now 18 months–3 years. Of even greater concern was the fact that the distinction between Carol's "good" moods and her depression was less clear. High-energy states were no longer pleasant; rather, they were high-energy mixed states in which she was often angry, irritable, and aggressive.

Treatment was initiated with lithium, and Carol did well for several months. Feeling well, she discontinued the lithium (compliance is the #1 problem in the treatment of bipolar disorders), as well as her psychotherapy, despite her therapist's repeated attempts to advise her of the need for continuation treatment. Sixteen months later, Carol came back to treatment, and started the lithium again. The lithium did not work, however; ultimately Carol was stabilized on synthetic thyroid hormone replacement (Synthroid), and Valproic acid, an antiseizure, antikindling medication frequently used as a mood stabilizer.

This case illustrates the phenomenon of kindling (chapter 2), among other important factors in the diagnosis, natural history, and treatment of mood disorders. Studies are nearly unanimous in showing that "more psychosocial stressors are involved in the first episode, than in subsequent episodes of affective [mood] disorder, or psychosocial stressors appear to have less impact on episodes occurring after many recurrences" (Post, 1992; also see figure 2.4). It appears likely that episodes of depression or mania induce long-term changes in the structure of the cell and in the expression of genes via alteration in the types and/or quantity of proteins that are made by the genes (figure 3.1). These protein changes may last for days, months, or years and are only activated in the nerve cells involved in the particular reaction to stress. These proteins, some of which are nerve growth factors, help to sensitize nerve pathways to become more easily stimulated, and eventually become activated spontaneously! For this reason, the treatment of depression, mania, and quite possibly other types of psychiatric problems (PTSD, panic attacks) must be aimed at preventing recurrence of the symptoms. *It is no longer justifiable to allow a patient to suffer repeated episodes of a mood disorder in the name of working through a problem. All available interventions must be taken to prevent recurrence whenever possible.*

In Carol's case, we can see that the frequency of her episodes increased and, as predicted by the kindling model, they became less tied to psychosocial stresses. The failure to diagnose her mood disorder early on, along with her apparent response to therapy, allowed her to suffer repeated episodes, which very likely caused further harm to her nervous system via alterations in gene expression and therefore neuronal structure and function. The disorder was now more firmly wired into her nervous system.

Used to the comforting idea that someday her treatment would not be necessary, Carol stopped the lithium, and thereby suffered a three-fold problem. First, not surprisingly, she had another episode. Second, the drug that once worked no longer worked! In fact, 10–15% of patients who have experienced long-term and stable prevention of recurrences with lithium will fail to respond to lithium when it is reinstated after a recurrence of an episode! Third, Carol did not appreciate the fact that long-term lithium treatment in both depressive disorders and bipolar disorders reduces the mortality rate due to suicide quite significantly (a reduction on average of 82%, from about 9 suicides per 1000 patient-years to about 1 suicide per 1000 patient-years [Copen, 1994]). There is additional evidence that the mortality rate due to cardiovascular deaths is also reduced. These new facts are critical for therapists to understand and use.

Carol could have been helped in three ways: earlier diagnosis via accurate and thorough history taking, more successful education and psychotherapy oriented toward improved compliance, and family cooperation and support to report early signs of relapse.

The Course of Mood Disorders

While the rates of bipolar mood disorder are relatively stable across time and cultures, the rates of depressive mood disorder seem to be increasing with each passing decade (Klerman et al., 1985), and the age of onset seems to be decreasing into adolescence, and even childhood (Reich et al., 1987). Thus, the personal experience of depression is becoming more common, and the costs of depression are becoming more important on a societal scale.

Like the common cold, depressive mood disorders seem to come on slowly, in a mild form (dysthymic disorder), eventually culminating in a severe depressive episode, which if not cleared up in six months seems to linger on as dysthymia (Shea et al., 1992). Untreated depressive disorder and bipolar disorder are strongly associated with impaired achievement in school, work performance, family and social relationships, as well as absenteeism from work and unemployment. These disruptions are clearly worse for patients suffering from bipolar disorder. Psychosocial factors that support good outcome in depressive mood disorders include maintenance psychotherapy and pharmacotherapy, as well as a supportive marital relationship. Good outcome in bipolar patients is supported by maintenence pharmacotherapy and low levels of family criticism and overinvolvement. Unfortunately, the relapse rate in depressive mood disorders after treatment is terminated is quite high and approaches 80% after five years (Kupfer et al., 1992). The relapse rate in depressive disorder is significantly reduced (to about 10%) by maintaining full therapeutic dosages of medication for several years. Five to 20% of patients who are thought to have depressive mood disorder go on to a bipolar disorder of the manic or hypomanic type (Akiskal, 1983). This is more likely in those who show atypical depressive symptoms, have a familiy history of mania, and women who experience postpartum depression. Patients with bipolar disorder have a 20% chance of having a panic disorder (Chen & Dilsaver, 1995).

As a result of these and other long-term studies, it has become clear that both depressive and bipolar mood disorders, even in their mild forms, must be treated actively. The duration of treatment for depressive mood disorders must be determined on an individual basis, but the general consensus is that the higher the number of episodes, and the stronger the family history, the more necessary long-term treatment is likely to be. Bipolar mood disorder, when not due to a temporary medical condition, generally requires life-long treatment.

SCHIZOPHRENIA

Just as schizophrenic patients lack boundaries, so too does the concept of schizophrenia. The definition of schizophrenia has varied from an overinclusive American approach (Bleuler, 1950), in which any gross impairment in the ability to function would be sufficient for diagnosis, to the more restrictive, narrow European criteria (Kraepelin, 1919), which require the presence of hallucinations and or delusions. Generally speaking, schizophrenia is an amalgam of disordered thinking processes (e.g., poor abstract thinking and reasoning, impaired working memory, disorganized speech), perceptual disturbances (hallucinations, delusions), behavioral abnormalities (catatonia), social incapacity, and affective dysregulation.

Schizophrenia is a genetically transmitted disorder of brain development. It is debilitating, chronic, and may demonstrate subtle manifestations as early as the second trimester in utero (Bracha et al., 1992), but does not make its full appearance as a psychosis until early adulthood. The genetically transmitted vulnerability probably is clinically manifested as a spectrum of disorders, since schizophrenia is related to schizotypal personality disorder and schizoaffective disorder (Kendler et al., 1995), whose incidence is higher in families of schizophrenics than in the general population. Schizophrenia itself directly affects anywhere between 0.2% to 1% of the population. This figure is remarkably stable across cultures, although there are population pockets of increased incidence. The risk of schizo-phrenia is higher in winter births; however, the reasons for this are unknown.

Despite the very strong genetic component, it is clear that environ-mental factors are also involved in the manifestation of the disorder, since identical twins share the disorder only 50% of the time.

Classification of Schizophrenia

Debate continues about the best way to subcategorize schizophrenia. The classic subtypes (undifferentiated, catatonic, paranoid, and he-bephrenic) have given way in the literature over the past decade to the current research schema (McGlashan & Fenton, 1992), which delineates symptom domains that are probably semi-independent of each other: **positive** symptoms (hallucinations, delusions) and **nega-tive** symptoms (e.g., flat affect, poverty of speech). More recently a third domain, **thought disorganization,** has been added to cover the cognitive and attentional impairment (Carpenter et al., 1993). This subcategorization, which has been validated by studies of the natural history of the disorder, some brain imaging studies, neuropsycholog-ical testing, and differing drug response, seems to indicate that there may be different physiological processes involved in the symptom domains and certainly different time courses for the development of these symptoms (figure 3.6). It is thought that a patient with endur-ing negative symptoms has an increased risk of poor prognosis, chro-

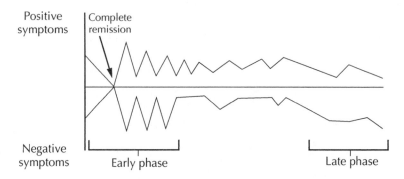

FIGURE 3.6. Schizophrenia: change in positive and negative symptoms over time.

nicity, neurological defects, and possibly increased genetic loading. Positive symptoms correlate with early phases of the disorder. Nevertheless, the DSM-IV (see DSM-IV for diagnostic criteria) has not fully adopted this in its classification schema, and relies on subcategories of paranoid, disorganized, catatonic, undifferentiated (those not meeting criteria for the first three subcategories), and residual types (in which there are no prominent positive symptoms). The latter is an attempt to build a bridge between the old and the new.

Where are we heading in the future classification of schizophrenia? If one reviews the history of subcategorization of other diseases, one can see that we are in the early phases of the process. With the advent of new technologies such as brain imaging, animal models, and neurochemical studies, we are moving toward the next step in subclassification. We will move from a subclassification system based on phenomenology (symptom profiles and course of illness) to one based on the ability to document abnormal physiology. Whether schizophrenia turns out to be the result of one abnormal physiological process or several is yet to be seen.

Despite years of research, we know relatively little about the biology of schizophrenia. According to Carpenter (1993), this is due to poor funding of research, inaccessibility of the live brain for study until recently, and a disorganized research approach. It appears now, however, that researchers are on the verge of rapid progress in understanding both the biology and classification of schizophrenia due to improved techniques for studying the brain in both live and postmortum subjects, improved organization of research, and recent validation of the concept of symptom domains. These domains include positive symptoms (hallucinations and delusions), thought disorganization (cognitive and attentional impairment), and enduring deficit or negative symptoms (inability to integrate sensory information, decreased social and physical pleasure).

The Biology of Schizophrenia

Biological theorists can be divided into two camps: "lumpers" and "splitters." The lumpers propose that the three symptom domains may be the result of one underlying abnormality. This would be analogous to how syphillis or lyme disease has different clinical appearances depending on which organ systems are affected by the common underlying infection. In schizophrenia research, the general consensus is that patients manifest a deficit in integrative functioning in the central nervous system. Wexler (1991) hypothesizes that the disorder is the result of one underlying defect, that is, when schizophrenics are presented with almost any task that activates a group of cortical neurons, there is a failure of those neurons to recruit, activate, connect, or link to additional cortical brain regions. It appears that this process is at least part of how conscious mental associations are made. Normally such linkage would help to prepare the individual for additional responses or to elaborate on a particular response. In this theoretical framework a symptom such as poor social interaction results from the inability to elaborate responses in a conversation (poverty of speech or thought). Another theory in the lumpers' camp is that frontal cortex dopamine activity is abnormally low (Weinberger et al., 1994a). Since frontal cortex neurons normally inhibit the deeper subcortical dopamine neurons, this low activity level results in a failure to supress dopamine activity in the subcortical regions. The result is hallucinations and/or delusions due excess dopamine activity in the subcortical areas. Supporting this theory is the fact that high doses of amphetamines can cause psychosis by increasing the amount of subcortical dopamine activity. The oldest theory in this camp is the almost 30-year-old dopamine hypothesis of schizophrenia (see Neurochemistry of Schizophrenia, below) which is currently viewed as too simplistic.

In the other camp, the splitters contend that it is also possible that schizophrenia is a syndrome in which a common clinical appearance is caused by several different disease processes (Crow, 1980). One could think of a schizophrenic as having the quite unfortunate inheritance of three semi-independent genes. These genetic defects would then cause a cluster of symptoms. Each of these genes would be responsible for the separate symptom domains of schizophrenia. Since these symptom domains occur in isolation from each other as well as together in the schizophrenic (e.g., schizotypy [odd speech and behavior; social aloofness, isolation, anxiety, and guardedness], attention deficit disorder [attentional, working memory, and other cognitive deficits], and affective disturbances [flattened, inappropriate affect and anhedonia]), the patient might be thought of as having a combination of genetic vulnerabilities.

The Genetics of Schizophrenia

That there is a genetic vulnerability to schizophrenia is not in doubt for a variety of reasons. It has been shown that the siblings of schizophrenic patients have an increased risk of the disorder only when they are biological siblings, not adopted. What this genetic vulnerability is, of course, is not known, as no single gene has been identified as a risk factor for schizophrenia. That the gene(s) involved interact with some environmental factor is clear since identical twins share the disorder only about 50% of the time. According to Schwartz and Africa (1988), an individual has an 8% risk of schizophrenia if his or her sibling is schizophrenic, a 12% risk if one parent is affected, a 14% risk of sharing the disorder with a fraternal twin, a 39% risk if both parents are affected, and a 47% risk when two individuals share the same exact genes. To explain the less than 100% concordance in identical twins, some authors (Barr, Mednick, & Munk-Jorgensen, 1990) hypothesize that viral, obstetric, and nutritional triggers may release the genetic vulnerability.

Neurodevelopmental Studies of Schizophrenia

Neurodevelopmental studies demonstrate strong, but not yet certain, evidence of central nervous system abnormality at birth (Hans & Marcus, 1991). These recent findings, which have been replicated, are resulting in an emerging reconceptualization of schizophrenia as a disorder of abnormal development of the neurons in the cortex of the brain. The abnormality of brain development is clinically manifested in infancy by low activity levels, extreme variation in alertness (dysregulation), poor motor maturity, and low muscle tone. Later in childhood there is clear evidence of lagging development and cognitive perceptual abnormalities (Marcus et al., 1993). Further support for these neurodevelopmental abnormalities is found in a number of recent studies. Conrad (1991) found that the cells of the hippocampus (which function in memory integration) are disoriented in relation to each other when compared to normals, and that the degree of cellular disorientation is related to severity of illness! Other studies (Akbarian et al., 1993, 1995) provide strong evidence that the normal orderly development of frontal lobe and temporal lobe cortex (including neurons of the hippocampus) which occurs early in development (day 40–125 of pregnancy) is disturbed. As a result, the cortical connectivity and associative functions (e.g., recruiting additional areas of the brain, as in Wexler's theory) may begin to go awry at that time. Theoretically, the final neurodevelopmental failure occurs during adolescence, when the cortex normally undergoes a reorganization. Animal models support this theory (see Animal Models, below) and would explain the clinical appearance of the disorder in adolescence. Is this neurodevelopmental abnormality caused by a virus and/or genetic malfunction? Once again, this remains to be determined.

Neurochemistry of Schizophrenia

On a molecular level, it seems likely that whatever abnormalities are transmitted and activated, they involve dopamine, serotonin, and GABA neurotransmission. The dopamine hypothesis of schizophrenia, which has been studied for almost 30 years, suggests that excessive dopamine function causes psychosis, and that the traditional antipsychotic medications work by binding to the dopamine receptor, thereby inhibiting or blocking the action of dopamine and reducing psychosis. Despite numerous attempts to confirm the dopamine hypothesis, a consensus is emerging that it is inadequate. More recent studies indicate that abnormalities of dopamine systems may in fact be the result of a decrease in the activity of the ubiquitous inhibitory neurotransmitter GABA (Reynolds, Czudek, & Andrews, 1990), a result of abnormalities in the conversion of the excitatory amino acid neurotransmitter, glutamate, to GABA (Akbarian et al., 1995). If confirmed by additional studies, this could change the pharmacologic approach of first breaking schizophrenia with dopamine blocking agents (the neuroleptics) to using agents that stimulate GABA activity, which might treat both the negative and positive symptoms more effectively and be closer to the source of the problem.

It is now known that there are five dopamine (DA) receptor types (DA1–DA5). Older antipsychotic medications seem to bind to the DA2 receptor, while the newer "atypical" antipsychotic clozapine

(Clozaril) binds preferentially to the DA4 and serotonin receptors. This is interesting to researchers since it is quite clear that patients who do not respond to the standard neuroleptics do respond quite well to clozapine! Could this indicate that this subgroup of patients have a different disease process?

Brain Imaging Studies in Schizophrenia

On a larger scale, new brain imaging studies indicate that patients with schizophrenia of the deficit type (i.e., enduring negative symptoms) have enlargement of the ventricles in the center of the brain. This enlargement is commonly thought to be a result of tissue loss in the brain's temporal lobes and prefrontal area. It is also possible, however, that the enlarged ventricles are the result of a failure of tissue development rather than tissue loss or degeneration. These decreases in temporal lobe tissue (e.g., the hippocampus) correlate with the hallucinations and memory problems seen in schizophrenia, while the decreases in prefrontal cortex activity are thought to correlate with the cognitive and negative symptoms of schizophrenia. When given a neuropsychological task (e.g., the Wisconsin Card Sorting Test), which requires abstract reasoning and working memory skills (the ability to temporarily hold information while assessing other incomming data), brain imaging studies show clear decreases in prefrontal cortex activity in schizophrenics and their affected twins, but not their unaffected twins (Berman et al., 1992; Weinberger et al., 1992). This test is a very sensitive measure of prefrontal lobe dysfunction.

Markers of Schizophrenia

As with the other psychiatric disorders, there is no signature marker that is specific and present only in schizophrenia. Nevertheless, researchers have found a number of abnormalities in various aspects of brain function in schizophrenic patients that are slowly helping to shed light on what aspects of the thinking process are abnormal. Future research will use a variety of techniques, each sensitive at a different level of observation (i.e., gross structure and function to microscopic), that can break down the component sequences in the thinking process. All of these techniques will be used in concert to evaluate the dysfunction in the schizophrenic (Pfefferbaum, Roth,

& Ford, 1995). I will briefly describe these techniques and the current findings in schizophrenics.

Magnetic resonance imaging (MRI) is a technique that enables us to look at the structure of the brain in fine detail. MRI studies have shown decreased tissue volume in the brains of schizophrenics (see Brain Imaging Studies, above), but these structural abnormalities are really only the end result of some abnormal process and do not tell us much about what that process may be. Functional MRI (fMRI) is another brain imaging technique, which is used to assess how blood flow changes or how much oxygen is used in specific areas of the brain during a particular task. This method of observation studies the changes in the gross structure and functioning of the brain over relatively long periods of time (seconds). These studies are fairly consistent in showing "hypofrontality"—decreased metabolism in different parts of the frontal lobes.

In addition to these techniques, investigators have been studying measurements of changes in electrical brain activity called event-related potentials (ERP). ERPs reflect changes on a time scale that is more appropriate to the microseconds time scale of neurons. ERPs reflect a summation of the electrical changes in neurons when exposed to a given stimulus. Different phases of this electrical response reflect different phases of the thinking process. Thus, the early parts of the response (1–8 milliseconds) reflect on the brain's automatic registration of the stimulus and do not require that the individual pay attention or make decisions. The later phases of the response (50–500 milliseconds) reflect processes that require attention and thinking. A variety of studies (Catts et al., 1995; O'Donnell et al., 1995; and Swerdlow et al., 1994) are showing subtle but widespread abnormalities in the later phases of information processing of schizophrenics.

One abnormality of ERPs is impaired "mismatch negativity" (Catts et al., 1995). Mismatch negativity is "an automatic alerting mechanism designed to stimulate individuals to explore unexpected environmental events" (Javitt et al., 1995). In order for an individual to be alerted to out-of-sequence or aberrant events in the environment, he or she must have the ability to retain some memory trace (i.e., temporary neural changes) of the recent events or stimuli. As a result of ERP research, this working memory is currently thought to be a central defect in the information processing of schizophrenics.

Animal Models of Schizophrenia

In humans, long-term sleep deprivation induces deficient sensory filtering, sensory overload, and psychosis. Thus, it follows that one of the animal models used in schizophrenia research is deficient "sensory gating" or "filtering" (Judd et al., 1992). In rats, this deficiency results in cognitive fragmentation due to sensory overload (figure 3.7) and can be measured by ERPs. Deficient sensory gating is a very powerful animal model that may prove to be useful in studying the neural circuits involved in one aspect of schizophrenia. It may also be useful in screening medications for antipsychotic potency.

Swerdlow (1994) induced this deficiency in rats by injecting dopamine into the nucleus acumbens and then blocked it by the use of

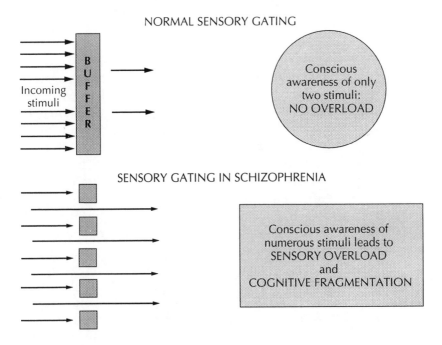

FIGURE 3.7. Impaired sensory gating (filtering) in schizophrenia.

antipsychotic medications. The nucleus acumbens is a site of convergence of neurons from the prefrontal and limbic cortices and is thought to play a central role in the activity of all antipsychotic medications. Lipska (1993) and Weinberger (1994b) actually induced lesions in the limbic-prefrontal connections in very young rats and thereby developed a model in which a syndrome analogous to schizophrenia developed after puberty, just as it does in humans!

Summary of the Biology of Schizophrenia

Despite the clear evidence from genetic studies that there is a strong heritable predisposition to schizophrenia, no hallmark symptom or marker of any type has been identified. Neither the much heralded brain imaging studies nor electrical and biochemical studies have identified a clear pattern of deficits that could be used as the sine qua non of schizophrenia.

The current consensus is that schizophrenia represents one or more core biological (very likely genetically transmitted) vulnerabilities that interact reciprocally with psychological, social, and developmental processes (table 3.2) including environmental factor(s) (e.g., virus, malnutrition, obstetrical complications) in early life. Current evidence suggests that this interaction begins during the early development of the surface layers (cortex) of the frontal and temporal lobes of the brain, during the second trimester of pregnancy and then again during adolescence. The result is disturbed function of one or more cortical brain circuits. Which circuits are affected, and to what degree, may affect the clinical presentation. The resultant impaired connections between various areas of the brain seem to affect a variety of brain processes, including the ability to filter incoming irrelevant stimuli and to process information (after it is received). These neuronal functions seem to involve dopamine, serotonin, and GABA neurotransmission. These deficiencies very often make their subtle appearance in childhood, but do not become clearly evident until after puberty. Psychosocial processes may be somewhat protective, in that a supportive family can delay relapse (Hogarty et al., 1991). All too often, however, a vicious mutually interacting cycle of deteriorating cognitive, vocational, and social function develops, which probably contribute further to the neurological dysfunction and negative symptomatology.

TABLE 3.2
Interaction of Factors in Schizophrenia

FACTOR	VULNERABILITY (TRAIT)	TRANSIENT CHANGES (STATE)	OUTCOME
BIOLOGY	Abnormal neural development	Sensory gating defect Hyperarousal Inability to recruit proper brain regions to assist in generating solutions Impaired reward systems Dysregulation of neurotransmitters	Impaired function of neural pathways Anatomic defects and neurochemical changes
PSYCHOLOGY	Working memory and cognitive processing defects lead to impared problem-solving skills and self-esteem	Inadequate learning opportunities and/or ability to process experiences	Psychosis, delusions, and cognitive disorganization
SOCIAL	Inadequate social and occupational skills and relationships	Stresses and life events (expressed emotion)	Nonsupportive social network, inadequate research and support agency funding; poor social functioning

Antipsychotic medications may act at the level of the nucleus acumbens, via neuromodulation (chapters 1 and 2) to compensate for the abnormal connections of these circuits. The new agent, clozapine, may act preferentially at the DA4 and serotonin receptors in the prefrontal cortex, when compared with the older antipsychotics, and thus may be acting closer to the site of the presumed defect. Research regarding nonpharmacologic treatment is lacking and funding is being reduced. New, more effective medications with fewer side effects are on the horizon, while researchers are finally reaching some consensus about symptom domains that have predictive value. Finally, and most importantly, clinicians are beginning to recognize that the treatment of schizophrenia must be multimodal and continuous to be effective at reducing relapse and human suffering.

A CLINICAL ILLUSTRATION   In the early 1980s my training provided me with few voices of reason in the treatment of my patients with schizophrenia. Aside from acute hospitalization and pharmacologic management, there was no standard of care for schizophrenic patients. Some pioneers advocated family therapy; others, milieu therapy; and still others, psychodynamic therapy. As a result I was witness to one of the most tragic patient outcomes of my career.

In 1980, Randy was a dapper, 20-year-old Vietnam veteran who had been discharged on psychiatric disability six months earlier. Randy had never functioned well in school, and never had more than a few friends. Randy's mother brought him to the emergency room and reported a several-week history of his living in his bedroom all day long, talking out loud to no one, avoidance of social contact, and an irregular sleep schedule. He had been hallucinating actively for at least three months and exhibiting inappropriate laughter, but had maintained his dapper, neatly kept appearance (a misguided source of hope for me in the early treatment phases). Randy's records revealed a prior schizophrenic episode while in the army.

I hospitalized Randy, medicated him with an antipsychotic, met with his family several times, and attempted to establish a supportive relationship with him. Eventually Randy improved and I followed him in individual supportive therapy, with occasional fruitless forays into the psychodynamic arena, over a seven-year period. Randy received disability income from the army, which his parents handled. He had two additional hospitalizations over the next four years, was only briefly employed, and lived with his parents, who would not become involved in the treatment process. I met with the patient's mother separately on two occasions in the fifth year of his treatment, when she informed me that she was having an ongoing affair. She never was willing to address the marital problem in therapy. In the sixth year of his treatment, Randy was hospitalized twice. He seemed less stable, and I felt there might be some relationship to the family tension, but could never get sufficient information or involvement of the family members to make an assessment, not to mention an intervention of some type. That year Randy's compliance with medication and office visits decreased. In the seventh year of treatment, perhaps as an attempt to improve things for the family, Randy's parents built a new vacation home. After three years of supervising the building process it was completed. On the third night in their new home, Randy's parents went out for dinner. Randy stayed at home. When they were gone, he set the house on fire, burning it to the ground.

A more successful case involves Fran, a 27-year-old single, very pleasant, friendly woman who was severely obssessive-compulsive as a child, but quite functional socially and academically. She said her father was emotionally abusive and depressed. In her late teens and early twenties, Fran had the abrupt onset of three psychotic episodes. These episodes were marked by bizarre and inappropriate sexual and social behavior, lack of sleep, auditory hallucinations, and delusions. Despite the tremendous upheavals in her life caused by these episodes and subsequent hospitalizations, Fran was able to recover and return to work, almost always retaining a positive outlook.

She has not been hospitalized since her early twenties. Fran's family and employer are quite supportive. As part of Fran's treatment, I have had regular educational and supportive contact with her employer, particularly during times of stress. This has helped her to maintain her job, since she continues to have ideas of reference, innapropriate affect at times, delusional thinking of a paranoid nature, and a clear disturbance in her ability to fully attend to and interpret social stimuli. She will frequently absorb parts of a conversation, recalling only one or two words, which she then neatly fits into her delusional system. Although the delusional system is quite disturbing to her, attempts to rationally help her disect and analyze her faulty thinking are grasped briefly, then lost to her within seconds. Despite her ongoing disabilities, with the support of her family, her employer, low-dose antipsychotic medication, and much contact between different parts of her system, Fran is able to live independently in a small group house, maintain friendships, continue her employment, and usually maintain a quite impressive and inspiring positive outlook.

Both of these cases unequivocally fulfill criteria for the diagnosis of schizophrenia, yet the outcomes are significantly different. Randy's outcome was worse for a number of reasons, including the fact that he was a young male, had a gradual onset, had poor support from his family (who frequently expressed disappointment in him) and his physician (who only provided medication and "supportive" individual therapy), received no rehabilitative support from social agencies, and had an enduring "deficit syndrome," as described by Kane (1993), including flat affect, low social drive, decreased spontaneity and curiosity, and decreased sense of purpose.

It is not surprising that Randy's inadequate support system failed to maintain his initial improvement. While it is impossible to determine whether his intractable illness actually resulted in his receiving minimal support, or vice versa, it is clear that his case supports the statististical predictors of poor outcome (Hogarty, 1993; Kane, 1993; Stein, 1993). In Fran's case we see the opposite: a woman with abrupt onset in her teens, rapid initial treatment, family support, physician support of her family and employer, employer support, and absence of deficit symptoms (despite persistence of positive symptoms).

At the current time, optimal treatment of schizophrenia is a continuous and seamless multidisciplinary team approach involving a neuropsychologist (assessment and possible future remediation of cognitive deficits), cognitive-behavioral therapist (social skills training), psychiatrist (pharmacotherapy and family, employer, landlord, and coworker education), social worker (coordination of medical, housing, and social supports), vocational trainer (retraining and placement). One individual must oversee the treatment to assure that the patient follows through with appointments, etc., and that all caregivers are integrated (the system must provide the integrating function that the patient cannot provide for him or herself). The immmediate environment of the patient (usually family, staff, and physician) must be educated regarding the disease process and supported in order to minimize expressed (critical) emotion. Excessive levels of expressed emotion (EE) has been repeatedly correlated with relapse in schizophrenia (Hogarty, 1993; Imber-Mintz et al., 1987). There is no evidence supporting the use of dynamic-oriented psychotherapies in the treatment of schizophrenia.

ATTENTION DISORDERS

Just as mood regulation may lie on a spectrum from depression to elation and mania, it is helpful to think of attention regulation on a spectrum (table 3.3). The attention spectrum may range from impaired ability to sustain focus (excessive distractibility and attention to extraneous stimuli) on one end, to hyperfocusing (inadequate disengagement of attention, such as uncontrolled obsession and stereotypical ritualized behavior) on the other end. Given this model, I will address attention-deficit/hyperactivity disorder (ADHD), and obsessive-compulsive disorder (OCD) under the heading of "disorders of attention." The reader should be aware that DSM-IV classifies ADHD under "disorders usually diagnosed in infancy, childhood, or adolescence" and OCD under "anxiety disorders." My presentation of these disorders under one heading of attention disorders is not meant as a substitute for DSM-IV, merely as another way of conceptualizing these disorders that might have some clinical benefit and stimulate your thinking.

TABLE 3.3
Hypothesized Model of Attention Disorders

ABILITY TO SUSTAIN ATTENTION	CLINICAL DISORDER WITH COGNITIVE SYMPTOMS ONLY	CLINICAL DISORDER WITH COGNITIVE AND MOTOR SYMPTOMS (IMPULSIVITY)
Low	Attention-deficit/ hyperactivity disorder– inattentive type (ADHD–i)	Attention-deficit/ hyperactivity disorder– hyperactive-impulsive type (ADHD–h)
High	Obsessive-compulsive disorder–obsessive type (OCD–o)	Obsessive-compulsive disorder–compulsive type (OCD–c)
Both	ADHD–i and OCD–o	ADHD–h and OCD–c

In this model, at the "underfocused" end of the spectrum, the purest form of an attention disorder is attention-deficit/hyperactivity disorder–predominantly inattentive type (ADHD–i). Currently classified under ADHD, and the syndrome which has been the primary focus of most research, is attention-deficit/hyperactivity disorder-predominantly hyperactive-impulsive type (ADHD–h). In the model presented here, ADHD–h is ADHD–i with a significant additional component of motor hyperactivity and/or impulsivity, possibly related to differences in serotonin regulation (Halperin et al., 1994). The "hyperfocused" end of the attention spectrum is somewhat less consistent with DSM-IV. Here, new subcategories of OCD are required, analogous to those in the current typology of ADHD. In this model OCD–predominantly obsessive type (OCD–o) would be the purest form of attention disorder at the "hyperfocused" end of the spectrum; when accompanied by motor impulsivity, the clinical picture would be OCD–predominantly compulsive type (OCD–c).

Just as some patients with mood disorders may be depressive only, while others are bipolar, so it may be with dysregulation of attention. Therefore, it is not uncommon to see some patients who exhibit states of both "underfocusing" or inattention (ADHD) and "hyperfocusing" or inability to shift focus (OCD). In fact, patients with tic-like OCD often have accompanying ADD, as do patients with Asperger's syndrome (right hemisphere deficit disorder) (Greist & March, 1995).

Diagnostic Issues in ADHD

Attention-deficit/hyperactivity disorder is a concept that has been around for many years under different names (attention-deficit disorder with and without hyperactivity, minimal brain dysfunction, hyperkinetic disorder). The DSM-IV diagnostic criteria present a number of difficulties for the clinician working with adults, including the fact that the disorder must have begun in childhood. This is a criterion that is often quite difficult to satisfy due to unreliability of patient history and frequent absence of other data sources in adults (Shaffer, 1994). Whenever possible, collateral history from the spouse, parent, coworkers, teachers, and old school records should be obtained, as the retrospective history of adult patients is less reliable than these sources (Wender, Reimherr, & Wood, 1981). It is often useful to have the patient and spouse read about the disorder, in order to facilitate a discussion regarding the likelihood of diagnosis.

Other diagnostic problems include the frequent co-occurence of ADHD with other disorders (comorbidity), such as conduct disorder, mood disorders, and substance abuse, and the overlap of ADHD symptoms with those of other disorders. (Once again the fuzziness of boundaries between diagnostic groups is apparent).

There are three myths (Zametkin, 1995) about ADHD that make diagnosis confusing. First is the myth that a positive clinical response to stimulants confirms the diagnosis. In fact, stimulants can improve the ability to focus in both ADHD and normal subjects. Second is the myth that ADHD will be outgrown, and therefore it is a disorder of childhood. In fact, it seems clear that teenagers and adults with ADHD continue to benefit from stimulant medication, and long-term follow-up studies seem to indicate that a significant number of children with ADHD continue to have symptomatology of the disorder as adults. The third myth is that, if the child does not exhibit the signs of ADHD in the physician's office, the child must not have ADHD. Because of the prevalence of these myths, the diagnosis has not even been considered in adults until recent years.

Confusion aside, the diagnostic criteria fall into three subtypes (see DSM-IV for full criteria). These subcategories distinguish the attention deficit from the hyperactivity/impulsivity, as well as note the combined type. The attention deficit is essentially manifested by symptoms of easy distractibility, difficulty sustaining attention, avoidance of tasks requiring sustained mental effort, tendency to make careless errors, difficulty listening to people, as well as disorganization factors, such as forgetfulness. The hyperactivity/impulsivity is manifested by excessive activity (as if driven by a "motor"), increased speech, fidgetiness and difficulty sitting still or waiting in line, as well as difficulty completing tasks (although this last factor may be caused by attention problems as well).

The most common mimics of attention disorders in adults are anxiety disorders and mood disorders, and these must be carefully ruled out to make the diagnosis. The list of other mimics includes eczema, mental retardation, schizophrenia, learning disabilities, developmental disorders, lead poisoning, thyroid hormone dysregulation, seizure disorders, sleep apnea, lyme disease, multiple sclerosis, and head trauma. Thorough evaluation is necessary to assess the possibility that one of these disorders is primarily responsible for an attention disturbance. Common comorbid disorders, such as conduct disorder, antisocial personality disorder, bipolar disorder, substance abuse disorder, must be ruled out as well (see associated disorders, below).

There are a number of computerized continuous performance tests (CPT) available as diagnostic aids. One of the more commonly used CPTs is the "test of variables of attention," or TOVA. This test requires that the patient (caffeine free and well rested) play a type of video game on a computer screen, hitting a button when a target appears and refraining from pressing the button when a nontarget appears. The test measures inattention, impulsivity, response speed, and consistency of results across different parts of the test. Universal Attention Disorders, Inc., who developed the test, claims that if the test results are positive there is a 90% chance of having the disorder, and if the test is negative there is a 40% chance of having the disorder. Thus, this tool cannot be relied on to make or exclude the diagnosis in and of itself, and should only be used as an aid. While there is dispute over the usefulness of this test, my clinical impression, after using the test on over 150 patients, is that it is a useful additional tool in diagnosing the disorder, assessing the response to medication, and determining appropriate dosage (which as you will see is very important). However, the TOVA cannot substitute for careful clinical assessment and history gathering.

Still other issues in the diagnosis of ADHD exist. There is some controversy over whether or not it is actually a bona fide disorder. Hartmann (1993) believes that what we call ADHD is actually a normal variant of human behavior that doesn't fit in with current cultural norms. He divides people into hunters (ADHD) and gatherers/farmers (obsessive-compulsive personality disorder). His idea is that people who have ADHD have qualities that would be quite adaptive, if not essential, to a hunting society. For example, if one were hunting with someone with ADHD, the distractibility would enable him to spot the subtle movements of prey from the corner of his eye, the impulsivity would allow him to initiate attack (motor) behavior rapidly, and the general decreased reliance on social relationships (people with ADHD are low on intimacy needs and often have conflict with authority and social standards) would serve him well as he would be away from the main social group much of the time. The farmer/gatherer person who is more rigid, rule bound, and can only act in stereotypic ways would clearly be at a disadvantage when hunting. He would ploddingly move through the forest, looking for game, bothered by the unpredictability of it all, and anxious about leaving behind the people he is attached to. When this person spots an animal (which he is less likely to do because he is less distractible), he will consider whether to attack, weighing options carefully, while the prey is likely to move away (perhaps this type would be better as a trapper).

This theoretical approach is useful on several accounts. It improves patients' self-esteem and corroborates their long-term experience of not fitting in. It seems to support the ADHD/OCD polarity and is consistent with the data on temperamental styles. It seems to make intuitive sense that the fabric of the human species is strengthened by the fact that it is composed of different strands, or temperamental styles, which allow for flexibility in the larger sense.

Diagnostic Issues in OCD

OCD was considered for many years by Kraepelin and Freud to be the prototypical psychological disorder, while schizophrenia was considered to be clearly a disease of the brain. Now, perhaps ironically, OCD is probably the best understood and most clearly demonstrated biologically based psychiatric disorder, according to Judith Rapoport. OCD is currently defined by DSM-IV as an anxiety disorder; however, research seems to clearly indicate the fact that the unwanted repetitive movements of OCD are a function of abnormal activity in multiple neural circuits between the frontal cortex and the striatum of the basal ganglia. The fact that the disorder is consistent across cultures, occurs in animals, and 25–30% of the time has its onset by age 15 helps strengthen the case that this disorder is strongly determined by genetics.

While a strong genetic component is present, there are estimates that as many as 10% of childhood cases of OCD are related to Sydenham's chorea (Swedo, Rapoport, & Cheslow, 1989). Sydenham's chorea is a disorder in which children exhibit multiple motor tics following rheumatic heart disease, which is itself a complication of untreated or treatment resistant streptococcal infections (strep throat). Fifty percent of children with Sydenham's chorea have OCD, and were previously normal (Swedo).

Recently, the concept of OCD spectrum disorders has arisen. In this concept any disorder that exhibits repetitive, unwanted behavior would be included under the OCD heading. In this schema (Hollander, 1993), compulsive shopping, compulsive gambling, substance abuse, nail biting (onchyphagia), hair pulling (trichotillomania), delusional disorders, Sydenham's chorea, Parkinson's disease, epilepsy, autism, anorexia and bulimia nervosa, body dysmorphic disorder, hypochondriasis, depersonalization disorder, paraphilias, ADHD, posttraumatic stress disorder, stuttering, and tic disorders are all considered variants of OCD. The validity of this hypothesis has not been tested, although most of these disorders have been shown to be selectively responsive to the same medications that work for classic OCD.

Genetic studies are consistent in showing that OCD usually clusters in families (Greist & March, 1995). OCD and Tourette's syndrome may be genetically related and are currently thought to be transmitted by a single gene, which is not always completely expressed. When incompletely expressed, a milder, subsyndromal form of OCD (which doesn't meet duration and distress/insight criteria of DSM-IV) occurs. When fully expressed, girls present with OCD and boys present with tics (Pauls et al., 1995). Rates of OCD are higher in women. The prevalence of OCD is remarkably consistent across a variety of nationalities and varies between 1.1–1.8 per 100, although some population pockets with lower or higher prevalence may exist (Weissman et al., 1994). ADHD also seems to aggregate in families, and according to at least two studies this seems to be consistent with the idea that a single gene is involved (Deutsch et al., 1990; Faraone et al., 1992). ADHD has a higher concordance rate in identical twins (50%) than fraternal twins (33%) (Goodman & Stevenson, 1989).

Associated Disorders

A large variety of disorders co-occur with both ADHD (Biederman et al., 1991, 1995; Jensen, 1993; West, 1995; Zametkin, 1995) and OCD (Greist, 1995). A number of clinical syndromes can exhibit attention dysregulation as part of their clinical picture, including schizophrenia, drug abuse, head trauma, thyroid imbalances (Hauser et al., 1993), mood disorders, lyme disease, etc.

Commonly comorbid with ADHD (not OCD) are conduct/oppositional defiant/antisocial disorders, substance abuse, and learning disabilities. (I can't resist noting that we do not call them System Inflexibility Disorders [SIDs] or Societal Teaching Disabilities [STDs!]). Disorders associated with both ADHD and OCD include neurological disorders (such as Tourette's syndrome, Huntington's chorea, Sydenham's chorea, and tic disorders) and mood disorders (both bipolar and depressive mood disorders).

OCD (not ADHD) is associated with anorexia, bulimia, and post-traumatic stress disorder (Greist, 1995).

Biological Theory and Brain Imaging Studies of Attention Disorders

Despite a great deal of research, the exact cause(s) of ADHD remains unknown, as does the mechanism of action of its treatment of choice. In fact, dysfunctions in at least seven different areas of the brain have been proposed (Voeller, 1991). As with other psychiatric disorders, it is unlikely that only one neurotransmitter or brain location is involved or can account for all of the findings of the disorder.

Recently, some emphasis in the literature has been placed on the idea that ADHD involves abnormal function of the dopamine-mediated neural pathways of the frontal lobes (Giedd et al., 1994) and striatum (a deeper structure involving movement); however, this is far from established. The evidence for this comes from brain imaging studies that have been replicated in at least three laboratories (Giedd et al., 1994; Hynd et al., 1991; Semrud-Clikeman, Filipek, & Biederman, 1994). The frontal lobes of the brain (the primary suspects) are involved in so-called "executive functions" such as the ability to plan, organize, and follow through. The frontal lobes also mediate socially appropriate behavior and are involved in working memory. Another researcher (Rogeness, Javors, & Pliska,

1992) suggests it is likely that norepinephrine may also be involved, as a regulator of dopamine-dependent behaviors, and that the balance between dopamine and norepinephrine may be the essential issue. However, this is still speculative. It is likely that ADHD involves multiple neural pathways and multiple neurotransmitters.

In keeping with this idea, Voeller (1991) suggests that ADHD involves three anatomically separate neural systems: the sensory-attention (helps process incoming stimuli), motor (helps control the threshold of motor responses), and arousal-activation systems (which control the general levels of excitability of specific neuronal systems). Interestingly, according to Voeller, the sensory attention system includes five separable components of attention: *detection* of novel stimuli, *vigilance* (the ability to sustain interest in detecting novel stimuli over prolonged periods of time), *selection* of the stimulus to attend to, the ability to *disengage* attention (which is mediated by the parietal lobe), and, once disengaged, to *shift* attention to the next stimulus. In keeping with the attention disorders concept I have advanced in this section, OCD might relate to the ability to disengage and shift. OCD, with its motor component (compulsive behavior), would involve the motor system, which has four components: *initiation, sustaining, inhibition*, and *termination* of movements.

It may be, then, that in ADHD and OCD, aspects of this motor system are dysregulated to produce the motor component of each disorder, while the attention components of ADHD and OCD are produced by abnormalities of the subcomponents of the attention systems. Brain imaging studies of OCD, as in ADHD, implicate aspects of the frontal-striatal circuits (Insel, 1992).

In OCD, the most commonly implicated areas of the frontal-striatal circuits are the orbitofrontal cortex, the cingulum, and the head of the caudate nucleus. The exact cause(s) of the disorder is unknown, and it is debated whether the increased blood flow in these areas is related to the cause of the disorder or is perhaps a compensatory response. Interestingly, it has been shown that both serotonin drug therapy (clomipramine) and, to a lesser degree, behavior therapy (exposure to the feared stimulus with prevention of response) normalize the blood flow to these parts of the brain (Baxter, Schwartz, & Bergman, 1992)! This proves for the first time that effective psychotherapeutic interventions in OCD actually cause changes in the same areas of the brain as effective drug therapy.

The main neurotransmitter involved in OCD seems to be serotonin. It is well-established that drugs that act on the serotonin systems of the brain are significantly more effective in OCD than drugs that affect the dopamine or norepinephrine systems, which are no more effective than placebo (Leonard, Swedo, & Leane, 1991).

Psychosocial Factors in the Attention Disorders

The person with ADHD is uncomfortable due to a poor fit with societal expectations. As a young, school-age child he or she would quickly become aware of the "wrongness" of sitting at a desk for hours at a time. She would experience continuous frustration — except at recess. As a child recognizes that she cannot conform to the expectations of parents and teachers and society at large, as the other children do, the "undiagnosed" or, better yet, unidentified child is faced with two possible resolution paths (although we now can offer a third option: medication). The path taken probably depends on psychosocial, hereditary, and other genetic factors. First, the child can accept societal/parental expectations and the fact that she cannot meet them. This leads inevitably to some degree of loss of self-esteem, helplessness, and depression. This is the route more commonly taken by females, and is less disruptive to society. Second, the child may decide that society is "wrong" and develop an antisocial attitude. Substance abuse may be used in either case to self-medicate what is a difficult path.

In addition to these early impacts on self-esteem and the ability to fit in with society, my clinical experience is that patients with ADHD seem to have a decreased ability to relate on an emotional level and they seem to remain in relationships at a more superficial level. They seem to have decreased dependency on relationships, and seek less intimacy. This can have significant impact on a marriage, and the diagnosis and treatment of ADHD can help both partners understand some of the dynamics of what is often a difficult relationship.

In the case of OCD, there may be fewer effects on self-esteem in childhood, especially when tics or motor behaviors are not present, since the structure of society is more consonant with the obsessive approach to life. Perhaps as a result of this, there is possibly less risk of substance abuse and antisocial behavior in OCD. Severe problems can arise, however, between parent and child when the parent attempts to interrupt compulsions. Severe isolation and relationship problems in childhood and adulthood can develop due to shame about the disorder (the compulsions of OCD relate to three areas: danger to self/others, cleanliness and safety, and acceptability to the group), inability to relate due to contamination fears, judgmental attitudes, perfectionism, etc. Job performance can be affected due to excessive attention to detail and inability to disengage from a task and shift focus, as well as difficulty relating to people with "flaws."

A CLINICAL ILLUSTRATION   Eric was referred to me by his therapist of three years' duration. He was a 51-year-old carpenter who had never married, and had a long history of substance abuse until one year before his referral to me. Upon evaluation it became clear that Eric was suffering from ADHD, and had obsessive-compulsive behaviors as well. Historically, he never was able to complete high school until much later in life because of a long history of academic failure and, ultimately, substance abuse. As a carpenter he had been able to support himself and his drug habits. However, for over 25 years Eric's compulsive substance abuse ran his life. His compulsiveness showed up in his work as well. He would, at times, get so involved with his work that he would neglect the time, missing other commitments he had made for the day.

Eric was quite reluctant to consider stimulant medication because of his history of substance abuse and the warnings of fellow Alcoholics Anonymous and Narcotics Anonymous members about using any substance to deal with life. They had saved his life and Eric was inclined to follow their advice.

In fact, Eric had a history of abusing amphetamines in high school, and the thought that a doctor would now be prescribing "speed" was quite disturbing to him. With a good amount of discussion and education, I was able to convince Eric to give the medication a trial so that he could make a fair analysis. If after trying the medication the benefits were not sufficient, or if there was any inclination or evidence of abuse, it would be discontinued at either his or my discretion. In this case, the use of the TOVA test was instrumental, since it documented in an objective way that there were clear abnormalities in Eric's function. When the test normalized with a medication trial, Eric was willing to continue the medication.

After three weeks on Dexedrine, Eric came into my office for a session that I will remember for a long time. While still ambivalent about the concept and the fact that he was using "speed," he broke down in tears of relief, thankfulness, and grief. He was immensely thankful because he felt normal for the first time in his life. He felt tremendous grief for the 51 years of suffering and loss that he had never understood. Being a very intelligent man, Eric could have achieved a number of professional degrees that were of interest, and this was very disturbing. His decades of substance abuse were also very disturbing. Over the subsequent six months, Eric continued in group and individual therapy and began to focus on inner conflicts. He began to notice that when he felt an emotion, he could actually identify it and think about it before acting on it. This presented a dilemma for him since new options were now available to him. Eric was able to work through this and face other issues about his personality and emotional makeup which, while difficult, enriched him as a person and clearly enabled him to develop the ability to be intimate, which he was very interested in.

In describing what it was like to have ADHD treated with stimulant medication, one patient said "It's like Casper the Friendly Ghost. The Ritalin enables me to slow the bastard down so that I can see him." While I had difficulty understanding this at first, it finally became clear and captured the essence of his experience: His thoughts were ghosts that would appear and disappear so rapidly that he could never grab hold of them.

Treatment Considerations in Attention Disorders

It is clear from the above discussion that when someone is treated for ADHD the diagnosis itself can be both upsetting and liberating. It is also clear that this disorder, if we consider it one, has a strong impact on the ability of the individual to fit in with societal norms, mainstream careers, and the ability to establish both working and intimate relationships. The result is anxiety and depression as well as decreased self-esteem, with or without antisocial behavior and substance abuse. I find it useful in counseling individuals and couples to use the hunter/farmer metaphor, and to point out to spouses that the person with ADHD can bring positive elements to the relationship, including spontaneity, fun, exploration, and lightness. These qualities are often what attracts the spouse to the ADHD individual. When married to an OCD personality type, their traits can be diametrically opposed, causing friction. When such a couple is willing to be taught to view themselves as a unit, the individual traits give the couple unit a great advantage in getting through life. The couple can learn to respect and appreciate the different approaches and when to use them. Medication, education, and psychotherapy can help these individuals and couples to develop improved relationships and career satisfaction.

What about Eric's concern? Is his doctor prescribing speed? Will he abuse it? Will he become dependent on it? Clearly there are risks associated with the use of stimulants. Stimulants may be abused, sold on the street, induce tics, raise the risk of seizure, and temporarily retard growth in children. In order to prescribe stimulants effectively, the use of them must be monitored carefully; height and weight must be monitored in children, as well as the development of tolerance, which would indicate that inappropriate use, misdiagnosis, or substance abuse is likely. Finally, it is important to assess the dosage via the TOVA test or another CPT when possible. The clinician should always question the patient about any tendency toward overfocused, stereotypic behavior (e.g., becoming so engrossed in an activity that other important activities are neglected), which would be an indicater that the dosage is excessive. With increasing doses of stimulants, the number of activities an individual engages in decreases, but the rate of behavior within a given activity type increases (Le Moal, 1995).

Addressing the recent widespread increase in the use of stimulants in ADHD as well as other conditions (e.g., to improve antidepressant response, to treat depression in the elderly medically ill patient, to treat narcolepsy, and even to treat negative symptoms in well-controlled schizophrenics), Volkow (1995) noted the similarities between cocaine and Ritalin. Ritalin has a relatively low rate of abuse when compared to cocaine. Both drugs act in the same parts of the brain (the striatum), increasing the amount of dopamine. The rate of initial increase of dopamine after administration seems to parallel the subjective high caused by both drugs. But, while cocaine leaves the striatum quite rapidly, Ritalin leaves the striatum slowly. Volkow concludes that despite the fact that both Ritalin and cocaine seem to act at the same sites in the brain, the risk of reinforcing the high (addiction) caused by these drugs is different: The Ritalin high cannot be recaptured, while the cocaine high can. Volkow postulates that this is because Ritalin remains in the striatum over an extended period and is cleared from the brain slowly, whereas cocaine is cleared rapidly, allowing a new dose to cause another dopamine rise.

In both ADHD and OCD, education about the disorder is paramount. Support groups for both family and patient are very helpful, and the family environment can be a significant factor in minimizing or worsening the disorder. Parents who are not permissive and who offer good structure in a calm, supportive manner will help a child with ADHD. Parents who encourage tolerance of anxiety and exposure to feared stimuli in a supportive and calm manner will be a clear advantage to a child with OCD. There is no place for individual psychodynamic therapy as it relates to the treatment of the symptoms; however, a good therapeutic relationship can help the patient and family with education, medication compliance, and problem solving. Individual dynamic therapy cannot replace support groups and therapies directed at the specific problems (e.g., behavioral response prevention for OCD and alternative strategies, training, and vocational assessment for ADHD).

EATING DISORDERS

Diagnostic Considerations in the Eating Disorders

Anorexia nervosa is characterized by four criteria: refusal to maintain a minimally normal weight, fear of gaining weight or becoming fat, a disturbed body image, as well as amenorrhea (loss of mentruation) for three consecutive cycles. The criteria used for subnormal weight is 85% of the normal weight for a person's age and height. Research studies use a number called a body mass index which is a ratio of weight (kilograms) over height (meters squared). In these studies, a body mass index of 17.5 kg/m^2 or less is considered subnormal weight.

Anorexics may be subtyped as either restrictors (patients who restrict their intake via dieting, fasting, or excessive exercise) or bingers-purgers (patients who utilize vomiting, laxatives, enemas, emetics (e.g., ipecac), or diuretics to maintain the subnormal weight). Often, the binge-eating/purging subtype has other impulse control problems such as drug or substance abuse, increased mood lability, and increased impulsive sexual activity. This makes sense considering the fact that the binge eating or purging is an impulsive act in and of itself.

There are five criteria for bulimia nervosa. First, patients diagnosed with bulimia must binge, taking in significantly greater than normal amounts of food in short periods of time. DSM-IV includes a frequency requirement, which seems to be arbitrary, of at least two binges per week for a three-month period. The patient must have a sense of lack of control over the binge eating, must indulge in some type of compensatory mechanisms, and, finally, must have a sense that his or her self-esteem is quite dependent on body shape and weight.

Bulimics are subdivided into two categories, both of which include binge eating and the above-mentioned factors as the core symptoms: The purging type uses vomiting and laxatives as compensatory mechanisms for the overeating; the nonpurging type uses mechanisms such as compulsive exercising. In general, most bulimics have a normal or slightly above normal weight; bulimia does not account for a very large percentage of morbidly obese patients.

Prevalence

The exact prevalence of eating disorders is uncertain. Garfinkel (1995) recently assessed over 8,000 subjects for bulimia nervosa and determineded a lifetime prevalence of 1.1% for females and 0.1% for males. Various other studies estimate a prevalence that ranges between 1% and 3%. Prevalence estimates depend on the narrowness or broadness of the definition used in the study, as well as the population studied. The prevalence of anorexia nervosa ranges between 0.5% and 3.7% (Walters & Kendler, 1995), depending on how narrow or broad the definitions are.

Comorbidity

Mood disorders are particularly frequent with the binge eating and purging types of anorexics. OCD, panic disorder, alcoholism, social phobia, and body dysmorphic disorder are also comorbid with anorexia nervosa (Hollander, 1993; Thiel et al., 1995). Mood disorders, such as dysthymia, bipolar disorder, and major depressive disorder (which may be primary or secondary to the bulimia); anxiety disorders; panic disorders; phobia; alcohol, stimulant, or drug abuse; and OCD are comorbid with bulimia nervosa.

Physical and Laboratory Findings

Anorexia nervosa is associated with numerous physiological abnormalities (Work Group on Eating Disorders, 1993) which are generally a reflection of the state of starvation. These include anemia, decreased white blood cells (the cells that fight infection), decreased platelet count (the cells that help clotting of blood), abnormal kidney function, increased cholesterol and liver function studies, decreased trace elements (e.g., magnesium, zinc, etc.), decreased potassium and chloride due to vomiting, and low to normal thyroid function. Other abnormalities found in anorexic patients include decreased heart rate, delayed sexual maturation, infertility, occasional arrhythmias or abnormal rhythms of the heart, decreased blood pressure on standing, and generalized abnormalities of the brain wave pattern — a result of metabolic abnormalities, which impair the brain function.

Individuals with bulimia are generally within the normal weight range. Their frequent binge-eating and purging behaviors can cause the following physical findings: electrolyte abnormalities (e.g., potassium, sodium, chloride), elevated amylase (an enzyme in the blood secreted by both the pancreas and salivary glands), loss of dental enamel, chipped or ragged teeth, calluses on the hands (due to rubbing the hands against the teeth to induce vomiting), and, rarely, tears in the esophagus, abnormal cardiac rhythms, and hiatal hernia (a bulging of the upper portion of the stomach through the diaphragm muscle). Abuse of ipecac can cause disturbances of cardiac function and sudden death.

Hormonal Abnormalities

In addition to the above physical and laboratory signs of starvation in anorexics, the hypothalamic-pituitary-adrenal (HPA) axis of a female patient who is anorexic is one that has regressed to the prepubertal state. The output of follicle stimulating hormone (FSH) and luteinizing hormone (LH), which stimulate the ovaries to produce eggs (ova), is reduced, as is the output of estrogen. In essence, this is probably a compensatory mechanism to adjust for starvation so that the reserves of the body are preserved. In a state of starvation, it would hardly be healthy or even possible to become pregnant, and certainly it would not be healthy to lose a significant amount of blood and its associated nutrients on a monthly basis. Therefore, this regression of the HPA axis can be seen as a conservation mechanism in which the patient's body is preserving resources. It is also a sign of starvation.

Numerous neuroendocrine challenges have been studied to evaluate the hypothalamic pituitary hormonal axes. Numerous abnormalities that are generally associated with the state of starvation have been found (Halmi, 1995; Krieg et al., 1988). Also demonstrated were increases in adrenal hormones (Gwirstman, Kaye, & George, 1989) and, as mentioned above, decreases in estrogen, and, in anorexic males, reduced testosterone levels. In bulimic patients the findings of hormonal dysregulation are much less compelling, even in the areas where there are some positive findings of hormonal dysregulation. This may be due to the fact that most bulimics are relatively normal in weight.

Neurotransmitter Abnormalities

In contrast to the hormonal abnormalities just discussed, the evidence for neurotransmitter abnormalities in the eating disorders is equally strong for both anorexia and bulimia. It is unclear, however, whether the abnormalities reflect a preexisting abnormality, a result of the disturbed eating patterns which themselves may leave neurochemical traces, or both. There is a fair amount of evidence suggesting serotonergic dysregulation in anorexia nervosa (low serotonin activity in low-weight restricting anorexics and high serotonin in restored-weight anorexics), and decreased serotonergic function in bulimia (Kaye & Weltzin, 1991). Additionally, women may be more vulnerable to dysregulation of the serotonergic aspect of the appetite control mechanism than men (Goodwin, Fairburn, & Cowen, 1987). This may account for the high prevalence of these disorders in women.

The norepinephrine system does not seem to be implicated to a significant degree in the eating disorders, while the dopamine system is hypothesized to be related to decreased satisfaction after eating

(Halmi, 1995). The few studies of dopamine in eating disorders (Halmi) do support a role for dopamine in the disturbed eating patterns of both anorexics and bulimics.

Brain Imaging Studies

While not consistent, brain imaging studies have shown increased ventricle-to-brain ratios that seem to be related to starvation (Datlof et al., 1986). Accrding to Krieg (1988), more than 50% of anorexic women have abnormal brain scans! As mentioned earlier, increases of ventricular-brain ratios have also been found in schizophrenia and occasionally manic depression. This seems to reflect some degree of tissue loss within the brain itself. I have found no brain imaging studies of bulimic patients in the psychiatric literature.

The Biology of Eating Behavior

The body provides two general mechanisms to help keep the internal body environment in balance with the external nutritional environment. One group of these mechanisms is located in the brain. This central eating-control mechanism involves two nuclei, one in the hypothalamus and one in the lower area of the brain stem. The second general group of mechanisms is located primarily in the gastrointestinal tract (peripherally) and involves the secretion of a variety of substances from the gut that help regulate a sense of hunger or satiety. Peripheral mechanisms of satiety seem to be mediated by the gastrointestinal hormones CCK, glucagon, somatostatin, and bombesin. Most of these substances exert their influence via the vagus nerve, one of the most widely distributed nerves in the bodily organs, which sends input, ultimately, to the paraventricular nucleus. It does not appear that this second mechanism is disturbed in patients with eating disorders. However, the first mechanism does seem to manifest abnormalities. In this section, I will review the biology of normal eating control followed by some of the abnormalities that are present in the eating disorders.

Normal Eating Behavior

Central eating control is influenced by two nuclei in the brain. In the hypothalamus, the paraventricular nucleus (PVN) helps to regulate the sense of hunger and fullness. If you will recall, the hypothalamus is an integrating and translating station that takes in information acquired through the senses as well as emotional information and translates that into physiological output that affects the functioning of the body in general. The hypothalamus influences basic functions such as eating, reproduction, sexual activity, and temperature regulation. The ventral tegmental nucleus (VTN), a nucleus in the brain stem, is also involved in the regulation of appetite.

The substances that have been identified as involving and affecting eating behavior include the common neurotransmitters, norepinephrine, serotonin, dopamine, as well as the opioids (endorphins), corticotropin-releasing factor (CRF), and vasopressin (VP).

It appears that the appetite is generally in a state of inhibition which is interrupted by norepinephrine. Norepinephrine, which is increased by stress and tricyclic antidepressants, stimulates alpha-2 receptors in the paraventricular nucleus, which in turn increase appetite for carbohydrates.

Serotonin suppresses carbohydrate cravings. Serotonin suppresses norepinephrine-induced eating. A general mechanism then, which is quite limited in scope and very simplistic, involves increased norepinephrine leading to increased carbohydrate cravings; increased carbohydrate cravings in turn lead to increased absorptions of tryptophan, which ultimately convert into serotonin in the brain; serotonin in turn then induces feelings of satiety, bringing the system back in balance.

Dopamine seems to act at the ventral-tegmental nucleus (VTN) and the nucleus accumbens, and seems to be involved in the rewarding aspects of eating. However, again defying simplicity, the brain responds to low doses of dopamine by increasing the desire to eat, and to high doses by decreasing the desire to eat. Nevertheless, it can be assumed that dopamine mediates rewarding effects of food as it does mediate other types of stimulation such as drugs of abuse.

Disturbed Eating Behavior

It can be useful to think of three types of disturbed eating behaviors.

1. *Stress-induced eating* would be related to increased norepinephrine (or tricyclic antidepressants, which increase norepinephrine activity). Stress-induced eating is also probably mediated by the opioid endorphin (endogenous morphines)

system (substances produced in the body that relieve pain and produce pleasant sensation). However, blockers of the opioid system do not necessarily decrease food consumption in humans. These endorphins act in the paraventricular nucleus (PVN) to increase eating. States of starvation reduce alpha-2 receptors (a presynaptic norepinephrine receptor whose activation acts as a brake, decreasing activity of norepinephrine neurons in the brain) in the PVN. However, as you have probably become aware from reading this book, things are never so simple in the brain. In fact, the brain is exquisitely sensitive and well-balanced, and so in response to starvation there is an increase of alpha receptors in the lateral parts of the hypothalamus despite the decrease of alpha receptors in the PVN. Thus, merely giving a drug that would decrease activity of the alpha-2 receptors would not necessarily be sufficient to alter appetite since other centers in the brain involving alpha receptors would also be affected.

2. *Abnormalities in the sense of fullness or satiety* are caused by dysregulated serotonin. Increased or decreased serotonin activity could be related to either anorexic or binge-eating behavior (see Neurotransmitter Abnormalities, above).

3. *Abnormalities of dopamine receptor function* could increase or decrease the reinforcing characteristic of eating.

It can be useful to try to sort out what aspects of the binge-eating or restricting behaviors are involved and thereby try to determine in some sense which neurotransmitters are involved, always remembering that this is simplistic, but potentially useful in addressing the source of the eating abnormality. These different experiences in disordered eating can help the patient understand more about their disorder.

Clinical Implications

Given the complexity of the feeding mechanism, which probably has only been understood by researchers to a very minimal degree at this time, what use can we make of this information?

Patients with eating disorders can be assured that they are dealing with strong, powerful biological determinants of their behavior. The impulsivity involved or the increased satiety involved in an anorexic experience are clearly mediated by abnormalities in the regulation of hunger and fullness; thus, this is not a character flaw. Control of the binge eating clearly should be addressed as something the patient must learn to deal with on a long-term basis. Patients with eating disorders have increased mortality rates. Anorexia in particular, is associated with an increased mortality rate of 5.6% per decade, a substantial difference from controls (Sullivan, 1995).

Anorexics have a difficult problem in that their sense of fullness in response to fats in the diet seems to be consistently abnormal, and so they become satiated much more easily than a patient with normal or bulimic controls. It seems clear that there are abnormalities in the pleasure responses to food in both anorexia and bulimia and that these are related to dopamine function (Kaye & Weltzin, 1991). Abnormalities in the dopamine pathways can lead to decreased satisfaction after eating (anorexia) or may facilitate binge eating. Patients with eating disorders have difficulty distinguishing between perceptions of hunger and satiety. High-fat meals may provoke hunger in bulimic patients, but not in anorexics. High-fat meals seem to cause an increased sense of satiety in anorexics, in particular, the restricting type.

In summary, there is a great deal of evidence that the processes that help to integrate information about nutrients available in the environment and the perceptual capacities that control eating behavior are markedly disturbed in both anorexics and bulimics. These are long-term disorders that require pharmacologic intervention as well as ongoing psychotherapy aimed at improving the patient's relationships and altering his or her sources of self-esteem.

Psychosocial Factors in Eating Disorders

It appears that aside from dealing with the biology of the dysfunction, patients in psychotherapy do best with cognitive therapy and interpersonal therapy. Behavioral therapy seems to be ineffective in the long term. Patients must be taught to dissociate self-esteem from appearance and this is difficult because of cultural factors. Patients who are bulimic must try to identify stresses that are temporally related to their binge-eating behavior. Often the relationship between a female and her mother has a significant bearing on the clinical state. At other times, the patient's relationship with her father is also important (Root, Fallon, & Friedrich, 1986). Large-scale studies have indicated that sexual abuse is more prevalent in bulimic patients (Garfinkel et al., 1995).

SUBSTANCE ABUSE AND ADDICTION

Pleasure is an essential part of life; it assists in learning and motivation and counterbalances the stresses and hardships we encounter. The brain appears to respond to reinforcing, pleasure-inducing substances and experiences by causing enduring changes in neuronal structure and function. These changes are designed to increase behaviors that will result in access to the source of pleasure. Life without pleasure or the possibility of pleasure (as in the case of severe depressive disorders), becomes tenuous and the survival instinct loses its predominance. When the environment does not provide sufficient sources of pleasure to maintain the survival instinct, or if the pleasure mechanism is for some reason not able to connect, associate, or become conditioned to available sources of pleasure due to prior experience (e.g., trauma or shame), impaired function of the brain or body, then alternative sources of pleasure are required. In that sense, substance abuse, although in the long run damaging, can be thought of as an "end-stage" survival mechanism.

Tolerance, Sensitization, Dependence, and Addiction

When discussing substance abuse, the concepts of tolerance, sensitization, dependence, and addiction are often used. *Tolerance* refers to a situation where repeated administration of a drug at the same doses has lessening effect, and increasing doses of the drug are required to produce the same initial effect — if it is recoverable at all. *Sensitization* is actually the reverse of tolerance and occurs when repeated doses of the same substance elicit increasing effects (see Kindling, chapter 2). It is possible for one drug to cause tolerance of some effects and sensitization to other effects. *Dependence* may be physiological or psychological. It is defined as the need for continued access to the drug in order to avoid a withdrawal syndrome. The withdrawal syndrome itself may be physical or psychological: When physical it can result in a physical withdrawal syndrome; when psychological it can result in motivational or psychological disturbances upon withdrawal of the drug. It is clear that tolerance, sensitization, dependence, and withdrawal are associated with many drugs that are not addicting. Drugs of abuse, however, are unique because they have very strong reinforcing properties that lead the drug user to seek access to the drug. This leads to a state of *addiction*, which can be understood as the sensation of craving and the compulsive seeking of a drug despite serious negative consequences in psychological, social, economic, or health areas.

The ability of a substance to produce addiction seems to be related to the following factors:

1. The degree to which the substance has an impact on the reward circuitry of the brain (discussed below).
2. The speed with which the substance causes a subjective rewarding effect. The speed of effect is important; drugs that have a rapid rewarding effect are conditioned or associated more easily with pleasure and therefore self-administration becomes much more likely. For example, both alcohol and nicotine are highly addictive because the subjective high closely follows ingestion of the drug. In fact, nicotine may be the most addicting substance known to man, since inhalation is followed within seconds by a subjective reinforcing high.
3. The genetic vulnerability.
4. The functional level of the family and environment.

Dependence on a substance is influenced by the following:

1. Dosage of the substance. In general, small doses are less likely to cause dependence since they have less physiological effect.
2. Duration of substance use. The longer a substance is used, the greater the degree to which the various systems of the body have adapted to its presence. Like a domino effect,

removal of the substance will require the realignment of those systems.

3. Mode of administration. Substances are more likely to cause dependence when the route of ingestion causes a rapid pleasure response. Thus, an orally ingested substance will take longer to reach the reward centers than an inhaled or intavenously injected substance.

Tolerance and its reverse, sensitization, are influenced by four factors:

1. Frequency of exposure to or ingestion of a substance. The more frequently a substance is ingested, the more rapidly tolerance or sensitization will occur.
2. The ability of the body to adapt to the presence of the substance. There is a variety of homeostatic mechanisms that are directed toward the reestablishment of the pre-drug equilibrium. Individuals vary in the efficiency with which they can break down (and thereby neutralize) a substance or adjust the "set-point" of other systems in response to a substance. With more efficient mechanisms comes more rapid tolerance to the drug effects, the need for higher dosage to achieve a given effect. With inadequate or absent mechanisms, the likelihood of sensitization becomes greater (see The Neurochemistry of Alcoholism, below).
3. Time. Both tolerance and sensitization are much more likely to occur with repeated exposure to a substance over time.
4. Dosage. Tolerance and sensitization are influenced by the rate of escalation of the dosage.

The Neural Circuitry of Addiction

Despite the fact that all drugs of abuse initially influence different neurotransmitter and receptor systems in the brain, ultimately it appears that all can produce addiction by a common long-term effect on the reward circuitry of the brain. The reward circuitry seems to involve the mesolimbic dopamine system as a major neural circuit mediating reinforcement. This system, which has been implicated in the deficit syndrome of schizophrenia where a blunted affect is manifest, seems to involve the prefrontal cortex, the nucleus accumbens of the limbic system, and the ventral tegmental area of the brain stem. It appears that the initial high experienced by a drug user is related to the speed of occupation of dopamine receptors in this area. Drugs, such as cocaine, that occupy these receptors quickly and then detach from them allow for a rapid high that is repeatable. Drugs, such as Ritalin (methylphenidate), that occupy these receptors somewhat less quickly and maintain attachment to them over a longer period of time, produce less of a high and leave less opportunity for repeating the high via repeated drug stimulation since the receptors remain occupied.

In the long term, reinforcement seems to be connected with altered function of receptors in this circuit, not of receptor numbers. It appears that chronic drug exposure alters the second and third messenger systems within the neuron itself; in fact, there is evidence that the structure of the neurons themselves as well as the production of proteins and the activity of genes are altered on a long-term basis.

Brain Imaging Studies

Brain imaging studies of substance abusers consistently indicate that while acute, small doses of substances of abuse may increase or decrease blood flow, chronic use of alcohol, sedatives, antianxiety medications, caffeine, marijuana, inhalants, and solvents are all accompanied by a decrease in blood flow to the brain (Mathew & Wilson, 1991).

Withdrawal states from substances of abuse and dependence are most likely related to a rebound increase in blood flow following a state of chronic decreased blood flow (Hemmingsen et al., 1988). In an interesting study (Modell & Mountz, 1995), blood flow on the right side of the brain, in particular in the caudate nucleus, was increased in individuals experiencing the compulsion to drink. This is interesting because individuals who suffer from obsessive-compulsive disorder also show increased blood flow in this area. This lends support to the common clinical assumption that both obsessive-compulsive disorders and substance abuse disorders are compulsive in nature.

Neurochemistry of Addiction

It seems clear that while one-time use of a drug will cause changes in receptors that are specific to that drug, long-term use causes changes within the neurons of the above-mentioned reward circuit. Amphetamines initially stimulate norepinephrine and dopamine receptors; alcohol stimulates NMDA, glutamate, GABA, serotonin, dopamine, and opiate receptors; nicotine, nicotinic receptors; marijuana, cannabinoid receptors; hallucinogens, serotonin receptors; and PCP, NMDA glutamate receptors (as alcohol does). After repeated administration of reinforcing drugs, long-term changes occur in the neural circuitry. It seems likely that most of these long-term changes are related to internal changes in G proteins, second messengers, third messengers, and ultimately in expression of genes. These cause adaptive changes in neuronal function and long-term changes in gene expression. The bottom line is that use of reinforcing drugs causes changes in gene expression and protein production, which ultimately are reflected by changed neural function and altered behavior, which seems designed specifically to obtain the source of reinforcement and pleasure.

Alcoholism

Alcoholism is the most common mental disorder and substance abuse disorder among men in the United States. The DSM-IV divides alcohol related disorders into alcohol use disorders (alcohol dependence and alcohol abuse) and alcohol-induced disorders (a variety of 13 subtypes, such as alcohol-induced delirium, dementia, mood disorder, sexual dysfunction, and sleep disorder). In this section I will use the term alcoholism to refer to the presence of any of these DSM-IV disorders.

While questions remain, it does appear fairly certain that alcoholism is a heterogeneous disorder and can be subdivided into two types (Bohman et al., 1987). It appears certain that *type I alcoholism*, which is the most common and accounts for 75% of male alcoholics and 100% of female alcoholics, occurs at a later age (greater than 25 years of age), and is not marked by inability to abstain from alcohol, is unassociated with antisocial behavior and lack of control during drinking, is frequently associated with psychological dependence, perhaps related to a general level of increased anxiety, and is frequently associated with guilt and fears of dependence (Cloninger). In addition, it seems that this type of alcoholic is low in the novelty seeking area, but high in the harm avoidance and reward dependence areas (see chapter 2, Temperament). *Type II alcoholism*, which seems to account for 25% of male alcoholics, is limited to males. Essentially, these patients are alcoholic and antisocial, and generally have the onset of alcohol abuse and dependence before the age of 25, have frequent inability to abstain from alcohol, and frequent histories of sociopathy and loss of control in drinking. In addition, type II alcoholics are less likely to be anxious and demonstrate less psychological dependence. They also exhibit much less guilt and fear of dependence. In terms of temperamental style, they tend to be very high in the novelty seeking area, but low in harm avoidance and reward dependence.

These subtypes have been replicated and are by and large accepted as being valid, although attempts at further refinement are ongoing (Cadoret et al., 1995). The subtypes seem to differ in the degree to which they are genetically determined and this subdivision has implications in terms of treatment. In order for a person who is a type I alcoholic to become alcoholic, a nonfunctional family seems to be required in addition to a genetic risk. A well-functioning family seems to protect despite genetic risk. Type II alcoholics seem to be associated with a very strong genetic component (Cloninger et al., 1981). In fact, these two types were originally called "milieu-limited" (type I) and "male-limited" (type II) (Cloninger). This referred to the observation that some adoptees, whose biological parent — mother or father — was alcoholic, were influenced by the environmental effects in the adoptive family (type I). This group demonstrated a later onset of alcoholism, minimal criminality, aggressivity, and antisocial behavior. In contrast, the other group of alcoholic adoptees demonstrated "father to son" genetic transmission only, and minimal influence of the adoptive family. According to Linnoila (1994), however, environment also plays a significant role, even in type II alcoholics. Fewer than 20% of the biological sons of antisocial alcoholics become alcoholic themselves.

The Neurochemistry of Alcoholism

Alcoholism of the type II variety seems to be clearly associated with decreases in serotonin activity in the brain (in the dorsal raphe nucleus and nucleus accumbens). In fact, even family members of these patients have low levels of serotonin when compared to patients who are not alcoholic. Low serotonin levels are associated with violence and suicide (see Impulsivity, chapter 2; Markers of Suicide, this chapter). In fact, the second most common diagnosis in suicide victims is alcoholism. Therefore, one could conclude that a low serotonin trait may be characteristic of young male alcoholics and their relatives. Depressed patients with alcoholic relatives are likely to have lower serotonin activity as well. Because of the association with violent behavior, clinicians must evaluate the suicide risk of all alcoholics. Clinicians must also be sure to evaluate the suicide risk in young male alcoholics with antisocial traits as well as depressive patients with family members who are alcoholic.

Extensive evidence links the body's own opioid system (in the pituitary gland) and dopamine (in the nucleus accumbens) and serotonin systems to the reinforcing, pleasure inducing properties of alcohol (O'Brien, Eckhardt, & Linnoila, 1995). On the other hand, alcohol-induced changes at ionophore (GABA and NMDA) receptors (see Receptors, chapter 1) seem to account for the amnesia and impaired coordination associated with alcohol use.

The toxic effects of alcohol are thought to be related to alcohol's interference with neurotransmission of glutamate neurons, through the NMDA receptor (Tsai, Gastfriend, & Coyle, 1995). It seems that recurrent, untreated, or inadequately treated withdrawal from alcohol leads to long-term brain damage in alcoholics, and therefore liberal use of benzodiazepines in the withdrawal phase should be undertaken. Tsai has shown that brain atrophy of a diffuse nature is often caused by chronic alcohol use. Over the long-term, alcohol can cause brain injury, which is manifested in various ways: alcohol intoxication, alcohol withdrawal, withdrawal seizures, delerium tremens, blackouts, Wernicke-Korsakoff syndrome, and alcoholic dementia. Blackouts and Wernicke-Korsakoff syndrome can be associated with memory impairment, which seems to be related to disturbed neurotransmission in the hippocampus (which, as has been discussed, is essential for memory formation). In addition, chronic use of alcohol can lead to degeneration of other brain areas and, in pregnant women, fetal alcohol syndrome.

Two liver enzymes (ALDH-2 and ADH-2) seem to be more prevalent in alcoholic patients (Higuchi et al., 1995). When the genes that control the production of these enzymes are inactive, they seem to protect against alcoholism by allowing high levels of alcohol metabolites (acetaldehyde) to accumulate in the blood, causing adverse side effects such as flushing and nausea. Theoretically, this discomfort inhibits chronic use and the development of tolerance and dependence is less likely. While these studies were done in a Japanese population, it is encouraging that the risk for alcoholism was predictable on the basis of the presence of the genes that control the production of these enzymes.

Comorbidity and Alcoholism

According to Rosenthal (1995), many alcoholics — particularly those in the middle class under the age of 35 — are polysubstance abusers. Thirty-seven percent of people with alcohol abuse or dependence will have an additional mental disorder (Regier, Farmer, & Rae, 1990). In addition, according to Linnoila (1994), 40% of men and 88% of women who are alcoholics experience major depression and dysthymia; 10–15% percent of male and female alcoholics experience generalized anxiety disorder; 10% of male alcoholics experience panic disorder; 21% of female alcoholics are phobic. Because of this comorbidity, it is clear that any treatment of an alcoholic needs to involve a differential diagnosis of psychiatric conditions.

Physical Findings Associated with Alcoholism

According to the DSM-IV, repeated intake of high doses of alcohol can affect nearly every organ system resulting in gastrointestinal (gastritis, ulcers, liver degeneration, inflamation of the pancreas, gastrointestinal cancers), cardiovascular (high blood pressure, abnormalities of the heart muscle, increased levels of fats in the blood), central nervous (mental disorders, degeneration of brain tissue, cognitive deficits, memory impairment, degeneration of the cerebellum), and peripheral (bodily) nervous (tingling, muscle weakness, decreased sensation) system dysfunction. Those who abuse or are dependent on alcohol are also at high risk for vitamin and nutritional deficiencies (e.g, B vitamin, protein).

The effects of alcohol on these systems accounts for the physical signs and symptoms of alcoholism, including upset stomach, belching, bloating, hemorrhoids, blotchy and puffy complexion (gastrointestinal system); headaches, heart attacks, and strokes (cardiovascular); insomnia, depression, poor memory, falls and fractures, seizures, job and relationship problems (central nervous system); and tremor, impaired coordination, and impotence (peripheral nervous system).

Chronic alcohol abuse is associated with changes that are measurable in blood, including elevated liver enzymes (GGT and SGOT), increased size of red blood cells (called mean corpuscular volume or MCV), high normal levels of uric acid, and high levels of fats (triglycerides and cholesterol).

The Treatment of Alcoholism

Treatment of the alcoholic must be directed at abstinence. All well-controlled studies of alcohol abusers indicate that controlled drinking is only possible in the short run. The optimal treatment team would involve a psychiatrist, an internist, a psychotherapist, and support via Alcoholics Anonymous. Interestingly, the subtype of alcohol abuse (type I or type II), seems to make an important difference in determining the effectiveness of clinical intervention (Litt et al., 1992). Type I, late onset alcoholics, have good outcome when given interactional psychotherapy aimed at relationship issues. Type II alcoholics, with the early onset of psychopathic traits, have better outcome when given coping skill training. When these types of therapies are reversed, both groups have poor prognosis. Therefore, in choosing the type of psychotherapy, the clinician must try to assess the alcoholic type.

Treatment of the alcoholic is advancing on the pharmacological end. In the past, the only treatment involved disulfiram (Antabuse), which caused very painful and sometimes fatal reactions when alcohol was ingested during use of this drug. As discussed above (Neurochemistry of Alcoholism), it seems clear that the euphoria of alcohol abuse is significantly related to the opiate receptors. New drugs now target these receptors to reduce the craving for alcohol among abstinent alcoholics. Naltrexone (Revia) has been found to be useful in reducing the loss of control that type II alcoholics seem to manifest. It seems clear that using selective serotonin reuptake inhibitors, which act in the serotonin system, will decrease the amount of compulsive alcohol use over time, although they do not eliminate alcohol use. There is evidence that dopamine inhibitors such as Haldol can reduce the cravings that seem to be associated with the dopamine receptor function. Finally, medications are being investigated to help neutralize or at least diminish the neurotoxic effects of alcohol that are mediated by the glutamate and NMDA receptors. There is also some evidence that serine and glycine (amino acids) can be protective against these neurotoxic effects.

Other Drugs of Abuse

Much less research has been done on other drugs of abuse as compared with alcohol; however, there are a number of promising leads. First, cocaine seems to exert its stimulant and reinforcing effects by binding to the dopamine system in the neural circuitry (described above). It exerts its adrenaline-like effects by binding to norepinephrine nerves in the brain. The acute effects of cocaine, as with other substances of abuse, are different than the chronic effects of cocaine. The chronic use of cocaine is associated with the mesolimbic pathway (described above). Controlled trials of pharmacologic agents in the treatment of cocaine abuse and dependence reveals only a few promising agents. These include amantadine, bromocriptine, carbamazepine, and desipramine (Withers et al., 1995). Psychotherapeutic interventions seem to indicate that psychotherapy aimed at improving coping skills can cause lasting change (Carroll, 1994).

PANIC DISORDERS

Panic disorders include panic with and without agoraphobia, and should not be confused with other anxiety disorders associated with panic, such as specific phobia, social phobia, and posttraumatic stress disorder. The controversy over whether these disorders are closely related, and in what way, is not addressed since the research in this area is inconsistent and inconclusive. The focus here is on the current understanding of the biological underpinnings of the panic attack itself, and how that understanding can help you clinically.

Diagnostic Considerations

Panic disorder, according to the DSM-IV, consists of recurrent unexpected panic attacks followed by at least one month of persistent concern, worry, or change in behavior as a direct result of the attack. The symptoms of the attack itself include at least four or more of the following symptoms: a subjective sense of terror, going crazy, losing control, or dying; symptoms of hyperarousal of various body systems, including cardiovascular (rapid heart rate, palpitations, lightheadedness), respiratory (sighing, hyperventilation, shortness of breath, subjective sense of difficulty breathing or breathlessness), gastrointestinal (dry mouth, nausea, vomiting, diahrrea), cognitive (trouble thinking clearly), dermatologic (sweating, clamminess, flushing), and neurological (tremulousness, tingling, trouble with speech, dizziness, dissociation).

There seem to be primarily three types of panic attacks:

1. Situationally cued panic attacks (here referred to as "phobic" panic).
2. Situationally predisposed panic attacks. In this case, a panic attack is more likely to be induced by a situation or cue, but does not necessarily occur in association with the cue.
3. Unexpected, uncued panic attacks (here called "spontaneous" panic).

Associated Features of Panic Disorders

Once a person has experienced a panic attack, a series of consequences may follow. If agoraphobic, he is likely to worry (anticipatory anxiety) about another panic attack; avoid situations that he believes would trigger panic (as in phobic panic); avoid situations where help might not be available. (In spontaneous panic, shortness of breath and suffocation feelings are a first symptom, therefore he or she would be fearful of being in any situation that would impair his ability to either get help if he felt he was suffocating or to get fresh air.) The result of these responses to panic is a progressive narrowing of his world, activities, and relationships.

Patients with panic disorder have a higher likelihood of having mitral valve prolapse (MVP), a weakness of one of the valves of the heart. It is relatively benign, but does occasionally produce abnormal sensations including pounding heart, rapid heart rate, lightheadedness, dizziness, fainting, fatigue, difficulty breathing, and chest pain. In one study, 34% of panic disorder patients had MVP (Liberthson et al., 1986).

Panic disorder is associated with an increased risk of suicide, major depression (Fawcett, 1992), and other anxiety disorders (Barlow, 1988). Patients with panic disorder have a significantly higher rate of gastrointestinal complaints, such as irritable bowel syndrome (Lydiard et al., 1994).

In general most panic disorder patients tend to describe themselves as having discomfort with aggression, low self-esteem, and of being fearful and shy as children (Shear et al., 1993). (This description is reminiscent of the discussion on temperament, chapter 2).

Biological Theory of Panic Disorder

The prevailing theory of panic disorder states that there are two types of panic attacks, spontaneous (nonphobic) and cue-induced (phobic). DSM-IV addresses a third type of panic (situationally predisposed panic attacks), but as this is not addressed by the current theories, it is not included in this discussion. Spontaneous panic attacks are thought to be the result of abnormal oversensitivity of a brain alarm system whose function is to detect early signs of suffocation (figure 3.8). This theory is called the *suffocation alarm theory*. The cardinal symptoms of spontaneous panic are respiratory: shortness of breath, chest discomfort, palpitations, and choking or suffocation sensations.

Normally, carbon dioxide (CO_2), the waste product of respiration, is exhaled from the lungs. In the event of suffocation, the levels of

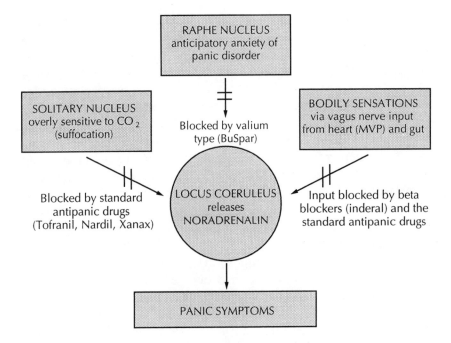

FIGURE 3.8. Brain mechanisms in panic disorder; people who have spontaneous panic attacks may have increased sensitivity in any of three areas: the solitary nucleus, the raphe nucleus, and bodily sensations.

CO_2 in the blood, and particularly the brain, rise. Neurons in the solitary nucleus of the brain stem, which are constantly sampling the blood in the brain for levels of CO_2, become activated about two minutes after an actual or misperceived drop in CO_2. This causes a deep sigh and sensations of smothering (respiratory distress: "Hey, you're not breathing big fella!"). About 1½ minutes following activation of this phase of the alarm, signals are sent to the locus coeruleus. This nucleus is the switch for almost all of the norepinephrine-containing neurons of the brain. Following this, the second wave of symptoms occur, involving the nonrespiratory systems listed above (fight/flight response: "You better act now if you want to live!") as well as compensation mechanisms in the respiratory system itself (hyperventilation: "Pick up the breathing pace, big guy!"). Thus, the panic itself is a time-limited episode of short duration (about 4 minutes). Nonphobic panic will occur whenever CO_2 levels build up. This usually occurs when respiration slows or CO_2 builds up due to excercise. Spontaneous (nonphobic) panic will often occur during sleep or relaxation training because respiration has slowed, allowing CO_2 levels to rise. This triggers the overly sensitive suffocation alarm system (solitary nucleus). Patients with this type of panic chronically hyperventilate and sigh, keeping the levels of CO_2 low, as a way of preventing sensations of respiratory distress and suffocation. Interestingly, women are more vulnerable to panic attacks premenstrually and just after childbirth. These are both times when the levels of progesterone drop suddenly. Since progesterone decreases the levels of CO_2 in the brain by increasing respiratory rate, the loss of progesterone at these points in time would lead to increased CO_2 and more vulnerability to panic.

The second and more common type of panic, phobic (cue-induced) panic, is fear-induced. It is manifested primarily by symptoms of pounding heart (palpitations), sweating, and trembling. In this type of panic the *separation alarm* is activated directly by the fear-inducing interpretation of a stimulus (a thought or a situation). This alarm resides in the cells of the locus coeruleus of the brain stem. The locus coeruleus is activated by separation from the group, an individual one is emotionally or physically dependent on, or life itself (i.e., one's own death). This separation alarm triggers the flight-or-fight response via the release of noradrenalin (more commonly called norepinephrine) in the brain and adrenalin (epinephrine) in the body. According to Klein (1993), fear-induced panic activates the stress response system (the hypothalamic-pituitary-hormonal axis) immediately.

Brain Imaging

Studies of panic disorder patients generally support the idea that there are abnormalities of brain function in the structures surrounding the hippocampus and areas of the brain stem (Baxter, 1995), including the locus coeruleus and raphe nucleus (involved in anticapatory anxiety). However, findings are not consistent and more brain imaging studies need to be done.

Clinical Differentiation of Panic Subtypes

In treating patients with panic attacks, the clinician should ask questions aimed at differentiating the type of panic attack from which the patient suffers. Table 3.4 will assist you in that process. Ask about the cognitions associated with the panic. Is it phobic? Does the panic wake the patient from sleep? Does it occur as he or she is falling asleep or relaxing? When it started, had the patient been premenstrual, just given birth, or weaned her child (when progesterone levels are falling)? Have there been recent separations or losses, which might activate the separation alarm?

Clinical Implications

Treatment must be tailored to the type of panic. The phase of the disorder must also be considered since over time complications such as anticipatory anxiety, agoraphobia, substance abuse, or depression may have developed.

Spontaneous, nonphobic, panic attacks, marked by respiratory distress, respond better to imipramine (Tofranil) than alprazolam (Xanax). It is thought that imipramine as well as the newer selective serotonin agents such as fluoxetine (Prozac), sertraline (Zoloft), paroxetine (Paxil), and fluvoxamine (Luvox) decrease the sensitivity of the suffocation alarm (the solitary nucleus). Theoretically, cognitive therapy would be useless in this group, since the panic is unrelated to cognitions. (In the clinical world, however, spontaneous panic attacks seem to generate anticipatory anxiety and — perhaps via kindling or cognition — cue-induced, phobic panic.) Relaxation training would be harmful, since it would slow respiration and increase CO_2, which would lead to panic. Excercise, and the premenstrual and postpartum period would also increase vulnerability to these panic attacks.

Cue-induced panic responds preferentially to alprazolam (Xanax) and clonazepam (Klonopin), since these medications work on both the anxiety (raphe nucleus) and the norepinephrine-induced terror (locus coeruleus). The anticipatory anxiety component of panic disorder is not treatable with imipramine. It requires other medications, such as buspirone (BuSpar), which acts on the serotonin receptors

TABLE 3.4
Differences between Spontaneous and Cue-induced (Phobic) Panic Attacks

	SPONTANEOUS PANIC	CUE-INDUCED (PHOBIC) PANIC
Initial symptoms	Respiratory distress: breathlessness, chest discomfort, feelings of choking or suffocation	Adrenalin response: rapid heart rate, lightheadedness, sweating, trembling
Brain nucleus involved	Solitary nucleus (monitors CO_2): suffocation alarm	Locus coeruleus (responds to perceived danger with fight/flight response): separation alarm.
Vulnerable periods	Relaxation, falling asleep, nondream sleep, exercise	Threatened separation from a relationship perceived as essential, from social group, and from life itself.
Naturally occurring human models	Ondine's curse (an inborn defect in serotonin neurons of the solitary nucleus: in these infants when breathing slows, the increased CO_2 does not activate the suffocation alarm); infants with this disorder stop breathing when asleep—the opposite of and absence of panic.	Separation of infant from mother
Psychotherapy type	Education	Cognitive and behavioral exposure therapy
Effective medications	Tofranil, Anafranil, Prozac, Zoloft, Paxil, Luvox, Nardil	Klonopin, Xanax, Nardil Inderal, Progesterone
Chemical inducers	Lactic acid (exercise), CO_2, bicarbonate, Isuprel (heart medication)	Caffeine, Yocon (used for sexual dysfunction)
Anticipatory anxiety	Yes	Yes
Activation of hormonal axis	No immediate activation; activated later as disorder becomes chronic	Immediate activation

of raphe nucleus neurons, or benzodiazepines, such as clonazepam (Klonopin), which acts on other brain regions that mediate general levels of anxiety via the GABA (inhibitory) neurons and receptors.

Cognitive therapy and behavioral exposure should be effective in cue-induced panic. Buspirone (BuSpar) works on the serotonin neurons in the raphe nucleus to reduce anticipatory anxiety, but does not have any effect on the norepinephrine-induced terror (locus coeruleus).

Treatment and Long-Term Outcome

No outcome studies have yet subtyped panic attacks according to the dichotomy discussed above (cue-induced vs. spontaneous panic). As with other disorders, a combination approach of appropriate medication and therapy are most effective. In a recent study (de Beurs et al., 1995), Luvox (a serotonin reuptake inhibitor), when used in combination with exposure to the panicogenic situation, was twice as effective in reducing self-reported avoidance behavior, depression, and anxiety.

Cognitive therapy aims to correct the misinterpretation and catastrophic thinking that result in disturbing feelings. The cognitive model of panic assumes that panic attacks develop as a result of misinterpretation of bodily sensations (such as palpitations) as dangerous. Black (1993) compared the effectiveness of cognitive therapy and Luvox, and found 81% of medication-treated patients were panic-free at 8 weeks, versus 53% of the cognitive therapy patients. However, relapse rates upon discontinuation of medication are high and are reported as being between 20% and 90% (Rickels et al., 1993). This indicates that, as in the mood disorders, there is a need for maintenance medication. Despite the sense that panic disorder can be chronic, there is evidence that a large number of panic disorder patients are significantly improved on long-term follow up (Nagy, 1993). Nevertheless, future studies will help sort out the best type and length of treatment.

POSTTRAUMATIC STRESS DISORDER

While most DSM-IV anxiety disorders present with some form of worry, anxiety, or panic as their main symptom, posttraumatic stress disorder (PTSD) does not. It clearly involves a persistent overarousal of multiple neural circuits as a direct result of a traumatic event. At some point following the trauma, the event is reexperienced in an uncontrollable and unpredictable way, again and again via any of a number of pathways (e.g., nightmares, intrusive thoughts, cue-induced memories, etc.). As a result, the person avoids any situation that could lead to reexperiencing the event. Despite a state of hyperarousal, or perhaps because of that, the individual gives the appearance of being numb in both emotional/social function and intellectual function.

Prevalence and Course of PTSD

The prevalence of PTSD is estimated at about 1% in the general population (Helzer, 1987), but may be as high as 20% in Vietnam veterans (Nemiah, 1995). The prevalence rises to as high as 53% in survivors of disasters (Smith & North, 1993). PTSD may be the result of one single event, or the result of chronic repetitive events (Foa, Riggs, & Gerhuny, 1995). If a single event results in PTSD, it is likely that the reexperiencing of it via uncontrolled flashbacks and nightmares effectively transforms it into a chronic recurrent trauma. Why some individuals experience trauma and develop PTSD while others do not is unknown. It is possible that intelligence level may facilitate adaptive coping, as decreased levels of education and IQ correlated highly with the likelihood of developing PTSD (McNally & Shin, 1995). Approaching the issue from a different angle, Breslau, Davis, and Prabucki (1995) found that the risk for PTSD was positively correlated with factors that increased the risk of exposure to trauma: high neuroticism (a general emotional overresponsiveness and liability to develop neurotic disorders under stress) scores, extroversion (outgoing, sociable, uninhibited, and impulsive inclinations), and African-American race. It appears that events capable of producing PTSD are more likely to occur in socially disadvantaged groups.

PTSD is a chronic disorder that increases a person's vulnerability to illness and death at a young age. In a 50-year prospective study of men who faced heavy combat in WWII, well over 50% were chronically ill or dead by age 65 (Nemiah, 1995). It also appears that PTSD causes permanent changes in the functioning of the hypothalamic-pituitary-adrenal axis (stress response system) (Yehuda et al., 1995, 1993) and quite likely decreases in the size of the hippocampus (Bremner et al., 1995).

Biological Mechanisms and Neurochemistry of PTSD

A CLINICAL ILLUSTRATION   Mr. Fine was a 45-year-old prison guard who was caught in a prison riot. On the afternoon of the riot he heard a phone ring and, in his memory, this was followed in quick succession by gunshots. He was injured in his shoulder. When the riot was quelled, he was taken to the hospital for treatment of his wound. Following this event, Mr. Fine began to have flashbacks of the event, accompanied by feelings of terror, full-fledged panic attacks, and a fear that he was "going crazy." These flashbacks were stimulated by a number of previously neutral events, such as the sound of his phone ringing. He was unable to control these responses, and began to be more and more frustrated. In addition, he was unable to reenter the prison because a variety of visual and auditory cues evoked the same panic response. Mr. Fine also felt that his peers had lost respect for him, thinking he was using excuses to get out on disability since he had a conflict with his supervisor. Soon, Mr. Fine became depressed. He was unable to sleep due to recurrent nightmares, from which he would often awaken in panic. He was placed on disability, and soon his emotional well-being and work life quickly unraveled.

In assessing this case, the therapist might choose to focus on a number of issues (using any number of approaches), including depression, loss of job, loss of role function, loss of peer acceptance, panic attacks, existential issues of life and death, Mr. Fine's fears of "going crazy," traumatic precursors in childhood that hadn't been worked through, etc. The therapeutic approaches might vary from a more passive psychoanalytic stance to cognitive therapy, interpersonal therapy, pharmacotherapy, career counseling, or spiritual counseling.

Some of these approaches are more likely than others to help the client, and some may be destructive and have no place in treatment of such a case. After discussing the biological mechanisms and neurochemistry of PTSD, I will apply these to this case, and then follow with a discussion of appropriate treatment based on these mechanisms. This is not to be read as an absolute indication of how Mr. Fine should be treated, but rather as an indication of the understanding the therapist must have at hand, or have access to, in order to define an overall therapeutic plan. (The therapy should be dictated by the problem, not by the method available to the therapist.)

PTSD seems to involve three symptom clusters (Foa et al., 1995): *high arousal* (e.g, panic attacks, terror, increased startle response, increased pulse, hypervigilance, and overstimulation) and *high avoidance* (anticipatory, phobic anxiety leading to avoidance of thoughts and situations related to the trauma), which lead to *psychic numbing* (uncontrollable stress leading to depression associated with social isolation, anhedonia, and blunted affect).

PTSD probably involves three mechanisms, which may be related to the three symptom clusters. First, there seems to be a strong association that is formed between the perceived environmental factors that are registered at the time of the trauma, and the actual emotional response and memory of the event. This is called *conditioning* and is a pairing of stimulus and response. Conditioning is dependent on an intact norepinephrine system. Just as moderate levels of anxiety and norepinephrine facilitate memory, so they may facilitate the synaptic transmission in PTSD. Once the strong emotional response and memory are linked to external or internal cues, the response is conditioned. Now, unpredictable exposure to stimuli cause a reliving of the emotions and memory of the event, upsetting the individual in an unpredictable but painful manner. This repetitive, intrusive elicitation of the memory may induce a *kindling* response (chapter 2). When repetitively stimulated by the cues, eventually the neural circuits involved in the memory begin to fire spontaneously, leading to flashbacks. Finally, living in a situation of uncontrollable, random pain, the person becomes *helpless*. He experiences emotional blunting, disturbed dream sleep, withdrawal from people, and anhedonia.

In theory, the panic and high arousal (e.g., panic, overstimulation, increased startle response, increased pulse, hypervigilance) are related to increased activity in the norepinephrine-containing neurons of the locus coeruleus and the amygdala (controls the level of emotional arousal). The avoidance and intrusive thoughts may reflect disturbances in serotonergic function (similar to recurrent obsessive thinking in obsessive compulsive disorder). Dopamine may be implicated in the late stages of the disorder, reflecting dysfunction in some of the same neural pathways that are thought to be involved in schizophrenia (nucleus accumbens and prefrontal cortex) and depression. Some theorists explain the addictive attraction to the remembrance of the trauma as due to activation of the body's opioid substances, perhaps as a pain control mechanism, during the initial event. This might explain why victims of sexual abuse may experience an exciting high with a sexual experience that recalls the abusive event — because of the linking of the pain and pleasure as part of the memory.

Mr. Fine, in a familiar environment, was stressed by a sudden gunshot and personal injury. His noradrenalin system was stimulated by the gunshot, as modified by the meaning of that gunshot; if the gunshot had been expected as part of the routine in the prison, it would hardly be perceived as a stress or danger. If the gunshot was thought of as a surprise, the event was more likely to set off the alarm system of the locus coeruleus. Mr. Fine clearly was surprised by the gunshot, and an alarm, a panic response, was activated, putting him in the fight-or-flight mode (high arousal), and sending more blood to the vital organs, such as the brain.

At the same time, the neurons in various other nerve networks were activated, including the vision, hearing, and memory systems. These higher centers sent signals to both the learning center in the hippocampus, which bound the events registered in the separate higher centers into a whole memory, including the association to the ringing phone which was almost simultaneous with the trauma, as well as to the emotional learning center in the amygdala. The sound of the phone was quickly linked to the fear response in the amygdala (conditioning).

This neurotransmission or activation of the quick-response chemical system described in chapters 1 (Neuromodulation) and 2 (Plasticity, Learning, and Memory) caused immediate firing, sensitization, and, in turn, activation of the slower, long-term response system (neuromodulation) in the various parts of the brain that were discussed above. A variety of transcription factors were produced within minutes and bound to the appropriate place on the DNA, initiating production of the appropriate proteins, which caused new nerve connections to be made, changed the number and/or type of receptors on the cells themselves, and altered the type and/or amount of neurotransmitters made, etc. Connections were made between certain nerve cells that evoked the sound and visual images related to the perception of the event, and between the other systems that were involved and stimulated at that time. These connections may be made when the transcription factors cause the production of nerve growth factor, which causes arborization to occur. The cells involved in the nerve network of this memory may become more sensitive to stimulation as the transcription factors cause the production of more receptors. Thus, the cells that evoke the memory, by cues from the auditory or visual systems, become more sensitive. These cues, or stimuli (e.g., the phone, the prison, the sound of his peers on the phone etc.), which were neutral before the event, began to take on emotional significance, and this emotional memory trace was made in the amygdala. By their new or strengthened connection to the locus coeruleus, some or all of these neurons became able to evoke the alarm or panic system in the locus coeruleus, which constituted a flashback. Mr. Fine's flashbacks occurred within days of the event, but in other cases flashbacks can suddenly erupt years later, as in the delayed posttraumatic stress reactions of Vietnam veterans or victims of sexual abuse. No explanation for this delay has been proven. Charney (1993) explained the delayed onset by suggesting that the original memory is masked by new associations and distractions, but when the context changes it is possible to remove the mask, restoring the original memory to its original magnitude.

Treatment Considerations

In therapy, repetitive, intense, emotional reliving of the event would only strengthen the vulnerability to future flashbacks, by reinforcing the stress, the production of transcription factors, and strengthening the new nerve connections. It may be critical that the stress response be minimized during discussion of these events with pharmacologic stabilization of the neurons (with antianxiety medications or antikindling medications), and/or discussion of the events in small increments in a therapeutic context that is perceived as safe. The patient must have some mechanism of controlling the flashbacks, or further damage will be done. The use of a variety of techniques, including dissociation, hypnosis, hospitalization, and, of course, a strong therapeutic relationship, might be used if they add a sense of control for the patient. An educational approach that could outline the biology of the event would be useful to the patient, alleviating fears and increasing understanding. It would support the notion of reducing uncontrolled exposure to significant flashback triggers.

The therapist must be aware of the principles of nervous system functioning, and that in the immediate and short-term, existential issues, other past trauma and free-running emotional catharsis do not have a place in the therapy. In the long term, of course, these issues might be explored without inducing the flashback experience. In the example of Mr. Fine, there is also a depression present, which implies other treatment considerations as well.

PTSD and Dissociation, Dissociative Identity Disorder, and Other Dissociative Disorders

Is dissociation a tool that traumatized individuals develop in order to cope? As reviewed in this and the previous chapter, uncontrollable stress results in increased vulnerability of the hippocampal nerve cells to toxins. This memory center helps bind memory fragments registered in different parts of the brain into a whole memory. If these cells are not fully functional, might not the patient present with fragmented memories of the trauma? In more severe cases, might not the ability to integrate even day-to-day experiences be compromised, causing at least an increased vulnerability to dissociative identity disorder (DID), if not a disintegration of the sense of self? In this view, the common psychotherapeutic view of dissociation as a defense might miss the essential damage that occurs to the memory cells of the hippocampus. Since the memory fragments may be partially stored in various parts of the cortex (e.g., visual, kinesthetic, sound), could they be systematically explored under hypnosis (to minimize recurrence of the trauma) in each sensory modality, and then reconstructed consciously?

What about the role of the current environment in inducing delayed memory of sexual abuse? I have treaated several cases in which abusive marriages or abusive employers were causing memory of the earlier events. Based on my understanding, I would strongly consider recommending removal of the patient from such an environment in order to decrease the repetitive stress, which could cause potential damage to the hippocampal cells. (Such a recommendation certainly would be seen as unorthodox by most therapists.) From the vantage point of the biological psychiatrist, however, this recommendation would be no different than telling a construction worker to change jobs because his lungs were being damaged by asbestos. PTSD is a serious, chronic, disabling disorder associated with increased rates of illness and early death. Therapists must be sure that they are not overlooking current triggers of sudden onset of PTSD, DID, or other dissociative disorders. Do not spend too much time in the past if the patient continues to be traumatized by the present abuse and disrespect.

CHAPTER 4

Medical Mimics of Mental Disorders (and How To Spot Them)

INTRODUCTION

As YOU READ THIS BOOK, you are becoming more aware of the biological aspects of brain function and mental disorders. This is to your client's advantage. In this chapter you will learn how to spot medical problems that masquerade as mental or emotional disorders, the so-called "medical mimics." While it is not feasible to cover all, or even most, of the medical mimics of mental disorders in one chapter, it is possible to cover the most common mimics and to learn some simple rules that will enable you to keep the possibilites in mind. If you review these rules in your mind with each new client, each new symptom, and even each case that is at an impasse, you will gradually develop a sixth sense. You will also be rewarded with a sense of deep satisfaction when you spot your first mimic.

You may be wondering, "Why not just have each and every new patient get a physical exam?" Although this may seem like a good idea, meeting with someone on a continuous weekly basis over a period of time gives you, the therapist, a different quality and quantity of information about symptoms—if you listen—than a busy internist can possibly obtain in one interview. You can supplement

181

the function of the family doctor, not replace it. This chapter is designed to help you do that.

In this chapter you will read about, and experience vicariously, the patient's thoughts when she finds out that a medical mimic has been missed. Then I will take you into my office to review a situation in which one of my patients begins complaining of a new symptom; I want you to experience my thought process, which will help you to understand what the biopsychiatrist does. Then, I will present you with a mnemonic to use as a self-training tool with each new patient. Using this mneumonic as a guide I will review the most common medical mimics. Finally, I will present three cases that will illustrate the process of spotting some common medical mimics.

THE BIOPSYCHIATRIST'S APPROACH

Imagine, if you can, that you are a 44-year-old married woman and mother of two grown children. You have had some marital difficulties over the past year or two and in your own mind you have associated this with the fact that your children are grown, out of the house, and your life is lacking a focus. Over the last several months, you have begun feeling that life has become meaningless and you have been feeling sluggish and depressed most of the time. You have become less tolerant and more irritable with your husband and, quite naturally, he has been spending less and less time at home with you. Things just seem to be spiraling down and you are worried about the marriage and the possibility that he may be having an affair. After all, you have not had sexual relations for seven months. You just feel very, very tired and have noted in the last several weeks that despite psychotherapy, which you have been engaged in for approximately 18 months, you are beginning to feel quite hopeless and even suicidal. You just don't have any energy left for living; even the smallest chores, such as brushing your teeth, combing your hair, pulling on your boots in the winter, take enormous amounts of energy and are a sheer act of will. You have mentioned this to your internist, who did some routine blood testing but found no abnormalities. It was at his suggestion that you entered counseling to decide what you wanted to do with the rest of your life. At that time you had thought it was a good idea, but here you are, a year and a half later, getting worse. Your therapist has been quite helpful, but the problems continue to escalate and you find yourself not knowing where to turn. Your life seems empty, only a shadow of what it once was. Ultimately, your therapist decides that perhaps medication would be of some help to you and reluctantly (you really don't want to start going through this all over again) you agree to see a psychiatrist for medication evaluation.

In the psychiatrist's office, you realize that this is a different approach. The psychiatrist asks you what seem to be hundreds of questions. By the end of the evaluation, it becomes clear, at least in his mind, that your main complaint is fatigue, specifically muscle fatigue. This, the psychiatrist tells you, is preventing you from being active and leaving you feeling frustrated and helpless. He describes to you that this is a perfect paradigm for what he calls "learned helplessness." You are not sure exactly what he is talking about, but you follow his directions and get some additional blood work. This just seems like one more stress, yet you feel a certain sense of hope.

Ultimately, a diagnosis of myasthenia gravis is made. (This is a disorder of the immune system in which the cells of the immune system actually attack parts of the muscle, leaving you in a very weakened state. It is not uncommon to have such profound weakness that combing your hair or walking up stairs would be very exhausting, if not nearly impossible.) As it turns out, you undergo treatment and begin to notice an improvement in your energy. A meeting with the psychiatrist and your husband, about one month after the diagnosis has been made, helps both of you to understand what had really happened: A medical disorder had robbed you of your strength. Not knowing what was going on, you began to feel helpless and spiraled into a depression. Your husband, also feeling helpless, began to work longer and longer hours and wondered about the possibility of separation. Now, with the diagnosis and treatment, there is renewed hope for your relationship and you feel quite relieved that your life, your marriage, and your self-esteem have been salvaged.

This case indicates how what appeared to be a psychosocial problem causing consequent depression was actually a medical problem causing a psychosocial problem. Unfortunately, as clinicians, we are trained so strongly in the psychosocial arena that we often assign a causal role to psychosocial factors. It is always possible that psychosocial stresses might have taxed the physical organs, in this case the immune system, to the point of breakdown. However, it is clear that all aspects of the patient's life (biological, psychological, social) must be evaluated.

This afternoon, I met with Angela, a 47-year-old remarried woman who had a history of family and marital problems as well as depression. She has been in therapy with me for approximately eight months. After briefly telling me her agenda for the session, she interrupted herself and told me she had a concern that she wanted to run by me. Here is how the conversation went:

"Dr. Hedaya, last Tuesday morning, the day of our last session, I woke up feeling a strange sensation, a tingling or vibration, in the lower half of my body. This morning, I woke up again with that same tingling feeling and I wonder if it's related to our sessions. I have been feeling kind of down and a little anxious, but I haven't been feeling very depressed at all."

Is she correct? I wondered. Could it be some anxiety about the sessions? Is it anxiety at all? Is she having a return of her depression? If it is anxiety, what could it be related to? And what if it is not anxiety or depression? Could there be some type of pressure on the spinal cord, or nerves? Could it be multiple sclerosis? No, I answer myself. She is too old. Could it be a B vitamin deficiency? That's certainly possible since the B vitamins are necessary for nervous tissue to function normally. The case of a 55-year-old housewife who had no history of psychiatric disorders, discussed earlier in this book, flashed through my mind. She had come to me with panic disorder, which she had for several years, and a secondary depression due to her frustration with the panic. Despite numerous attempts at therapy and medication, I could at best get a partial response. Upon investigating further, I found that she had a B-12 deficiency. When this was treated, all of her symptoms cleared. How about her thyroid, I wondered as I looked at her previous laboratory work. Interestingly, these tests, while normal, were tending to the high side. Could she be hyperthyroid? I had never heard of any correlation of thyroid problems and tingling sensations. As these possibilities buzzed through my mind, I began to formulate my questions, cognizant of the need to make some type of determination while allowing time for the therapy. I then asked Angela all the usual questions:

"Angela, when was the first time you ever felt this? How long does it last?"

"Once, about a year ago. It only lasts a few minutes."

"Do you have any other symptoms with it? Are there any thoughts associated with it? Do the thoughts precede it? Does the feeling wake you? Do you recall any dreams? Have you started or stopped any medications?"

"Yes, I started 800 units of vitamin E about one and a half years ago. I just cut it in half about two weeks ago."

Well, I thought, that's one possibility, since vitamin E plays a role in neurologically mediated movement disorders. Perhaps it's some type of withdrawal syndrome. I never heard of that, however.

After more questioning, I developed a list of diagnostic possibilities, including mild anxiety (breaking through), unsuccessful avoidance of some conflict, early recurrence of her depression, B vitamin deficiency, excessive thyroid activity, spinal cord disease (specifically disk disease, which she had in the past), or, more remotely, some adaptation response to the change in vitamin E.

I asked Angela to get some blood work to check the vitamin blood levels and general metabolic function as well as tests of her thyroid function. I also had her make an appointment with her family doctor for a physical examination. We moved back to the therapy, having spent 10–15 minutes on her symptom.

From her test results and physical exam, it became clear that Angela indeed was having a spinal problem with narrowing of the spinal canal in the very early stages (called spinal stenosis). She eventually underwent surgery (three years later), which relieved these symptoms.

GENERAL PRINCIPLES FOR SPOTTING MEDICAL MIMICS

Obviously, it is not possible to be cognizant of all medical mimics of mental disorders. What, then, can a therapist do? Most importantly, during your initial meeting, before attempting to begin the actual psychotherapy, allow time for structured questioning. This will allow you to apply the following principles to the evaluation process and have the significant added benefit of reassuring your patient. Here are several rules to keep in mind to help you spot most medical mimics:

1. *Never assume that an emotional symptom has a psychosocial cause until physical causes (or contributors) are fully investigated.* The above two cases demonstrate this first rule of thumb. Your first presumption should be that symptoms are medically caused until proven otherwise. This is the opposite of how most professionals think, including those who have been medically trained. Adopting this rule as a working assumption will result in the uncovering of hidden physical factors before psychosocial treatment is initiated — when the disease process is less advanced — rather than after the psychosocial therapy has failed to produce improvement or, worse, the underlying disease process has become so advanced that it demands medical attention. There are well over 100 disorders that can mimic mental illness. As a therapist you may be the first one in the health care system to be alerted to the presence of a disorder. In order to be attuned to the first signs of illness, you must broaden your view of your role: You are no longer only interested in the psychosocial part of the person; you are treating the whole person, and that encompasses the entire biopsychosocial model.

2. *Always have your patients get a very complete physical examination if they haven't had one since their symptoms began.* The same applies in the case of marital therapy. It is reasonably common for one or both members of a couple to have some type of emotional disorder, such as a drug problem, attention deficit disorder, dysthymia, or an anxiety disorder. These disorders are destructive to self-esteem, affective stability, communication, and empathy. Each spouse must be fully evaluated to rule out medical mimics and then treated pharmacologically if appropriate.

3. *Look for a history that doesn't fit.* When a patient comes

to you with a series of complaints, you must be a detective. As an example, I recall Mrs. Able, who was 48 when her husband of 23 years left her. She was quite functional and felt fine for the first 18 months of her separation. Gradually, however, she became fatigued and depressed. She began to complain of low back pain. Her physician told her it was stress related to the separation and referred her to a trusted psychotherapist for counseling. After six months of counseling, she fractured her thigh. X-rays revealed a suspicious area that turned out to be cancer, which was also present in her lower back and thus the cause of her pain. Mrs. Able died one month later. In this case, the therapist might have questioned the internist's diagnosis, since the 18 months of good functioning after separation does not fit with the conclusion that she was psychologically stressed by her separation. That this history does not fit is common sense, requiring good listening skills and an openness to medical mimics. Her physician lacked the former, and her therapist the latter. As a therapist, you must develop trust in your own medical common sense.

4. *Check personal and family history thoroughly.* Take a careful history. Look for depression, gambling, alcohol and drug use, suicide, obesity, panic, agoraphobia, institutionalization, etc., in three generations. If thorough assessment of an extended multigenerational family history fails to reveal biological relatives who have the same or related mental disorders, be suspicious of a mimic. It is rare for someone presenting with depression or anxiety to have a family history that is absent of any comorbid disorders. If the symptom pattern is not consistent with the family history, be suspicious.

    Mrs. Garth, a 52-year-old married female, was described by the referring psychiatrist as having loose associations and hallucinations. She was admitted to the hospital with a diagnosis of schizophrenia. A family history (obtained from her husband) revealed some obesity but no major mental disorder. Close examination of her speech pattern revealed difficulty naming objects and substitution of incorrect words, as opposed to classic loose associations. A neurologic work-up revealed a brain tumor, and she was transferred to neurology.

5. *Be suspicious if the onset of the disorder is late in life, and/ or there are no stresses present.* The age of Mrs. Garth illustrates this point well. Tohen, Shulman, and Satlin (1994) found that patients who had first-episode mania in the older age brackets were twice as likely as younger patients to have a neurological disorder.

In addition to the case of Mrs. Garth, this reminds me of a 72-year-old woman who came to me with a psychotic depression. Her first episode began when she was 45. She had since had five episodes and was treated with psychotherapy and marital counseling, but never received medication. When I referred her for both a neurological and cardiac evaluation, she was found to have a blockage in her carotid artery (one of the main arteries leading from the heart to the brain) on one side. Furthermore, there was evidence of multiple small infarcts (clotting or small strokes) on an MRI scan. It became clear that her psychosis was at least exacerbated, if not caused, by these infarcts. The cause of these infarcts was eventually traced to the buildup of carotid artery disease. She eventually underwent surgery to repair the carotid blockage.

6. *Be suspicious if there is a history of recent onset of headaches, loss of function, unusual perceptions (tingling, dissociation, visual disturbances, paranormal experiences, or hallucinations—especially visual, olfactory, or tactile) or weight loss of a severe nature.* Interestingly, the woman whose panic attacks were eventually found to be due to a B-12 deficiency sent her daughter to me several years later. Her daughter was having paranormal experiences that turned out to be related to a B-12 deficiency as well.

7. *Drugs, drugs, drugs!* Ask every patient about over-the-counter drug use (which patients often consider harmless), when new medications were started (heart medications, birth control pills, homeopathic remedies), and how these medications correlate with the chronological onset of symptoms. Also get a careful history on alcohol and illicit drug use,

which are very often underreported, hidden (e.g., patients with chronic pain often abuse pain medications), or assumed to be irrelevant. Remember that most over-the-counter or prescription medications can cause psychiatric symptoms.

About one year ago, I received a call from my mother, who casually informed me that she was on a new heart medication. Since she had always been in good health, I questioned her and found out that she had a recent onset of palpitations. The medication seemed to be helping. After getting more information, I decided it would be appropriate for her to have a cardiologist evaluate her. She was given a Holter monitor, which monitors the heart rate over 24 hours. It turned out that her palpitations were most common one to two hours after falling asleep. At first, this piece of information did not ring any bells, but soon she called me quite delighted, stating that she thought she had figured it out. Apparently, she had been taking a homeopathic medication (ginkgo biloba) that she thought was harmless. When she stopped this, the palpitations stopped and she was able to discontinue the heart medication.

Farther from home is the case of a 38-year-old woman recently referred for evaluation by her seventh therapist. After very thorough—and for the patient, anxiety provoking—history gathering, and actual charting of her moods and life events, it became clear that, while she had some mild to moderate depression intermittently throughout adulthood, her mood disorder became very significantly worse—and an anxiety disorder first developed—after her hysterectomy and estrogen replacement therapy (ERT) 10 years earlier. Discontinuation of her ERT resulted in a sharp reduction in psychiatric symptomatology.

MAJOR CATEGORIES OF MEDICAL MIMICS

My personal mnemonic is THINC MED. This mnemonic, if reviewed in appropriate situations, can train you to broaden your thinking.

T = Tumors

Tumors in the brain often present first with psychiatric symptoms. Tumors of the frontal lobes often present with abrupt personality change, flat affect, and/or euphoria; occipital lobe tumors present with visual hallucinations; parietal lobe tumors, with sensory disturbances, agnosia (difficulty naming objects), and lack of awareness appearing as denial (e.g., the 52-year-old women who left her husband during a TV commercial and was found eight days later, living in her car parked on the side of the road. In response to questioning by the psychiatrists-in-training, she saw nothing wrong: "I just went out to the store and got lost." Until her tumor was discovered, she was unempathically nicknamed "The Queen of Denial"); and temporal lobe tumors, with mood and memory disturbances, hallucinations (all types), and paranoid delusions. If the brain tumor is growing rapidly, headaches may be the first complaint; if it is growing slowly, memory loss, difficulty with concentration, and mood disturbance may be the first symptoms. Relatively sudden personality change is common.

In addition to brain tumors, tumors of other organs can present as emotional disturbances. Of all malignant tumors, pancreatic cancer presents most commonly as severe depression (most common in men between the ages of 50 and 70) accompanied by abdominal pain radiating to the back and weight loss. One clue that this is not a typical mood disorder is the absence of both a sense of guilt and a previous psychiatric history. Pheochromocytoma (a tumor of the part of the adrenal gland that produces adrenaline) can often present as anxiety or panic attacks. These tumors are associated with episodic releases of large amounts of adrenaline into the blood stream and result in physical manifestations of the fight/flight response that can easily be misinterpreted as anxiety or panic (e.g., sweating, rapid heart rate, tremulousness). With detailed questioning, these episodes can be differentiated from panic or anxiety disorders by the presence of severe throbbing headache, hypertension, and the absence of catastrophic thinking (as in cue-induced panic) or a sense of suffocation (as in spontaneous panic attacks).

H = Hormones

Dysregulated or absent hormonal function is very intimately associated with mental disorders. As seen in chapter 1, the hypothalamus and pituitary gland (the primary regulators of hormonal activity) have strong input from the higher brain centers that are involved in thought, memory, and emotion (cortex and limbic system). The hormone levels in the blood, as seen in chapter 2, are in turn necessary for normal nerve cell function and adjustment of gene expression. Thus, hormonal dysfunction may cause, or be caused by, mental disorders. Among the most common hormonal mimics of mental disorders are dysregulation of thyroid, parathyroid, and gonadal hormones (such as progesterone, estrogen, and testosterone), and insulin.

Low thyroid function (hypothyroidism) is about four times more common in women than men and frequently presents with a history of gradual onset of fatigue, loss of energy, trouble thinking, and depression. Hypothyroidism is associated with physical signs and symptoms of sensitivity to cold, weight gain, muscle weakness, excessive hair loss, dry skin, brittle nails, hoarseness, increased cholesterol and blood pressure, B-12 deficiency, heavy menstrual periods, and infertility. Overactive thyroid function (hyperthyroidism) frequently presents as an anxiety disorder, depressive or manic episode, or psychosis, and is accompanied by physical symptoms of sensitivity to heat, weight loss, increased activity, oily skin (e.g., acne), tremor, and restlessness. In children, thyroid disorders can also present as ADHD, and in the elderly as dementia.

The parathyroid glands are embedded in the surface of (para) the thyroid gland in the neck, and control the calcium and phosphorus balance in the body (and consequently the function of nerve cells, muscles, as well as the remodeling of bone) via the release of parathormone. Patients with the sudden onset of low parathyroid function (e.g., after inadvertent removal of the parathyroid gland during thyroid surgery or neck surgery) may experience anxiety, irritability, or hyperactivity. In the case of the slow onset of parathyroid disease (e.g., in alcoholics due to severe malabsorption of magnesium) depression with gradual apathy and social isolation will be seen and, in more severe cases, a delirium (disorientation and confusion). In the case of hyperparathyroidism, anxiety, depression, fatigue, and irritability are common.

The cortex (outer layers) of the adrenal glands produce cortisol, while the inner part—the adrenal medulla—produces adrenaline. When secretion of cortisol is excessive (Cushing's syndrome) or steroids are being administered exogenously (e.g., in the treatment of a medical disorder or illicit use in athletes), patients may develop fatigue, anxiety, depression, irritability, or mania. Physical signs and symptoms that differentiate these conditions from mental disorders include purple streaks in abdominal skin, stomach ulcers, diabetes, elevated blood pressure, easy bruising, and increased weight in the face ("moon facies"), lower abdomen ("truncal obesity"), and back of the neck ("buffalo hump"). On the other hand, decreased production of cortisol (Addison's disease, which is commonly associated with withdrawal from steroids after chronic use and can be seen in autoimmune deficiency syndrome) is usually gradual in onset and is initially associated with low energy and weakness under stress; thus, without appropriate history and testing, it is easily confused with a dysthymic disorder and attributed to marital or job dissatisfaction. Eventually, as the disorder progresses to a life-threatening condition, restlessness, personality change, memory disturbances, and episodic irritability may develop, culminating in severe depressive symptomatology, including psychotic depression and paranoia. Associated physical signs and symptoms include gastrointestinal complaints (e.g., loss of appetite and weight loss), progressive weakness, and low blood pressure. Salt craving (see Dietary Management, chapter 5) and an unusually persistent or unexplained tanning of the skin clearly differentiate Addison's disease from the mental disorders.

The gonadal hormones (estrogen, progesterone, testosterone)—also called gonadal steroids or sex hormones—have a very direct influence on the emotional and behavioral functioning of the individual. You should consider sex-hormone dysregulation in the presence of sexual or reproductive problems, menstrual abnormalities, changes in hair growth patterns, and psychiatric problems that are associated with changes in the reproductive cycle (e.g., postpartum mood or panic disorder). In adults, progesterone tends to be calming and even sedating. It is implicated in late luteal phase dysphoric disorder (commonly known as PMS), the commonly observed normalization (or, more rarely, worsening) of mood disorders during pregnancy, and possibly the increased risk of postpartum panic disorder and mood disorders. Estrogen, on the other hand, tends to be activating and causes increased irritability of the central nervous system, perhaps via its effect on dopamine activity. Clearly then, the history of birth control use and estrogen replacement therapy (ERT) must be assessed carefully in women, as these hormones can be associated with virtually any mental disorder. In normal males and females, high levels of androgens (male sex hormones such as testosterone) are associated with increased physical aggression but not with increased sex drive. In contrast, decreased testosterone is associated with impotence and decreased libido, as well as depression. In males with decreased testosterone levels, testosterone supplementation reverses these symptoms. Interestingly, while males suffering from the paraphilias (e.g., pedophilia, fetishism, and voyeurism) have normal levels of testosterone, their sexual urges, fantasies, and behaviors can be successfully reduced with testosterone-lowering hormones (e.g., a type of progesterone).

Dysregulation of insulin secretion from the pancreas (or the ability of the body to use insulin) and consequent abnormal blood sugar levels can present in a number of ways. Low blood sugar (hypoglycemia) may present as anxiety, attention problems, irritability, nightmares, and night sweats. A history of morning headaches or worsening of symptoms when the patient is without food should alert you to this medical mimic. High blood sugar, as in uncontrolled diabetes mellitus, may present with complaints of drowsiness, lethargy, increased appetite, weight gain (mistaken as dysthymia or even a seasonal depressive disorder), or rapid heart rate (misinterpreted as anxiety). A family history of diabetes, complaints of increased urinary frequency, and increased thirst should raise this possibility in your mind.

I = Infectious and Immune Disease

Among the numerous infectious diseases that can affect any part of the central nervous system and therefore may present as a mimic of any psychiatric disorder, AIDS, syphilis (the "great imitator"), herpes, and tuberculosis are most commonly seen. However, because of the rapid rising rates of Lyme disease (a tick-borne infectious disease), its widely varying manifestations, and the need for rapid antibiotic treatment to prevent severe neurologic damage, the index of suspicion for this infectious disease should be high. Lyme disease is produced by an agent which is very similar in behavior to the agent causing syphilis. Ask clients about a history of exposure to wooded areas.

Mononucleosis (Epstein-Barr virus) and hepatitis (from various causes) have been associated with chronic fatigue and depression. Chronic sinus infections and allergy can lead to depression as a result of chronic low energy, headaches, and disturbed sleep. Untreated or unresponsive streptococcal infection ("strep throat") that has spread to the heart valves (rheumatic heart disease) is often followed by the onset of tics (Sydenham's chorea) and sometimes obsessive-compulsive disorder, which clears when the infection is eliminated.

There is much reciprocal intercommunication between the immune, nervous, and hormonal systems. It is not uncommon (particularly in females) for the immune system to "misperceive" various organs or systems in the body as foreign and then attack them, causing what are commonly referred to as the autoimmune (or connective tissue) diseases. Systemic lupus erythematosus (SLE) is a common example of such a disease. SLE may affect the central nervous system, causing cognitive deficits (which may be misidentified in young women as a previously undiagnosed learning disability or job-related difficulty), depression, migraine, psychosis, severe anxiety, and the inaccurate diagnosis of borderline personality disorder, hypochondriasis, or malingering. Physical findings associated with SLE most often include fatigue and weight loss. You can spot this mimic by listening for a history of joint problems, unexplained fevers, and a variety of rashes.

N = Nutrition

Vitamin deficiency or excess, mineral deficiency or overload, and protein depletion can all manifest as mental disorders. These mimics are most common in those who have serious gastrointestinal problems, drug or alcohol abuse, chronic illnesses (e.g., cancer and AIDS), or poor nutrition. However, states of malabsorption can occur without any of these conditions.

Cobalamin (B-12) deficiency, which is surprisingly common, can exist without abnormalities of the standard blood tests (aside from low levels of the vitamin itself), and can cause mood disorders of all types, as well as paranoia, hallucinations, panic disorder, and cognitive deficits. If prolonged and undetected, permanent neurological and psychiatric changes may occur.

Niacin (B-1) deficiency is common in chronic alcohol abusers and the rare disorders carcinoid syndrome and Hartnup's disease. It manifests as a triad of "three Ds": dementia, dermatitis, and diarrhea. This syndrome (pellagra) is often first manifested by fatigue, apathy, and insomnia—symptoms all too easily misdiagnosed as dysthymia, even in alcoholics.

Pyridoxine (B-6) deficiency is often caused by medications such as Nardil (an MAO inhibitor antidepressant) and possibly Effexor (venlafaxine). This can result in "electric shock" symptoms and seizures.

Excessive doses of vitamin C over the long term can interfere with the absorption of vitamin B-12 and cause increases in levels of estrogen in women taking birth control pills or ERT.

Excess blood levels of manganese (e.g., in miners) can present as asthenia, anorexia, apathy, impotence, headache, or psychosis.

Iron overload (hemochromatosis) is associated with disabling fatigue, anxiety, depression, obsessions, compulsions, and panic attacks. This is not surprising since iron plays an essential role in many of the brain's enzymes that facilitate the regulation of monoamine neurotransmitters (e.g., dopamine, serotonin, norepinephrine). Although laboratory diagnosis is sometimes the only way to detect this imposter, it can be suspected when bronzing of the skin or enlargement of the liver and spleen are detected.

C = Central Nervous System

The cause of abnormal function of the nervous tissue is not—from the therapist's point of view—as important as the very fact that functions of the brain are disturbed. Obviously, the more subtle the neurological disturbance the more difficult it is to detect, the more sensitive the therapist must be to the possibility, and the more likely it is that the symptoms will be attributable to psychosocial causes.

After even mild head trauma, which may not be remembered (a scenario that is particularly common in alcoholics and the elderly), a collection of blood may remain on the surface of the brain and present as senility.

Multiple sclerosis (MS) most commonly presents in women in the third and fourth decade of life, and is a disorder in which neurotransmission is hampered by destruction of myelin (see chapter 1). The manifestations of MS depend on the location(s) of the lesions within the nervous system. The most common emotional manifestation of MS is depression, but euphoria (mania), impaired cognitive function, impotence in males, and dementia are not uncommon. The emotional symptomatology may follow years of being labeled a hypochondriac (as with SLE, above), because there is often a previous history of episodic temporary loss of vision in one eye, muscle weakness and spasticity, tingling sensations, and bladder and bowel dysfunction. Alternatively, because these complaints are episodic, patients may not seek medical attention and may forget about them. Thus, even though the person may have had manifestations of the disease for years, the therapist may be the first health professional consulted when depression occurs.

Seizure disorders usually present to the therapist as mood disorders (depressive or bipolar), anxiety disorders (panic or dissociative), or schizophrenia. A history of head trauma, past seizure activity (e.g., febrile seizures as a child), frequent déjà-vu (the unfamiliar appearing familiar) or jamais-vu (the familiar appearing unfamiliar) episodes, micropsia (objects suddenly appearing far away and small), macropsia (objects suddenly appearing large and close up), out-of-body experiences, episodic rage (particularly, but not only, unprovoked), or irritability should prompt a neurological and psychiatric consultation.

Parkinson's disease, a movement disorder of the elderly caused by an impairment of dopamine neurons in the brain, often presents with depression. The slowed movements (bradykinesia) of the disorder are misinterpreted as the psychomotor slowing of depression and the decreased facial movements as flat affect or sadness. Parkinson's disease can be differentiated from depressive disorder by the stiffness of movement and frequently, the lack of negative cognitions.

Huntington's disease, also a movement disorder appearing later in life (fourth or fifth decades) will mislead the therapist with personality change, depression, or paranoia, long before the classic disordered movements occur. A good family history will eliminate the possible misdiagnosis as schizophrenia or a mood disorder.

Sydenham's chorea, discussed above under infectious and immune disease, affects areas of the brain closely associated with those of Parkinson's disease and Huntington's chorea.

Learning disabilities and dyslexia can cause a depressive disorder when they result in lowered self-esteem and academic failure or when the effort to succeed severely limits other pursuits. For instance, a student, Frances, recently presented as obsessive-compulsive personality disorder when with sheer persistence she worked twice as hard and long as other students to achieve academic success. This led to social isolation and a sense of inadequacy, as well as suspicion that her isolation was primarily related to poor social skills. Once her auditory processing problems were identified and the school pressure reduced, her social life normalized in less than one week. The earlier pattern of social success (she was school president in third grade) then reemerged.

M = Miscellaneous

Sleep apnea is a very common disorder caused by frequent decreases in blood oxygen levels during sleep, usually due to obstructed upper airways (nose and throat). Sleep apnea may be associated with obesity and hypothyroidism and frequently causes complaints of decreased energy, overeating, depression, and insomnia. Questioning both your patient and those he or she lives with about morning headaches, snoring, and a history of high blood pressure will usually uncover this mimic and clarify whether or not a sleep study is necessary. Without treatment, the initial complaints (decreased energy, etc.) will not resolve and the patient will have an increased risk of developing heart disease and dementia.

Other sleep disorders to consider in the fatigued or depressed patient are narcolepsy (severe daytime sleepiness with rapid onset of dreaming accompanied by brief loss of muscle control and a sensation of paralysis during sleep) and paroxysmal nocturnal myoclonus (twitching of legs during sleep, which prevents deep sleep, thereby promoting daytime fatigue).

Anemia is a general term for any number of disorders that result in decreased concentration of red blood cells and thus decreased ability of the blood to carry and deliver oxygen to the tissues. Patients with anemia initially complain of fatigue, trouble breathing, and palpitations, and thus can be misdiagnosed as mildly depressed or anxious. As the anemia worsens, pounding pulse, dizziness, headache, irritability, insomnia, impaired attention, menstrual abnormalities, impotence (in males) and loss of libido may develop, thereby supporting and validating the misdiagnosis. Physical findings associated with anemia that are clues to this include paleness of the skin, especially the creases on the palm.

One type of anemia—called acute intermittent porphyria (AIP)—is a great mimic in the spirit of SLE and MS. These patients have histories of episodic vague nervousness, emotional instability, and "psychosomatic" disturbances. Once an acute attack occurs (severe abdominal pain is most common, and can last hours or days), the condition is more likely to be diagnosed. Your tip-off here is the episodic nature of the disorder, with completely normal interepisode functioning, and of course, the severe abdominal pain. Laboratory diagnosis, particularly during an episode, is essential.

Other causes of decreased oxygenation of the brain, aside from anemia, include heart failure and lung diseases. These chronic conditions are often accompanied by anxiety, cognitive disturbances, and impaired day-to-day function. It is not uncommon for an overweight elderly person with unsuspected congestive heart failure or a younger person with undiagnosed asthma to complain of difficulty sleeping, a feeling of not getting enough air, and an inability to carry out normal functions. Yet, the individual may be reluctant to seek out medical assistance, assuming that "it's all in my head."

Rarely, inborn errors of metabolism may present as mental disorders. As an example, Wilson's disease (an inherited disturbance of copper metabolism that begins in adolescence and leads to progressive destruction of the liver and part of the brain) frequently is indistinguishable from schizophrenia, bipolar mood disorder, and anxiety disorders. If diagnosed and treated early, all manifestations of the disease can be prevented. This diagnosis should be considered in any patient under 40 with an unexplained mental disorder that is associated with chronic hepatitis and/or a relative with the disorder. The Kayser-Fleischer ring, an essential physical sign that is present in any patient with Wilson's disease who has psychiatric manifestations, is a golden or brown ring of copper surrounding the cornea of the eye. Examination by an ophthalmologist will detect the Kayser-Fleischer ring, which confirms the diagnosis of Wilson's disease.

E = Electrolyte Abnormalities and Environmental Toxins

Abnormally high or low levels of electrolytes (e.g., potassium, sodium, chloride, magnesium) can cause psychiatric disturbances and are common in patients who are hospitalized for other serious problems, such as burn victims, those who have undergone major surgery, and the elderly who use diuretics. These electrolyte abnormalities can cause confusion, irritability, and dementia. Once laboratory testing identifies such abnormalities, treatment usually leads to rapid improvement of mental function.

We live in an environment that is infused with man-made chemicals, solvents, insecticides, aerosols, and pollution. These substances may be an unrecognized cause of mental disorders. Exposure to environmental toxins will have a variable effect, depending on the dose and potency of the chemical, coexisting illnesses, previous exposure, and individual differences in biologic reactivity to the chemical.

As one example, ethylene glycol is a colorless, odorless, rapidly absorbed solvent used in the manufacture of paints, plastics, cleaners, and antifreeze. A person ingesting antifreeze will appear drunk (slurred speech, trouble walking, nausea, lethargy). If the poisoning is not identified quickly by a history of exposure, a sweet smell of the breath, and appropriate blood work, it can quickly be fatal.

A wide variety of chemicals used in industry can reduce the oxygen-carrying capacity of hemoglobin (the molecule in red blood cells that carries oxygen). These chemicals include aniline (used in shoe polish, paints, varnish, and inks), nitrates (found in contaminated well water), and sodium nitrites (used as a meat preservative). Chronic exposure to these chemicals in the workplace leads to symptoms similar to those found in anemia, including fatigue, headache, dizziness, muscle weakness, and rapid heart rate. Associated physical findings are cough, nausea, vomiting, excessive sweating, blurry vision, and urinary frequency. The physical finding that should arose your suspicion is bluish skin (cyanosis) which, together with a history of exposure (usually occupational), can be quite helpful. Sudden or long-term exposure to insecticides (organophosphates) can result in anxiety and restlessness. In severe cases, tremor, confusion, weakness, and even death may occur. Some organophosphates are long-acting and may cause these symptoms for months.

D = Drugs

Almost all drugs, whether illicit, prescribed, over-the-counter, homeopathic, or dietary (e.g., caffeine) can cause psychiatric symptomatology. Because of this fact, every new patient or couple should be carefully questioned regarding substance use. Identification of a temporal link between the symptoms and ingestion of the substance will aid in the identification of the contributing agent. Some general drug categories that can cause symptomatology of a mental disorder include, but are not limited to, psychotropic agents themselves (e.g., antipsychotics can cause severe restlessness [akathesia] — a side effect that is often misidentified as a worsening of psychosis!), agents that treat heart disease and high blood pressure, pain medications, antibiotics, hormones, cold medications (e.g. Sudafed, antibiotics), aspirin, asthma medications, antitumor medications, food additives (e.g., MSG), and herbal preparations (e.g., ginkgo biloba).

SPOTTING MEDICAL MIMICS

The following cases are presented to help you understand the process patients go through when being evaluated and treated by a biological psychiatrist.

A CLINICAL ILLUSTRATION   Laura was a 47-year-old recently married, unemployed computer systems analyst. During the evaluation she complained of a lifelong history of anxiety and depression as well as numerous current stressors, including unemployment, family concerns, financial problems, her recent marriage to a manic depressive, health worries, and the potential threat of bankruptcy. Her list culminated with the death of her dog six months earlier. "Since then," she stated, "everything that could go wrong has gone wrong." Thorough evaluation revealed numerous symptoms suggestive of depression, hypomania, panic, and possible dissociative disorder, as well as other symptoms suggestive of a possible seizure disorder. Added to all this, she fulfilled criteria for obsessive-compulsive disorder. Reviewing her family history, it was clear that there was a strong history of impulsivity; in fact, a grandfather was described as quite impulsive, "squandering a fortune," and being suicidal at times. In addition, the patient's grandmother was institutionalized for a mental illness. Laura's parents apparently were quite unstable — she described her mother as being marginally functional, miserable, always negative, and hypochondriacal.

The patient entered into psychotherapy and ongoing evaluation of her problems. I asked her to keep a chart of her moods in graphic form so that any events or medication changes could be objectively reassessed later in the course of treatment. As part of her treatment, I started her on Depakote (valproic acid), which I felt would be useful for her mixed mood state, a dissociative disorder, panic disorder, and possible seizure disorder. She responded quite well to this, feeling calm, relaxed, and "unflappable." As the therapy progressed, she recalled having been abused significantly both emotionally and physically as a child. Also, despite her response to the Depakote, she continued to have significant amounts of anxiety and began to complain of twitching of the right side of her face. The twitching apparently was made worse by stress and fatigue and had been present for two to three years. At times it would be visible in sessions and at other times it would be absent. She tied it to the onset of her unemployment and interpreted the twitching as a sign of a fear of rejection and being unwanted. I initially suspected that the facial twitch was related to her obsessive-compulsive disorder and was really a tic (commonly associated with obsessive-compulsive disorder), but rejected that hypothesis because of its relatively recent appearance in her life.

I sent Laura for a neurological evaluation, which revealed an abnormal MRI scan of the brain. After multiple sclerosis was ruled out, the most likely culprit was Lyme disease. Because of the abnormal brain imaging, I sent her for neuropsychiatric testing to determine what areas of cognitive function were impaired. This testing revealed attention problems, which were then treated with stimulant medication (Ritalin). Ultimately she improved on a combination of three medications, Depakote, Effexor (an SSRI), and Ritalin.

This is a case in which a woman with numerous psychosocial stressors and a long history of psychiatric disorders was manifesting worsening mood swings and employment problems secondary to probable Lyme disease, which had influenced her brain structure. As a result of the treatment, Laura became gainfully employed and in fact did quite well in her position. She described being able to handle conflicts and problems in a way that she could not recall ever having done. She was able to get along with her peers and superiors, and traces of dissociative disorder evaporated. She remained somewhat obsessive-compulsive although it did not interfere with her functioning.

A CLINICAL ILLUSTRATION   Jerome, a 39-year-old business owner who was separated from his wife, was anxious, sad, and depressed. He was referred for psychiatric evaluation by a therapist who had been treating him during the previous two years. At the time of the evaluation, Jerome complained of a number of stressors, including the imminent divorce and financial settlement, which he felt would leave him in debt for years. He was in the process of abandoning his business. He had a great deal of guilt and was worried about his 7-year-old son. Three weeks before the evaluation he felt, that when he dropped his son off at his soon-to-be-ex-wife's new house, he had lost his relationship with him.

Evaluation revealed a history of one prior depressive episode a year before. At that point, Jerome had admitted himself to a local hospital for two weeks. He reported no other episodes of depression. Between the present episode and the previous one, he was "very up" for six to eight weeks, sleeping only five hours per day, having racing thoughts, pressured speech, extreme creativity, and a sense of euphoria. Clearly his judgment had been off during that period. As a result of this history, as well as a family history of severe depression in his older sister, cocaine abuse in his younger sister, possible alcoholism in his deceased father, and epilepsy in his deceased mother, alcoholism in his aunt and uncle, and depression requiring shock treatment in another uncle, the suicide of another uncle, and Parkinson's disease in a grandfather, the patient was diagnosed as probable manic depressive and treated with lithium. However, shortly after lithium treatment was initiated he became suicidal and was hospitalized.

During the hospitalization, Jerome began to stabilize and complained of a sore that was not healing on his neck. Visual inspection revealed a somewhat suspicious-looking lesion; however, I did not pursue this for several days. When he persisted, I referred him for a consultation with an infectious disease specialist, who diagnosed type II tuberculosis and cat scratch fever. He was placed on four medications for a period of 15 months. As a result of the treatment, his symptomatology diminished and his mood swings were eliminated. The patient was eventually taken off lithium and his antidepressant without any difficulties. In follow-up five years later, his moods were stable and he had no recurrence of mood swings. He remarried and joined another colleague in starting a new business.

I believed that it was unusual to see a case of tuberculosis in these times, particularly in a metropolitan area in the United States. If it were not for the persistence of the patient, the underlying infections would not have been diagnosed and he would have been treated incorrectly as having only a mood disorder. This case, which occurred early in my career, taught me the value of listening carefully to symptoms.

A CLINICAL ILLUSTRATION   Janet, a 52-year-old divorced computer programmer, was referred for a psychiatric evaluation by her therapist of two years. At the time of the evaluation she had been on lithium carbonate and synthetic thyroid hormone for seven years; she had also been taking estrogen replacement therapy for the previous two years. Her complaints indicated moderate depression, anxiety, and obsessive-compulsive features. When collateral interviews were done with her boyfriend, a number of possible factors emerged.

First, the patient clearly had a mood instability in the bipolar category. Apparently, in 1976 when taking a dopamine-active medication, she became highly energetic, "very effective — I did everything with less and less sleep." She was grandiose and had very bizarre ideation, including a sense of being possessed. At that point, she believed that killing herself would end the possession. She was hospitalized and placed on lithium. Since that episode, she had had no other manic experiences but had been hypomanic. This indicated the need for some type of mood stabilization.

Review of her endocrine system revealed that she was hyperthyroid and earlier had been hypothyroid. This, along with the possibility of her hormone replacement therapy making her feel worse, needed to be addressed. On the hormonal front, we deduced that she was at least reactively hypoglycemic, as she could not tolerate going without food for more than three hours before feeling very light-headed and faint. In addition to the above, it seemed possible that she could be suffering from a sleep disorder, attention deficit disorder, and a seizure disorder. She complained of a lot of daytime sleepiness and of always being distractible, disorganized, and restless. She also had a great deal of difficulty maintaining attention on a task, had difficulty listening, and did not like reading. These characteristics were confirmed by her boyfriend. The patient was scheduled for a sleep study, a study of her brain waves to rule out a seizure problem and a test of variables of attention to assess the ADD.

Janet's sleep-deprived brain wave test (EEG) revealed an abnormality on the right side of her brain. At her fourth visit she complained of having a great deal of difficulty organizing her diet to accommodate for increased frequency of meals and increased protein intake. Her test of variables of attention was abnormal and reflected inattention, mild impulsivity, and inconsistency of response.

At the current time, this patient's evaluation is incomplete. This case is presented to demonstrate the multifactorial nature of these problems and the benefits of a thorough evaluation in determining the most effective treatment.

SUMMARY

As these clinical illustrations show, it is important to listen attentively to your patient's complaints and descriptions of physicial symptoms, to evaluate all aspects of the patient's life, and to always be on the alert for a medical mimic, a medical problem causing a psychosocial problem. Integrating the rules and principles outlined in this chapter into your thought process will result in your broadening your diagnostic focus and developing an instinct for sensing something that doesn't fit and investigating clues to find the mimic. Be suspicious! Remember to THINC MED!

CHAPTER 5

Practical Considerations in the Use of Medications

INTRODUCTION

THIS CHAPTER WILL COVER three areas: the split treatment model with its associated pitfalls and promise, the therapist's role in both the referral process and the treatment phases, and practical questions that arise for patients on medication.

THE SPLIT TREATMENT MODEL AND THE THERAPEUTIC TRIANGLE

The now very common situation in which a patient is treated by both a therapist and a psychopharmacologist leads to what I call the therapeutic triangle. This therapeutic triangle is embedded in the larger systems that each of the three parties is a part of. Its possible impact on the treatment process is discussed under Effective Referral, below. Triangle dynamics have been discussed as a source of tension by family systems theorists (Kerr & Bowen, 1988). In general, triangular relationships may be described as being of low, moderate, or high anxiety.

In a low-anxiety triangle, there is little conflict and little need for moving in or out of the triangle and, in fact, there is a great deal of flexibility in terms of moving in and out of the triangle. In practical terms, this means that in a low anxiety therapeutic triangle, neither the therapist nor the psychopharmacologist would be offended by one or the other making a foray into the other's arena, and the patient would be able to utilize input from both of the treating parties without provoking significant anxiety.

In a moderate-anxiety triangle, the source of anxiety may come from any of the three parties. In this situation one or more parties may experience a fear of being excluded by the other two members of the triangle who are perceived as more closely bonded. Usually there is anxiety about being outside of the triangle. In the patient's case, this may be a result of a fear that both therapist and psychopharmacologist will reject him, as perhaps his siblings or parents had. From the therapist's or psychopharmacologist's point of view, this can be related to a fear of losing the patient, being criticized by the other mental health professional, or feeling inadequate. These fears are then responded to in ways that may be therapeutically damaging. Healthy coping in such a triangle requires that the therapist and psychopharmacologist discuss these tensions as openly as possible, acknowledging that it is not just the patient's anxieties causing what is commonly mistakenly attributed to the patient's "splitting." While the patient may indeed be percieving one therapist as all good, the other as all bad, and fostering that process via a number of conscious or unconscious behaviors, is is not uncommon for the therapist and/or psychopharmacologist to also foster this process. This may be due to a variety of problems in one or both of the treating parties, including narcissism, competitiveness, professional inadequacy, financial considerations, as well as the factors discussed in the next section.

In a high-anxiety triangle the patient is usually the source of the tension and, in practical terms, both treating parties want out of the triangle, while the patient desperately wants to keep one or both parties involved. Often, the patient may be suicidal, with both the therapist and psychopharmacologist feeling overwhelmed and burdened by the anxiety and fears circulating throughout the triangle. These dynamics are common and predictable in virtually any triangular system, and they must be addressed.

Sources of Problems and Pitfalls of the Therapeutic Triangle

Differences in Training and Theoretical Orientations

Psychiatrists are trained in what is called the medical model. This model is traditionally based on power: the healer and the healed. This type of training develops the habit of working long hours (e.g., 36-hour shifts), continuous availability (emergencies do not happen in accordance with one's schedule), immediate response to problems that are conceptualized as disease entities (as opposed to being an integral part of the whole person and their relationship systems). In this model, the physician is the active expert while the patient is the passive bearer of information and recipient of treatment. In its most pure form, a patient's complaint (e.g., cough) is diagnosed by objective standards and laboratory procedures (e.g., sputum culture) and the offending agent (pneumococcus bacterium) is eliminated. Modern psychiatry has, since the introduction of effective pharmacologic treatment of mental disorders in the 1950s, been identifying itself with this model. This is a very different model from the collaborative and empowering model used by many counselors and some physicians. In that model, the patient is an active participant in the decision making process, is kept fully informed, and is understood to be able to contribute to the success of the treatment via both the work with his physician-consultant and on his own. The treating party need not take on the responsibilities of full-time availability and success or failure. As a result of these differences, the psychiatrist's role can be perceived by the patient and/or the psychotherapist as authoritarian, dominating, and controlling or, conversely, comforting and anxiety relieving. On the other hand, the therapist may be perceived as too passive and laissez-faire or, conversely, as competent and offering the empathy and support that the physician and/or patient may need.

Aside from these differences in training, the problems in the therapeutic triangle are often compounded by different theoretical orientations toward the understanding and treatment of mental disorders. Historically, most theories of psychology have been rivals, each competing with one another to explain the human behavior in an all-inclusive fashion. The primary schools of psychotherapy have been psychoanalytic/psychodynamic; more recent schools include behavioral, cognitive, and interpersonal theories. Exploration of each of these theories in the course of training invariably reveals shortcomings. When the anxiety over conflicting theories is added to the anxiety about being a new therapist, a natural attempt is made to reduce the anxiety. The most pragmatic way of doing this is to choose one theoretical approach and then focus his or her energies on becoming an expert in that type of therapeutic approach. While this premature closure in thinking alleviates anxiety, it leads to fragmentation in the mental health field. This can affect the functional ability of the therapeutic triangle via a polarization of viewpoints between the treating parties: Despite objective shortcomings of every theoretical school of thought, practitioners often cling to their viewpoint as firmly as believers cling to religion. In the case of patients who are being treated by both a psychotherapist and a biological psychiatrist, this polarization can undermine the progress of the patient by impairing communication between the treating parties or, worse, by engendering confusion or distrust in the patient. In the worst case scenario, one treating party may consciously or unconsciously extol his theoretical approach and denigrate that of the other treating party. For example, the psychotherapist may say, "Improve your relationship with your wife; don't surrender to this narrow-minded drug-pushing modern society" or the authoritarian biological psychiatrist may unconsciously denegrate the benefits of psychotherapy: "You have a chemical imbalance." Often this will set up a need in the patient to reduce anxiety by choosing one treatment approach over the other, despite indications that combined treatment is often most effective. A patient who is being treated by both of these parties may easily be caught in a bind. If a patient is prone to splitting, the split that is already present in the mental health field can become present in the treatment. It is therefore essential that each of the professionals in such a setting approach the patient from a unified biopsychosocial spiritual view.

In general, a systems theory that encompasses the multiple levels of interaction and observation is the most useful in understanding an organism or a group of organisms. In the same way, mental health problems must be assessed at different interacting levels. Each theoretical approach to a problem is the equivalent of looking at a different facet of the same problem.

Communication Problems

There are a variety of reasons for problems of communication in the split treatment model. First, differences in training lead to differences in therapists' accessibility. While psychiatrists have been trained in the medical model and are accustomed to always being on call or having someone cover for them when they are away, most psychotherapists are not trained this way and may not be as readily available. This difference in availability can at times cause problems. On the other hand, biopsychiatrists may be inaccessible due to a high case load and thus be difficult to reach, which can be quite frustrating for therapists and patients.

A CLINICAL ILLUSTRATION: A CASE OF INACCESSIBILITY   I recall treating a woman for recurrent unipolar depression. When she became suicidal on a Saturday night, she was unable to reach her therapist and so paged me, which required me to intervene both as a psychopharmacologist and as a psychotherapist. After assuring her safety I urged her to contact her therapist. However, when I saw her in my office two days later, she had still not been able to reach him. This state of affairs raised difficult and negative feelings toward the therapist on both the patient's and my part. Fortunately, communication had been good between myself and this therapist and we were able to talk this through and understand the source of the problem. The patient was also able to work it through with the therapist; however, it certainly could have been otherwise.

When therapists lack knowledge of biological psychiatry, they may feel a great deal of anxiety when dealing with a biological psychiatrist (one of the reasons for this book is to decrease this anxiety). They may, of course, have authority conflicts or other anxieties about medication or physicians in general. These can be conveyed — either subtly or overtly — both to the biological psychiatrist and to the patient, causing difficulties in the therapeutic triangle.

When splitting occurs, it is usually on the part of the patient. In such a situation, a patient may cause both the psychotherapist and biological psychiatrist to take on attitudes about the other that reflect the patient's conflicting attitudes and which are rooted in the extant differences in training and orientation. In the case of poor communication or a poor working relationship between the treating parties, the patient may play on the inherent differences in views and approaches. This creates a vicious cycle, leading the therapist and biopsychiatrist to eventually develop negative, unexpressed feelings and, ultimately, decreased communication.

Blurred Clinical/Legal Boundaries

The therapeutic triangle or split treatment model can be difficult to work in due to blurred clinical, legal, responsibility, and risk boundaries. When the relationship between the treating parties is very good, with mutual respect and communication at a high level, there is no blurring of the clinical boundaries. It is permissible for the therapist to raise issues and make suggestions about medication and for the biological psychiatrist to inquire into the patient's life conflicts and responses. As we have seen, the latter may be useful because it provides the biological psychiatrist with information about the patient's response style which in turn can help in medication choice. However, during such discussions, patients can become confused about the roles of the treating parties. It is important to clarify this for the patient, explaining that the increased flexibility eventually enhances the patient's growth.

Legal boundaries, responsibilities, and risks inevitably become blurred. In any lawsuit, both treating parties are likely to be named and therefore both parties are at increased risk due to the actions of the other. This creates increased anxiety and a situation of dependency. The biological psychiatrist must rely on the psychotherapist for information about the patient's psychosocial status, how the patient relates to the medication, and, to a lesser degree, side effects. The therapist, on the other hand, must be able to spot serious adverse effects, and then warn the patient and insure communication with the psychiatrist.

Solutions

In essence, the solutions to the problems listed above are simple:

1. *The treating parties must adopt a biopsychosocial spiritual view of the problem.* They must realize that different approaches are complementary, not exclusionary. A useful analogy is the examination of a specimen under a microscope. Different degrees of magnification allow the viewer to see different details. In the same way, a therapist who takes a systems view takes the broad view while the biopsychiatrist takes the molecular view. In order to maintain the biopsychosocial spiritual view, therapists must educate themselves in different models.

2. *The psychotherapist and biological psychiatrist need to get to know each other.* It is important that the psychotherapist know what types of clients the biological psychiatrist prefers to work with and what type of settings (hospital, office, nursing home, health maintenance organization, preferred provider organization) the psychiatrist works in. The psychotherapist should ask the biopsychiatrist how he or she prefers referrals be made. Some prefer that the patient call and make an appointment, while others prefer that the therapist call to discuss the case first. Finally, both the therapist and the biological psychiatrist must clearly state their expectations for communication.

3. *Both parties must maintain active communication in order to successfully treat the patient.* Preferably, this communication is in person, but can be by phone, voice mail, or in writing. Both treating parties must provide updates of changes that occur in the context of the treatment. Medication changes, changes in mental status, side effects, major life changes, and observations about treatment are all important sources of information for both parties. In practice, conveying this information is time consuming and cannot be done with each and every patient. (For the full-time biopsychiatrist, who might see as many as 20 patients

in one day, this could theoretically involve contacting up to 100 therapists per week in addition to routine calls for prescriptions, appointment changes, insurance forms, and medication problems. For the therapist, who might see five split treatment patients per day, this would involve numerous phone calls as well.)

Thus, both the experience of working with the other treating party and the art of working within a triangle are important. Efficient and well-selected communication is quite helpful, but requires constant awareness of the potential need to communicate ("out of sight" cannot mean "out of mind"). When the communication system fails, an understanding relationship can weather the storm and often, but not always, repair the damage.

THE THERAPIST'S ROLE

Referring the Patient to a Biological Psychiatrist

While I advocate psychiatric evaluation of every new patient, couple, or family, I realize that this may not always be possible. Referral should certainly be made when medication may be needed, to rule out a medical mimic, and specifically in the situations outlined in table 5.1.

The Referral Process

Effective Referral

The therapist can ease the referral process for the patient in several ways.

1. The possibility of such a referral should be mentioned as a common part of the evaluation and intake and explained as a useful means of assuring that all the bases are covered in understanding the patient's distress: "You should know that at times I think it is very helpful to this process to have a thorough evaluation by a medically oriented psychiatrist

TABLE 5.1
When To Refer a Patient To a Biological Psychiatrist

Referral must be made in the presence of:

- Suicidal or homicidal thoughts
- Depression that does not begin to improve within two to four weeks after initiation of cognitive or interpersonal therapy
- Panic attacks (a strong risk factor for suicide)
- Hypomania (excessive activity, overextension, promiscuity, inappropriate financial overspending, rapid speech)
- Psychosis and/or delusions
- Drug or alcohol abuse
- Posttraumatic stress syndrome and dissociative disorders
- Sudden onset of psychological or emotional symptoms without previous psychiatric history
- Sudden personality change
- Family violence and abuse (abuser and abused often have comorbid mental disorders)
- Postpartum blues
- Eating disorders
- Chronic deterioration in functioning at work, home, and school
- Prolonged difficulty with decisions
- Significant problems with sleep
- Rapid unintended or unusually easy weight loss

Referral should seriously be considered in the presence of:

- Chronic obesity
- A job or marriage in jeopardy
- Significant problems with motivation
- Hypochondriasis
- Chronic pain
- Premenstrual worsening of emotional problems
- Loss of ability to play and enjoy
- Anxiety (yours or the patient's!)
- Ongoing therapy with little progress or a therapeutic impasse
- Personality disorders
- Unresolved grief reactions
- Marital and family problems that are not resolving in therapy

for a variety of reasons, which we can discuss, if that should seem appropriate in the future."

This is often very reassuring to patients since it implies thoroughness on the part of the therapist (if the referral is made later in the process of therapy, it can imply something is not going well in the therapy, which can easily lead to a split, with the therapist being the bad guy). Patients should be helped to understand that sometimes subtle medical problems, hormonal imbalances, or other biological problems can actually cause them to feel the way they do, and therefore these should be eliminated (there is an old saying in medical school: When you hear the sound of hooves outside your door, think of horses, but remember it can always be a zebra).

2. The meanings, myths, misconceptions, fears, and concerns of the patient should be addressed in the process of making the decision to refer for psychiatric evaluation. Usually the prospect of evaluation or treatment by a psychiatrist is perceived as a big step: Seeing a nonpsychiatric therapist is one thing to most people, but a referral to a psychiatrist is often seen as a step in the wrong direction. The meaning of referral depends on a number of factors: the timing of the referral (discussed in the preceding paragraph), the patient's context, and the manner in which the referral is made (hopefully the referral is made with confidence and presented as a choice as discussed later in this section).

A common misperception is the patient's belief that "I must be a hopeless case. You [therapist] can't help me anymore." The patient assumes that seeing a psychiatrist implies that his or her problems are quite severe since the stereotype is that a psychiatrist treats crazy people, while counselors treat everyday-type problems. The therapist should address this perception in the course of the referral so that it will not cause the patient undue shame, depression, and anxiety. This perception, of course, can lead to a resistance in the entire process, which can be acted out in a number of ways, including the patient's withholding of information during the evaluation, presenting a healthier picture to the psychiatrist, experiencing a worsening of symptoms prior to the evaluation, terminating with the therapist, etc. A useful reframing of this perception is to explain to the patient that years ago, such a perception may have been the case, but in today's world medical advances have been made that allow psychiatrists to work with different tools to help the patient progress toward his or her goal. The patient's personalization of the referral as evidence of his or her hopelessness and severity can be prevented by mentioning the possibility of such an evaluation at the start of treatment. Then, at the point when the referral seems appropriate, reference can be made to the earlier statement, and the referral can be framed as concern that a biological problem may be causing some of the difficulties and that addressing this problem biologically will help speed the patient's progress:

"When trying to solve any problem we encounter in life, we are constantly reevaluating what we need to do to achieve our goal. We try different strategies until the problem is successfully resolved. This referral does not mean you are hopeless. It means that we need more information, another perspective on something that I feel may be an important factor in how you are feeling, in understanding the nature of your problem."

Additional negative meanings attributed to the referral by the patient are: "You [therapist] want to get rid of me, I made you angry with me, my feelings must be bad or wrong; you must have failed or else this wouldn't be necessary; medication will definitely be prescribed; I will be drugged like a zombie; medication will cure me, change my brain, damage my brain, eliminate who I am; in 20 years they will discover that the medication causes cancer; medication covers up problems."

3. When possible, refer to someone you have strong confidence in and with whom you work well. Passing on this confidence to your patient will alleviate a great deal of anxiety and minimize splitting.

4. Allow reasonable time and discussion whenever possible (assuming you are not dealing with suicidal or homicidal behavior) for the client to process the idea. If safety is a concern, establish the referral as part of the evaluation or

parameters of treatment without which you will not enter into or continue treatment.

5. Call the physician first to pass on information and check the appropriateness of the referral if you have questions. Then have the patient call.

6. Let the patient know you will help oversee the process of evaluation and treatment.

7. Tell the patient what to expect when meeting and working with the biological psychiatrist (e.g., short sessions, numerous questions, the medical model).

8. Define for the patient the role of the psychiatrist. Clarify that the psychiatrist is not a therapist, but may inquire into life issues for the sake of gaining information.

9. Finally, assess the setting within which the psychiatrist works. In the 1990s, health care reform has come of age. Greater numbers of people are getting their health care in health maintenance organizations (HMOs), and preferred provider organizations (PPOs). These forms of managed care are becoming more prevalent. It is possible that fee-for-service medicine will no longer exist, but it is also possible that it will exist as a minor or alternative form of health care.

In a recent study, Rogers et al. (1993) found that depressed patients cared for by psychiatrists in most prepaid health plans (HMOs and PPOs) developed substantial new limitations in their ability to function. Patients treated in the traditional fee-for-service environment experienced an improvement in their ability to function. This has important implications for patients. As a therapist, you must realize that the quality of the psychiatric evaluation and treatment your client receives is significantly dependent on the setting in which that care is delivered. Some questions you and your clients should ask in deciding where to obtain psychiatric care include: Is the psychiatrist working in an environment where he is encouraged to see his patients as few times as possible, to administer the minimum care necessary? Is he working in an environment where he is paid on a capitation basis so that he is paid a fixed amount per year, regardless of whether he sees a patient once or 50 times? In these cases, the patient would probably be well-advised to seek evaluation and treatment outside his or her managed care setting. The costs of fee-for-service psychiatrists are higher than those in managed care; however, according to the above study and a recent report in *Psychiatric News*, ("Do You Put Yourself at Risk," 1995), patients are significantly more likely to regain normal function and maintain these gains in the traditional fee-for-service environment. In the future, as legislation and quality control improves, this imbalance may be addressed.

The Limits of Medication

When patients are concerned that medication will change who they are, I tell them, "It frees you from the weight of symptoms so that you can be who you are." In some situations, however, medication has limits. If the environment is a depressogenic one, as in the case of an abusive spouse or boss, then medication can only be of limited benefit and very often the patient will relapse into depression or anxiety. If biological defects are present but have not been understood and are not being treated effectively, then further evaluation — going back to the drawing board — is necessary.

The Therapist's Role in the Maintenance Phase of Pharmacotherapy

The therapist can play a crucial role in the success or failure of pharmacotherapeutic intervention.

1. The therapist can help the patient to integrate the biopsychosocial and spiritual factors into a holistic model (Ashbrook, 1995).
2. The therapist can monitor compliance and side effects, and inform the psychopharmacologist. The therapist can also alert the psychopharmacologist to any significant developments in the patient's life as well as problems on the horizon.

3. When side effects or questions develop, the therapist can encourage the patient to speak directly with the psychiatrist.

4. All patients with difficult histories (i.e., patients who have recurrent disorders, whether they be a psychosis, depression, or panic disorder) should be encouraged to keep records of medications they are taking, dosages, side effects, beneficial effects, and duration of treatment. Failure to keep records makes it difficult to assess the adequacy of previous medication trials.

5. One of the most important things you, the therapist, can do is to maintain a good working relationship with the psychiatrist.

6. Finally, use the therapeutic triangle as a teaching tool to observe interpersonal dynamics and to deal with conflict. The triangle can also be used as a model for family of origin transference.

PRACTICAL CONCERNS REGARDING MEDICATION

Dependency

Dependency refers to a state in which a person's functioning requires the presence of something external to him- or herself; dependency on a medication may be psychological and/or physical. Patients are concerned about dependency and have difficulty coming to terms with needing a medication. Even patients who abuse drugs or alcohol seem to recoil from the idea of needing a daily medication. Sometimes these feelings are so strong that the patient will resist pharmacotherapy completely, despite attempts to explore the emotions and thinking behind the feelings. Patients should understand that, aside from the benzodiazepines, barbiturates, narcotics, and possibly the stimulant medications, the risk of psychological dependence (i.e., craving) is minimal. This is because most medications used in psychiatry have delayed effects (see chapter 3, Substance Abuse) in addition to side effects. On the other hand, as a part of the physical adaptation to daily ingestion of a substance, a cascade of chemical reactions in the body will be adjusted to maintain homeostasis. Once this new state of equilibrium is reached, removal of the substance can result in physical withdrawal reactions, which should be differentiated from craving the substance.

Psychological dependence—the loss of independence inferred by taking a medication to assist or supplant one's autonomous function—can be such a powerful force that it can prevent the beneficial use of medications for years, increase noncompliance, and, if ignored, lower self-esteem. While patients must retain choice, they should be encouraged to make a cost-benefit analysis: "You know how life is when you feel bad, now try it feeling good—then you can weigh the benefits, risks, and potential costs and reassess your concerns about dependency." One way a biological psychiatrist can operationalize this is by having the patient document their symptoms daily, both before and after medication. Despite appeals to logic, however, these fears are not often alleviated by rational arguments alone; rather, repeated experiences of adversity without the medication (e.g., further bouts of depression or mania) or the experience of improved quality of life with medication is often necessary. In-depth discussions with the therapist along these lines can be very useful.

Medication Side Effects

The potential of any medication to cause short- or long-term side efffects is a major concern for virtually every patient who considers the use of medication. Every medication has the potential for side effects, and the patient should have a thorough understanding of the most common side effects to be expected, as well as any dangerous side effects that may be unique to that particular medication or combination of medications.

Often, the initial side effects (e.g., dry mouth, blurry vision, constipation, dizziness, sedation, agitation) are lessened considerably (when clinical circumstances allow) by slowly increasing the dosage, reducing the dosage, or dividing the dosage through the day, as well as the passage of time. Some patients, (obsessive-compulsive, hypochondriacal, paranoid) are virtually intolerant of side effects and one must procede extremely slowly, beginning with low doses that are specially compounded (e.g., 10% of the normal doasage). This must be done within the context of a trusting, communicative relationship. The therapist can aid this process by expressing her trust in the psychopharmacologist and encouraging the patient to communicate troublesome side effects to the psychopharmacologist.

Most medications used in psychiatry do not commonly cause serious long-term side effects. The common exceptions are: lithium carbonate, which can cause low thyroid function and abnormalities in the kidneys ability to concentrate urine (no one has ever lost a kidney due to lithium); Ritalin (methylphenidate), which can cause delayed growth in children; antipsychotics, which can cause permanent movement disorders (tardive dyskinesia); and Clozaril (clozapine is an antipsychotic with remarkable efficacy) and Tegretol (carbamazepine), which are associated with severe, potentially fatal, anemias. Most medications can cause abnormal allergic reactions and liver damage on occasion.

Less serious but troublesome long-term side effects that can affect compliance include weight gain, sexual dysfunction (decreased libido, impaired orgasm, difficulties with erection), sedation, and certain movement disorders (e.g., akathesia). These must be taken seriously by the treating parties and, when possible, addressed by dosage reduction, change of medication, or additional medication to treat side effects. Too often, however, these stubborn problems do not resolve and one is faced with a difficult choice requiring a careful cost-benefit analysis of the medication. All affected parties (e.g., patient, family members, coworkers) should be considered in the decision process.

Effective August 1995, the Food and Drug Administration announced new guidelines encouraging pharmacies to voluntarily provide handouts about a drug's approved usage, possible side effects, and incompatibilities with other drugs (Schwartz, 1995). This will help patients to be more knowledgeable.

Rapid Cycling of Mood

Rapid cycling of mood (defined as four or more mood episodes per year) is a long-term side effect that seems to be more common in women than men. Since the appearance is that of recurrent relapse of depression, this side effect can be difficult to detect in patients who do not have hypomania as part of the cycle. Careful evaluation of mood patterns before and during the use of antidepressants is imperative. Use of a daily mood and energy chart can be quite effective in detecting cycling (figure 5.1). It is generally thought that patients with low-grade thyroid disease or histories of hypomania (mild or moderate) or cyclothymia are at greatest risk for rapid cycling induced by antidepressants. The appropriate treatment is discontinuation of the antidepressant with or without addition of a mood stabilizer such as Tegretol, or Depakote (Hurowitz & Liebowitz, 1993). If an antidepressant is necessary, Wellbutrin may be less likely to induce rapid cycling, although this is not proven. High doses of supplemental thyroid hormone may help to reduce cycling as well. Lithium seems to be ineffective here, while valproic acid and Tegretol may be more helpful as mood stabilizers in rapid cycling. However, the treatment of choice for antidepressant-induced rapid cycling remains discontinuation of the antidepressant.

Some evidence exists for a role of estrogen and progesterone in rapid cycling bipolar patients (Parry, 1995), particularly during the premenstrual, postpartum, and menopausal periods. Progesterone may supress rapid cycling, while estrogen may increase it. Approximately two-thirds of rapid cycling bipolar patients are women, compared with an equal sex distribution in nonrapid cycling bipolar patients (Parry).

Tumor Promotiom

In 1993, L. G. Miller reviewed several studies that indicated a possible link between several antidepressants (e.g., Norpramin, Elavil, and Prozac) and tumor promotion in laboratory animals. Conflicting results (Bendele et al., 1992) indicated that these drugs do not cause cancer in laboratory animals. Depending on dosage, they may promote (low dose) or inhibit (high dose) tumor cell growth in vitro. No firm conclusions can be made about the absolute safety or risk of antidepressants in tumor promotion in humans at this time. Brandes and Cheang (1995) state:

> Although there is no disagreement that depression is a potentially serious illness for which antidepressant therapy is often both beneficial and required,* nonetheless on the basis of our

---

*The risk of successful suicide in unipolar depression is estimated at 3% (Black, Winokur, & Nasrallah, 1987) to 12% (Angst, 1988) and 3–7% in bipolars (in the same studies) with a weighted risk of successful suicide of 4% in both unipolar and bipolar affective disorder (Goodwin & Jamison, 1990).

1) Keep this form in a convenient place—taped to your bathroom mirror or inside your medicine cabinet.

2) Rate your mood and energy daily as a BAR GRAPH. Thus you can rate the RANGE of your mood that day. (while your mood was low your energy may have been elevated).

3) Note any events that may have affected your mood.

4) Note any sleep disturbances, caffeine, alcohol, or other substances in the lower area of the chart. Please be sure to note any changes in medications or dosage.

Date →		
Mood	Energy	
Mania	+5	
Euphoria	+4	
Very "Up"	+3	
"Up"	+2	
A Bit Better	+1	
A Bit Down	–1	
Down/Irritable	–2	
VERY down	–3	
Hopeless	–4	
Suicidal	–5	
Menses (M/m)*		
Weight		
HARD TO FALL ASLEEP		
HARD TO STAY AWAKE		
EARLY A.M. WAKING		
NEED TO OVERSLEEP		
ALCOHOL		

* M = heavy menstrual flow: m = light flow.

© R. Hedaya

FIGURE 5.1. Chart for patient monitoring of mood and energy.

findings, it is conceivable that, depending on drug dosage, duration of therapy, tumor type, and individual metabolism, some patients at high risk for developing cancer, or with a history of cancer, could be adversely affected by fluoxetine and tricyclic agents. In conclusion, as always, the potential benefits of a given therapy must be weighed against the potential hazards.

G. M. Miller (1995) states in response, "I do not believe that there is, by any means, enough information to alter our prescribing patterns, but we should pursue this information expeditiously."

Pregnancy

Psychiatric disorders may improve or worsen during pregnancy, and a history of this can be quite valuable. According to Dalton (1984), a history of mood improvement during pregnancy may indicate potential benefit for the later use of progesterone in the treatment of late luteal phase dysphoric disorder (commonly called PMS), although this is controversial.

The use of any medication, drug, or alcohol during pregnancy is seriously discouraged due to the high risk of fetal abnormalities. The risk is almost always highest during the first trimester of pregnancy, when organ systems are at their most primitive and underdeveloped stages. Abnormalities caused by ingested substances in the first trimester are more likely to have wide-ranging effects, just as impact at the root of any system will have wide-ranging effects (Wisner & Perel, 1988).

Nevertheless, various psychotropics have been used during pregnancy when absolutely necessary although dosage requirements may vary (Wisner, Perel, & Wheeler, 1993). If such use is contemplated, full research into potential risks for the compound in question should be undertaken. In the case of severe suicidal, manic, or psychotic patients, electroconvulsive therapy has been used successfully, eliminating the need for long-term drug exposure to the fetus.

Nursing

The postpartum period is a high-risk period for onset of psychiatric disorders due to changes in hormonal status, altered sleep patterns, and general adaptational changes in all organ and interpersonal systems. Because of these factors, the use of psychotropic medications are often considered. When women choose to continue breast feeding at this time, consideration must be given to the effects on the baby. Data on this subject are lacking, but the literature seems to indicate that tricyclic antidepressants are either undetectable or present in trace amounts in breast milk (Wisner, Perel, & Foglia, 1995; Wisner & Perel, 1988), with normal therapeutic doses in mothers. The only adverse effects of tricyclic use during breast feeding were reported for Doxepin (Sinequan); Matheson, Pande, & Alertsen (1985) reported respiratory depression in an 8-week-old infant with barely detectable serum levels. This raises the unanswered question of whether or not undetectable or trace blood levels of psychotropic medications might have behavioral effects of a gross or subtle nature in some infants. This should be taken into consideration when prescribing medication during the postpartum period.

Driving

Nearly all psychotropic medications are labeled by pharmacists with a precautionary label: "Warning: Do not use when operating heavy machinery or a motor vehicle." Unfortunately, this blanket statement is often ignored by patients and not addressed by physicians. There are numerous studies of impaired performance under laboratory conditions with various classes of psychotropic medications, but few studies evaluate the risks of driving under real conditions. No studies have sorted out the proportion of increased risk due to medication versus the proportion of increased risk due to the disorder itself. Depressed patients clearly have impaired motor performance in laboratory testing (Linnoila, 1992). In my practice, it is fairly common for me to hear about fender-benders in the parking garage at my building when a patient is depressed. This makes sense, given the fact that the basal ganglia, which control motor movement, are probably functioning abnormally in at least some depressive patients.

As a general rule of thumb, patients should be warned against operating machinery or motor vehicles until their symptoms have cleared and they have reached steady-state levels of medication, when performance can be assessed. BuSpar, selective serotonin-reuptake inhibitors (Prozac, Zoloft, Paxil, and Luvox), and Pamelor are in that order least sedating (with Pamelor being most sedating). Other medications have not been studied. Clearly, controlled studies of medications and psychiatric disorders are indicated so that rational decision making may be applied in these situations. Until that point, caution and discussion are the watchwords.

The Elderly

The elderly often have some impairment of function in one or more organ systems, are on multiple medications, are less able to metabolize drugs, are less tolerant of side effects, and have a narrower margin of safety with drugs. Because of all of these factors, exquisitely careful assessment of medical conditions and medications must be added to the normal procedures when treating and evaluating these patients. Close monitoring, small changes in dosage, reduced initial dosage (usually one-half the normal starting dose), and close follow-up and observation for worsening of concomitant medical conditions or emergence of new medical conditions are essential.

Medical mimics of mental disorders, particularly when there is no prior history of a mental disorder, are more likely to be present in this population. Mental disorders caused by medical disorders (e.g., depression secondary to heart attack, psychosis due to carotid artery stenosis [narrowing], and dementia and depression due to sleep apnea) are very common and must be evaluated thoroughly. Drugs for use in the elderly, as for the younger population, are chosen based on target symptoms and side-effect profile. In the elderly, the side-effect profile must be coordinated with the medical conditions and vulnerabilities of that particular patient.

Recovered Addicts

Numerous psychiatric conditions coexist in patients recovering from substance abuse and dependence. In patients with such a history, the question often arises as to whether or not treatment with potentially abusive substances, such as benzodiazepines, narcotic pain relievers, or stimulants, should be prescribed. Despite protestations of alcoholics anonymous and narcotics anonymous members to the contrary, psychotropic medications can be of enormous benefit in recovered addicts. Most psychotropics are not addictive.

In general, patients with a history of alcohol abuse should not be prescribed benzodiazepines or narcotics, since they act on the same neurotransmitter-receptor systems (GABA and endorphin) as alcohol. In these cases, anxiety can be treated with nonaddicting agents such as BuSpar, beta blockers (Inderal), antidepressants, trazodone (Desyrel) (Ansseau & De Roeck, 1993) and perhaps valproic acid and calcium channel blockers. Recovered alcoholics, however, do not seem at excessive risk for stimulant abuse. As an example, recovered addicts with attention deficit disorder treated with stimulants remain abstinent from alcohol and drugs for two to three years of follow-up (Schubiner et al., 1995). In my own practice, close monitoring of prescribed amounts of medications in these patients is essential. Of the approximately 100 patients with a history of polysubstance abuse I have treated with stimulants, three abused them. Close monitoring rapidly uncovered all three. In each case, the situation was addressed, the abuse was discontinued, and the stimulant was restarted with low doses.

The patient who takes excessive amounts of medication may have an addictive-behavioral pattern, a desire to escape emotional pain, an overdose attempt, an incomplete or inaccurate diagnosis, or problems with the actual medication compound itself that cause the patient to self-medicate in search of relief. These types of behavior are quite problematic if left unaddressed, and will harm the family and work environments of the patient as well as the psychotherapy and efforts at medication. The therapist must look for any signs of medication abuse and alert the biopsychiatrist so that the problem can be addressed.

A CLINICAL ILLUSTRATION   Jill, a 41-year-old housewife and teacher, had been diagnosed as having dysthymia, attention deficit disorder without hyperactivity, and a history of addiction to minor tranquilizers (clonazepam) for which she had been successfully treated. Prozac was prescribed for the dysthymia, and Ritalin, slow-release form, for the attention deficit disorder. It had come to the attention of the therapist and psychiatrist that she was taking excessive amounts of Ritalin, running out of the medication before the next prescription was due. The husband reported erratic, unpredictable behavior and the assumption was made by all parties involved, including the patient, that her addictive temperament was the cause of her abuse of the medication and that she was experiencing a relapse. The case was reffered to me for consultation, and after carefully assessing the motivation behind the patient's behavior, I concluded that the medication was ineffective. She had been on a slow-release form of the Ritalin and was taking nearly double the maximum standard dose. After reconsidering the situation, I placed Jill on a shorter-acting form of Ritalin, at one-half the previous daily dose. Her absorption of this form of Ritalin was much better, she had a good therapeutic effect, and was quite compliant with the new regime.

Patients with Personality Disorders

New medications available over the past several years have created a new area of controversy. Personality disorders, previously considered amenable only to psychotherapy, have now been proven to be responsive to medication (Ratey, 1995; Salzman et al., 1995). In fact, when treated with appropriate medication, many patients who were first diagnosed as having personality disorder no longer fit the criteria. Because of these changes, a diagnosis of personality disorder is not warranted until any biologically responsive disorder is considered and treated (see chapter 2, Temperament).

The impulsive personality disorders (borderline, hysterical, sociopathic) can benefit from mood stabilizers, antipsychotics (e.g., borderline personality disorder is treated with low dose Stelazine), stimulants, beta blockers (e.g., Inderal), or serotonergic and tricyclic antidepressants. Paranoid or schizoid personality disorders can benefit from antipsychotics, while intense unstable personalities can successfully be treated with anticonvulsants and antidepressants.

A CLINICAL ILLUSTRATION   Heather was a 34-year-old woman who had been in therapy for several years. Her therapist reported that the therapy was at an impasse. After an evaluation, I began treatment with Prozac and Heather had an excellent response. She felt the depression was gone, began to experience optimism, and reported that her intense, chronic, anger had dramatically abated. We all were quite pleased. After about six wonderful weeks, Heather relapsed. It was then that I first began to understand why her therapist had diagnosed her as a borderline personality disorder. I began to get frequent emergency calls during the week and Saturday evenings were suddenly punctuated by Heather's intense angry affect: wailing and rage were accompanied by suicidal ideation. The temptation to describe her as "borderline" was enormous; after all, she was exhibiting behavior that fit the criteria. However, based on the excellent response to Prozac, and the above-mentioned studies, I continued (for 1½ years) to assure Heather and her therapist that her initial response was an excellent indicator of what medication could do for her. In all likelihood the diagnosis of a personality disorder was probably not accurate since we had established the fact that she had a biologically treatable depression. As I had hoped and anticipated, we were eventually able to recapture Heather's response by using a combination of two antidepressant medications. As Heather began to have confidence that she would no longer be overreactive, she began to develop a clearer sense of identity. In the therapy, she began to tolerate the discussion of abuse. Two years after the successful medication regimen was begun, Heather was able to leave an unsatisfactory job, make solid plans for a new career, and relocate to an area closer to her imperfect, but important, family.

Over the years, I have seen numerous people like Heather respond to medication and begin developing themselves. I have also seen people use medication for symptom relief and avoidance of difficult issues they are faced with. In the latter case, the medication might be harmful in that it helps to stabilize a pathological state. An example of such a situation was the case of a 45-year-old widowed male who was raising his daughter alone. When he came to see me, he was depressed and an inadequate and neglectful parent. After a full response to an MAO inhibitor (Nardil), which fully alleviated his depression, he became more involved in his work and hobbies but did not change his parenting. The main difference was that he was now pain-free.

Life-style Issues

Patients often ask, "Is there anything else I can do to help myself?" The answer is a resounding yes! Aside from psychotherapeutic interventions, there are a number of life-style changes that should be evaluated by the biopsychiatrist. These include sleep hygiene, dietary issues, environmental issues (such as the amount of sunlight; see chapter 2, Seasonal Rhythms), exercise, and alcohol and cigarette use.

Sleep Hygiene

Sleep hygiene is a term that refers to the general habits that promote good sleep. These should be addressed in any patient for whom medication is being considered. Under this heading are included how long the patient lies in bed when sleepless (this should be no more than 30 minutes to avoid associating bed with sleeplessness), the color (soft pinks are most calming) and decor of the room, the comfort of the bedding, room temperature (cool is best), noise, and consistency of sleep/wake schedule (patients with shift-work experience greater degrees of helplessness). A thorough investigation of the patient's sleep hygiene and relevant education may be quite helpful. An inadequate amount of sleep is often associated with relapse of depression, and is one of the most likely ways of precipitating a manic episode. Having patients experiment with adequate sleep, and monitoring the effect this has on mood (figure 5.1) may convince them that a regular amount of sleep is essential to their well-being. In some cases a rearrangement of the sleeping area, the decor, or temperature can minimize or alleviate the sleep disorder. A minimum of six hours and a maximum of ten hours of sleep per day is considered healthy.

Dietary Management

Protein

Dietary management in the treatment of most psychiatric disorders is essential. It is clear from recent studies (e.g., Miller et al., 1992) that diets that are inadequate in tryptophan (an amino acid) can prevent a serotonergically-acting medication (an SSRI such as Prozac, Zoloft, etc.) from working and can even cause relapse once they have worked. Since neurotransmitters are made from amino acids (which are the breakdown products of ingested dietary protein), it follows that if a diet is deficient in protein, the neurotransmitter production will be abnormally low.

Many patients with depressive and anxiety disorders have exceedingly poor diets that are deficient in protein. Working with a nutritionist or the biopsychiatrist on improving the diet is essential, and should be part of all evaluation and treatment efforts by the biopsychiatrist and therapist.

Caffeine

Caffeine use is an integral part of our culture, but the effects of caffeine use are often not appreciated. Caffeine acts within minutes to increase adrenalin (epinephrine) and to cause the release of sugar into the blood. This results in increased energy, which peaks within an average of one to three hours. Following this peak is a rather sudden drop in blood sugar and adrenalin as the pharmacologic effect of the caffeine wears off. As the blood sugar and adrenalin drop, one experiences any number of symptoms. On the one hand, the person may actually suffer from low blood sugar and feel irritable, nervous, shaky, and have trouble thinking clearly. Others may experience a lack of energy and a craving of some source of quick energy. People with a history of a seizure disorder can have mild symptoms due to the irritating effect of caffeine on their central nervous system (in fact, caffeine is used to decrease the seizure threshold in patients being treated with electroconvulsive therapy).

One way of coping with this need for quick energy is another dose of caffeine. If the person resorts to more and more caffeine, eventually adrenalin and sugar stores are depleted and the caffeine has less and less effect by the end of the day (this is not tolerance to the effect of the caffeine, but rather a depletion state; tolerance to the effect of the caffeine builds up over weeks and months). In this scenario of escalating caffeine use, symptoms of anxiety, panic attacks, irritability, difficulty falling asleep, and gastrointestinal and urinary tract problems are common. Alcohol may then be used as a sleeping aid, causing the person to fall asleep with some ease. However, since alcohol lightens sleep in the second half of the night, the person wakes feeling tired and in need of a caffeine boost.

Another way of responding to the need for increased energy is to increase intake of carbohydrates, cookies, doughnuts, cakes, and chocolate. This of course leads to a rapid, but again brief, rise in blood sugar. However, the intake of these foods can lead to increased absorption of tryptophan (Hedaya, 1984), which is then converted into serotonin in the brain. Serotonin often causes the onset of sleepiness, and hence within an hour after the doughnut is consumed fatigue sets in (some people use this effect to help them fall asleep by eating a carbohydrate before bedtime). This, of course, is then countered with another doughnut, caffeine, or an attempt at a sensible meal. The hourly cycle of increased energy, depletion, and self-medication (via caffeine, starches, or alcohol) is familiar to many, and can often be a contributing factor to anxiety and depressive disorders as well as impaired work performance and alcohol abuse. Clearly, caffeine is not as innocuous as we think.

Salt

In my experience, the use of salt is of interest in four ways. First, in women who suffer from PMS, salt use can lead to a worsening of bloating and irritability. Salt causes increased water retention in the body and some of the symptoms of PMS seem to correlate with bloating. Second, when patients are taking lithium, the amount of lithium in the blood is affected by the amount of salt taken in the diet or lost due to excessive sweating, diarrhea, or vomiting. Patients must be made aware of this to prevent toxic reactions to lithium. Third, salt cravings can be a symptom of Addison's disease (see chapter 4, Major Categories of Medical Mimics). Fourth, although I know of no studies documenting this, I have noticed a correlation between salt cravings and bipolarity. A patient's acknowledgement of a craving for salt encourages me to carefully explore his or her personal and family history for bipolar disorder.

Alcohol

"How about a drink?" The effects of alcohol on the mind, body, and society are well-known and it is essential that we, as mental health specialists, educate patients about the effects of alcohol on specific mental disorders or medication. In particular, they must become aware that alcohol makes medical evaluation and treatment of psychiatric symptoms much more difficult, if not impossible. Alcohol can be a relaxant, a depressant, or an inhibitor of sleep. It can raise the risk of a seizure when taken with certain medications, cause excessive sedation when mixed with other medications, alter the blood level of various medications, prevent therapeutic responses to medication, and cause deficiencies of nutrients essential to the functioning of the nervous system and atrophy of the brain. It can also mimic other psychiatric disorders. In my opinion, all patients who are being evaluated for or treated with medication should be strongly advised against the use of alcohol. If a patient cannot comply with this, the use and safety of medication must be questioned. Often, it is helpful to explain to the patient that any attempt to evaluate or treat symptoms in the presence of drug or alcohol use is bound to fail. Treatment is best left until compliance with this requirement is met. This can bring an issue of alcoholism or drug addiction to the forefront rather quickly, while keeping hope alive for the patient and directing them to appropriate treatment. Generally speaking, once the patient has been stabilized, and assuming there is not an addictive history, alcohol use may be permitted with certain medications, in very limited amounts and frequencies, if it must be used at all.

A CLINICAL ILLUSTRATION   Nadine, a 28-year-old housewife, mother of four children, and former teacher, was referred for evaluation and treatment of a severe depression in the context of sexual abuse, both in her childhood and in her previous job. A series of medication trials were undertaken with little success and, in fact, a gradual but steady worsening of the symptoms occurred. Nadine and her family seemed to be coming apart at the seams. The patient's problems came to a head with a suicide attempt involving medication and a large amount of alcohol. Upon admission to a hospital and recovery of consciousness, she admitted to alcohol abuse over the preceding two-year period and related this to her anger toward several alcoholics in her past. This clarified the situation greatly, and appropriate measures were taken to address this problem. This was a case of a missed diagnosis and medication interactions. The patient withheld information critical to her treatment and was using a substance that would eliminate any possibility of successful alleviation of her symptoms by medication or psychotherapy.

Chocolate

"How about a chocolate?" Chocolate contains substances that are similar to caffeine. In addition, chocolate can be a causative factor in migraine headaches and may be used by a subclass of rejection-sensitive patients as a mood-altering substance. These patients (usually female), who have a cluster of symptoms including severe crashing depression when rejected as well as chocolate cravings, are thought to be more responsive to Nardil, an MAO inhibitor, and thus assessment of chocolate craving can have significance in medication choice.

Nicotine

"How about a smoke?" We are all familiar with the hazards of smoking. What we are less aware of, and only understand to a minor degree, is the role of cigarette smoking, specifically nicotine, on mental health. It is clear with cigarettes, as with other addictions, that the likelihood of successful abstinence from nicotine is improved when depression is absent. The frequency of relapse is higher when people have depression. Treatment of depression results in a more successful ability to stop smoking. In addition, the ability of the liver to process or metabolize a number of psychotropic drugs is affected by cigarettes and, in turn, the dosages of these medications may be higher than normal. Less clear, however, is the effect of nicotine on mood and appetite. The following case is an example.

A CLINICAL ILLUSTRATION   Claire is a 44-year-old overweight, married mother of three children who was diagnosed with bipolar disorder type II (mild form), hypothyroidism, and late luteal phase dysphoric disorder (premenstrual syndrome). She recalled a history of the spontaneous onset of severe debilitating anxiety 10 years earlier, that she associated with her withdrawal from cigarettes. This episode was so severe that it left doubts in her mind about her own emotional stability, which undermined her self-esteem. She sought psychiatric help and eventually recovered but was left with nagging doubts about her mental stability. She resumed smoking, only to quit again one year prior to her first appointment with me. That year she had visited several therapists and two psychiatrists. She was looking for someone who could understand the link between nicotine withdrawal, extreme, deep emotional pain and anxiety, and serious weight gain. I could offer no ready explanation at the time. However, I could offer alleviation of her symptoms as well as encouragement of work on psychosocial issues.

Over a period of time, the patient had trials of various antidepressants, including lithium. Eventually, she seemed to do best on thyroid supplementation and progesterone (a reproductive hormone). Her moods were stabilized, but her weight did not respond to weight-reduction methods. Her underlying fear of an innate emotional instability remained. Finally, in frustration with her significant weight problem, we decided to try appetite suppressants. The medication we tried was a combination of fenfluramine and phentermine. These medications act on the release of serotonin from nerve cells and improve absorption and usage of glucose by cells. The result was quite surprising. The patient reported a return to her normal mood and, most importantly, a sense that the underlying emotional instability was no longer a threat. Her weight decreased modestly.

This response clearly suggests that the contents of cigarette smoke are linked to the serotonin system in some way and indicates that many smokers may be self-medicating a mood disorder. The biopsychiatrist has a unique opportunity to help many smokers quit by prescribing a nicotine-substitute and substances (e.g., clonidine) that may alleviate some of the withdrawal reactions (such as increased appetite, anxiety, and depression) and treating the depression.

We now know that nicotine releases the stress response, causing a pleasant, calming effect. Eventually the release of stress response becomes dependent on nicotine. When Claire stopped her nicotine use, it abruptly caused the absence of a stress response. She had no way of turning her stress-response system on and therefore was left extremely vulnerable. With this new understanding it is not difficult to see why she felt such debilitating, nearly psychotic anxiety when withdrawing from cigarettes.

Compliance

"What can I, the therapist, do to help improve compliance?" Once the patient has decided to take medication, many practical as well as subtle factors come into play. Practical factors include the frequency of dosing, where to keep the medication, how to take the medication,

medication interactions to remember, remembering to take the medication at the same time each day, swallowing pills (an issue for children and some victims of sexual abuse), and how to deal with side effects. Both the therapist and biopsychiatrist should discuss practical ways of addressing each of these problems. The therapist can help by questioning the client in some detail about whether there are any difficulties with the medication and, if so, encouraging problem solving. The questioning must be done in a nonaccusatory manner, explaining that most patients miss doses and have difficulty complying.

The risk of compliance problems increases with the patient's anxiety about the medication, his general ability to be organized, the frequency of doses required, regularity of the patient's daily schedule, lack of disease education in the patient and family, failure of follow-up, and the presence of side effects. This all too often results in premature discontinuation of the medication with re-emergence of symptomatology. A good collaborative relationship between all three parts of the therapeutic triangle can clearly minimize the risk of noncompliance.

In general, chronic illnesses are associated with greater degrees of noncompliance (Fawcett, 1995). The very factors that prevent most psychotropics from being abused (the lack of any noticeable immediate positive effect and therefore the lack of clear emotional association of the benefits with the medication itself, as well as the usually immediate onset of side effects) are additional important factors promoting noncompliance.

Finally, the expertise of the treating parties in helping the patient integrate the various treatments into a comprehensible holistic approach to his or her problems may be an important factor in long-term issues of compliance. According to Fawcett (1995), compliance can be improved by doing the following in the initial visit:

1. Define the illness from the patient's point of view.
2. Define target symptoms and severity.
3. Convey empathy, support, and understanding of the patient's experience.
4. Provide rationale for the use of medication, mentioning beneficial side effects.

    5.   Disclose side effects; include education and reassurance.
    6.   Ellicit patient resistance to medication.
    7.   Explain the importance of taking the prescribed dose.
    8.   Convey hope and optimism.
    9.   Establish therapeutic alliance.
  10.   Discuss alternative treatments.

Drug Interactions

The new guidelines by the FDA (Schwartz, 1995) that will encourage pharmacies to provide handouts with each prescription about a product's usage, side effects, and incompatibility with other drugs will go some distance in solving this ubiquitous problem. New research on enzyme systems in the liver (called the Cytochrome P450 system), which break down drugs, are helping researchers and clinicians to understand the basis for these interactions and to predict with greater accuracy the likelihood of interaction (Hansten & Horn, 1990). Some of the more common drug interactions that biopsychiatrist's encounter are between:

    1.   *Tricyclics and SSRIs* (selective serotonin reuptake inhibitors, such as Prozac, Zoloft, Paxil, and Luvox). When used concommitantly, the dosage of the tricyclic must be lower and blood levels should be monitored to be sure that the tricyclic blood level is safe.
    2.   *SSRIs and Risperdal* (an antipsychotic medication). When used in combination, the SSRI will often ellicit extrapyramidal side effects (EPS, or abnormal, involuntary muscle movements). Lowering the dosage of Risperdal usually alleviates the problem.
    3.   *Serzone* (an antidepressant) *and Seldane* (an antihistamine used in the treatment of allergy). This combination should never be used since it can be fatal.
    4.   *Serzone and Xanax* (an antianxiety, antipanic medication). This combination may cause an increase in the sedative effect of the Xanax, and therefore the dosage of Xanax should be reduced.
    5.   *Lithium and NSAIDs* (nonsteroidal antiinflammatory agents,

such as Advil, Anaprox, Indocin, Motrin are commonly used for pain control and inflamation). The combination of an NSAID and lithium can result in serious and dangerous elevations of lithium blood levels. While the combination is possible, close observation is necessary.

6. *Lithium and diuretics.* This combination can lead to elavated levels of lithium, which is treated in the same manner as the lithium-NSAID combination.

Unfortunately, drug interactions are frequent, particularly in the elderly and other patients who are on multiple medications or have chronic medical conditions. Interactions may be immediate, or delayed (most common) over a period of several weeks after the initiation of a new medication. The therapist and biopsychiatrist must be aware of potential interactions and be alert to their occurrence.

Length of Treatment

In psychotic disorders without a definable cause, such as a metabolic disease, tuberculosis, or syphilis, medication is usually a lifelong prospect. This is particularly true in the schizophrenias, although recently this has been questioned (Baldessarini & Viguera, 1995; Greden & Tandon, 1995; Jeste et al., 1995), and in the psychosis of bipolar disorders (Post, 1993). The prospect of doing anything for life can be quite overwhelming and stir up resistance in anyone. Addressing compliance issues can be a major help in achieving a successful medication intervention. In psychoses caused by a medical disorder, such as kidney failure, open heart surgery, or intensive-care-unit stays, medication is used temporarily—this may also be the case in an acute, sudden onset psychosis that clears rapidly, if there is no prior history of similar episodes.

In depressive disorders, including manic depression, long-term ongoing maintenance medication may be necessary when there have been several episodes or when a depressogenic situation exists (a situation that perpetuates the tendency toward depression, such as a nonsupportive marriage or severe job frustration) (Fava & Kaji, 1994; Greden, 1993; Hirschfeld, 1994; Maj et al., 1992; Stokes, 1993). In 1990, Frank and colleagues published a three-year follow-up study of patients with recurrent depression. There were two main findings, which were later confirmed in a five-year follow-up study (Kupfer et al., 1992): First, the dose that gets you well, keeps you well; and, second, depression is a recurrent illness and episodes must be prevented. While it was previously thought that when one recovered from the depressive episode, a gradual decrease in the dosage of medication could be encouraged with eventual termination of the medication, this study showed that with reduction in dosage the risk of relapse increased from about 10% (with maintenance medication) to 80% (with no medication). The most effective way of preventing relapse of depression over the five-year period was a combination of maintenance medication (at the effective dose) combined with maintenance therapy (in this case, a once-a-month visit after initial short-term psychotherapy).

Often these studies need to be reviewed with patients in order for them to understand the serious recommendation of continued medication treatment for depression. Despite this information, many patients will wish to come off medication. If this course is chosen, I recommend that they discontinue medication very gradually when their life situation is most predictive of a sense of success and control and positive feedback in the areas that are of vital importance to them. I encourage resolution of basic depressogenic factors: development of improved relationships, work situations, and spirituality, whether through volunteer work or in a more formal individualized manner. These measures are likely to make the discontinuation of medication a more realistic possibility. The patient who has been depressed must realize that he or she will always have an increased vulnerability to depression, even after one episode.

In anxiety disorders of a mild nature, benzodiazepine use should be temporary since these medications are used to relieve temporary stress. Here, the object is to reduce the stress so that the generalized stress response, including release of excessive amounts of steroids and disruption of biological rhythms of sleep and appetite, is minimized. Medication need not be used in a prolonged manner or in the absence of development of additional coping mechanisms. If medication is used on a prolonged basis (more than six weeks) psychological and physical dependency may result.

Severe chronic anxiety disorders may require lifelong medication, unless there is some clear change in life circumstances. In these cases, nonaddictive antianxiety medications should be used. In some cases, long-term use with benzodiazepines is the only effective treatment that can be used safely.

Studies have shown that panic disorders (Pollack & Otto, 1994; Rickles, 1993) and obsessive-compulsive disorders (Leonard, Swedo, & Lenane, 1993) are very often recurrent when measured over the life span. Behavioral treatment such as desensitization and exposure therapy are quite effective. The need for continuing medication in these disorders is less clear than with the major disorders discussed above. There is no doubt that medication is helpful in the short term but the need for long-term medication seems to be related to compliance with the therapies that are recommended. Those who are less complaint probably need long-term medication. In one of the largest systematic follow-up studies on childhood obsessive-compulsive disorders, Leonard (1993) states, "A surprising number of patients (70%) continued to received medication at two- to seven-year follow-up. These results suggest that ongoing treatment may be required for this population. Recent treatment advances appear to reduce impairment from the condition." In these disorders many behavioral methods are helpful, but Leonard found that "behavior therapy was used by a minority of those for whom it was suggested."

Polypharmacy and Multiple Medication Trials

Polypharmacy is the use of more than one medication in a patient. Because of side effects, drug interactions, and compliance problems, polypharmacy is discouraged, as it increases the risks of negative outcomes; also, it becomes quite difficult to assess beneficial drug effects and which medication to attribute them to when multiple psychotropic medications are used.

Despite these caveats, patients with recurrent and chronic illness (e.g., hypertension, diabetes, seizures) and psychiatric disorders are quite commonly treated with more than one medication. Reasons for this include the frequent comorbidity of psychiatric disorders (e.g., a bipolar with OCD and panic disorder), excitement about new medications with more specific actions that target one receptor type with fewer side effects, the gradual development of tolerance when some medications are used on a long-term basis (Post, 1993), the desire to treat troublesome side effects when an effective medication is found (e.g., sexual dysfunction with selective serotonin reuptake inhibitors, akathisia with antipsychotics), and the nature of the disorder (Nichol, Stimmel, & Lange, 1995) that predicts polypharmacy (most common in bipolars and schizophrenics). Lithium, antipsychotics, and stimulants are the most likely psychotropics to be used in combination with others. Numerous studies document the ability of lithium to convert nonresponders to responders in significant numbers. There are no studies supporting (a) the use of multiple antipsychotic in the same patient, (b) the use of antipsychotic medication with or for treatment of depression or as an adjunct to an antidepressant for insomnia, or (c) multiple central nervous system depressants, such as benzodiazepines, barbiturates, and sleeping agents (Nichol et al., 1995). The most common medication combination seems to be benzodiazepine and antidepressants, which should only be necessary for brief periods when initiating treatment.

When a patient is taking multiple drugs, the therapist can be of enormous help in developing a strategy to improve compliance and record doses, side effects, etc. The patient and therapist should discuss the use of multiple medications with the prescribing physician. Defensiveness on the part of the physician or inability to explain the rationale clearly is cause to consider a second opinion.

CHAPTER 6

The Psychotropic
Medications

INTRODUCTION

PSYCHOTROPIC DRUGS include all drugs that have effects directed toward (tropic) the mind (psyche). Many drugs used in other fields of medicine have psychotropic effects (e.g., antihistamines make one drowsy) but are not usually used for psychiatric purposes. More than anything else, the discovery of these medications has propelled research in biological psychiatry over the past four decades. Many of the prototype drugs have been, and continue to be, used as research probes. A patient whose mood swings respond to lithium can be studied on and off medication to track down differences in physiology that account for his mood swings. The tools used to study such patients include laboratory studies of body fluids, brain imaging studies, and postmortum studies. Such studies have facilitated the remarkable progress in the neurosciences during these past four decades.

Our understanding of how psychiatric medications work is largely dependent on one principle: the principle of the receptor. *If one understands the receptor, it is relatively easy to understand, in a basic fashion, the hypothesized workings of nearly the entire range of psychiatric medications.* The exceptions to this rule are hormones (thyroid, estrogen, progesterone), which probably have their main action at the level of the cell nucleus, and lithium, whose site of

241

action is less clear, but may be at the level of the cell membrane or one of the internal proteins.

To review quickly (see chapter 1 for full discussion), the four main cell structures of concern are:

- the presynaptic (before the synapse) vesicles
- the synapse (the space between the nerve cell endings)
- the postsynaptic receptors
- the reuptake pump

The presynaptic vesicles are minuscule sacs of chemicals at the ends of the nerve cells. Different nerve cells have different chemicals in their sacs. When a nerve cell is stimulated enough to pass a signal on to another nerve cell, these sacs are emptied into the synapse. Most of the chemical neurotransmitters move across the tiny space and lock onto a receptor, which then changes the receptor's shape, just as the insertion of a fist into a sock changes its shape. The change in shape then causes a sequence of reactions inside the second, or receiving, cell. Any remaining chemical neurotransmitter is taken back up into the *first* nerve cell by a reuptake pump, and this clears the synapse of excess neurotransmitter. When the neurotransmitter is taken back into the first nerve cell, it is dissolved into its component parts by an enzyme called monoamine oxidase: mono (one) amine (containing one amino acid) oxidase (an enzyme type that "burns" or breaks down the substance by using oxygen). This important enzyme breaks down the main neurotransmitter chemicals we are concerned with: serotonin, dopamine, and norepinephrine.

THE MINOR TRANQUILIZERS

The medications in this category are used to alleviate moderate to severe anxiety, usually on a short-term basis, and to help with certain sleep disorders and seizures. Over 2000 medications in this class have been created by the pharmaceutical companies, but only a dozen or so have been marketed. They are called tranquilizers because they have a sedating, calming effect. These drugs are among the most commonly prescribed drugs in the United States. The fact that antipsychotic medications are also called major tranquilizers (discussed below) can be misleading. While both classes of medication are sedative in effect, their mechanisms of action, side effects, and potentially dangerous effects are totally different. *It is important to understand that the minor tranquilizers and the major tranquilizers are very different and are chemically unrelated.*

The individual medications in the minor tranquilizer class differ from one another in the manner and speed with which they are broken down and disposed of, as well as whether or not the breakdown products themselves have active effects on mental function. Table 6.1 lists the majority of medications in the minor tranquilizer class, as well as their dosage, speed of elimination from the body, and any information that is relevant to this particular medication.

Other classes of medication may be used to treat anxiety. These include barbiturates (such as Seconal), antihistamines (e.g., Atarax), antidepressants, and even some medications used to treat high blood pressure (e.g., Inderal and Visken).

The minor tranquilizers (also called the benzodiazepines because they contain a benzene ring structure with two [di] nitrogen [azo] groups) can be addictive both physically and psychologically, and generally must be withdrawn gradually. The length of time necessary for safe and comfortable withdrawal varies, depending on the half-life of the drug, the total dose of the medication, the length of time the patient has been on the drug, the patient's fears about discontinuation, and the patient's situation (has the source of the anxiety, seizure, muscle tension, hyperarousal, etc., been removed?). Withdrawal from these medications after prolonged use can be difficult. Often, the use of another medication may be necessary to facilitate the withdrawal process.

In general, the minor tranquilizers are quite safe when used on a short-term basis, and the risk of lethal overdose is minimal. Long-term use of these agents is fairly common but has not been well-studied. In the latter use, periodic blood work should be done to be sure there are no toxic effects. Since these medications can affect clarity and ease of thinking (in either a positive or negative manner), memory, coordination, and the ability to drive or operate machinery, as well as the response to alcohol, their use should be carefully assessed on a case-by-case basis. Use during pregnancy or breast feeding is strongly discouraged.

TABLE 6.1
Minor Tranquilizers

BRAND NAME (GENERIC NAME)	DAILY DOSAGE	DURATION OF ACTION, ONSET, ELIMINATION	COMMENTS
Ativan (lorazepam)	0.25–2.0 mg 1–3 ×/day	Long acting Slow onset Slow exit	Easiest major tranquilizer to tolerate for patients with liver dysfunction
Centrax (prazepam)	5–60 mg 1–2 ×/day	Moderate duration *Very* slow onset Slow exit	
Dalmane (flurazepam)	15–30 mg at bedtime	Long acting Rapid onset Slow exit	Used *only* for insomnia
Doral (quazepam)	7.5–15 mg at bedtime	Long acting Very quick onset Moderate exit	Used *only* for insomnia
Halcion (triazolam)	0.125–0.5 mg at bedtime	Short acting Quick onset Ultra-fast exit	Used *only* for insomnia Associated with amnesia
Klonopin (clonazepam)	0.25–10 mg 1–3 ×/day	Moderate duration Intermediate onset Slow exit	Psychologically less addictive than other minor tranquilizers
Librium (chlordiazepoxide)	5–25 mg 1–4 ×/day	Intermediate duration Moderate onset Slow exit	
Paxipam (halazepam)	20–40 mg at bedtime	Long acting Moderate onset Slow exit	Expensive
ProSom (estazolam)	0.5–2.0 mg at bedtime	Moderate duration Moderate onset Moderate exit	Used *only* for insomnia
Restoril (temazepam)	15–30 mg at bedtime	Short acting Fast onset Fast exit	Used *only* for insomnia
Serax (oxazepam)	15–30 mg 1–3 ×/day	Short acting Moderate onset Fast exit	Excellent safety profile
Tranxene (clorazepate)	3.75–30 mg 1–4 ×/day	Long acting Rapid onset Slow exit	
Valium (diazepam)	2.5–10 mg 1–4 ×/day	Long acting Very rapid onset *Very* slow exit	Slow exit eases withdrawal
Xanax (alprazolam)	0.25–2.0 mg 2–6 ×/day	Short acting Quick onset Fast exit	Antipanic activity Withdrawal difficult

How and Where Do the Minor Tranquilizers Work?

Minor tranquilizers work by binding to the GABA receptor (a type of brain receptor). When these medications bind to the GABA receptor, the nerve cells are actually inhibited from firing, and they become stabilized, less excitable, and less reactive to stimulation. These GABA receptors are located in five main areas of the brain, and the outcome of stabilization of the nerves depends on the function of the particular group of nerves affected by the medication. Unfortunately, at this time we are not able to target these medications to the specifically desired part of the brain, so all five functions are affected by any of these medications:

1. Calming of anxiety is achieved by activation of GABA receptors in the limbic system.
2. Antiseizure activity is enhanced by activation of GABA receptors in the cortex.
3. Impairment of memory (useful for surgical procedures) is achieved by activation of GABA receptors in the hippocampus.
4. Relaxation of muscles (useful in surgical procedures, and pain syndromes) is achieved by activation of GABA receptors in the striatum.
5. Reduction of arousal (useful for insomnia) is achieved by activation of GABA receptors in the base of the brain.

The antiseizure effect can be quite useful in psychiatry, as patients with dissociative disorders may actually have minor seizure-related symptoms such as perceptual distortions, including déjà vu experiences (e.g., due to physical trauma and resultant scarring of the brain), etc. These seizures occur when certain parts of the brain become more easily excitable. The symptoms one manifests is dependent on which area of the brain is more irritable. In the part of the brain involved with hearing, a source of irritability might cause auditory hallucinations; in another area, depression.

THE MAJOR TRANQUILIZERS (ANTIPSYCHOTICS)

In general, because of potentially damaging side effects, the medications in this category should be reserved mainly for psychotic conditions. When used consistently, in appropriate doses, and with monitoring of side effects and compliance, the major tranquilizers can significantly enhance the quality of life for many patients with psychotic disorders.

When these medications were first discovered in the 1950s, they created a revolution in the mental health field. Patients who were institutionalized for years were able to function more independently. It was natural for psychopharmacologists to test the efficacy and limits of these medications in other conditions. For a time they were thought to be useful in the treatment of depression and anxiety. There was a need for medication in both these states. Barbiturates, such as Seconal and phenobarbital, were often used to treat anxiety, but were very easily abused; therefore some psychopharmacologists took to using the major tranquilizers in the treatment of anxiety. In present day psychiatry there is no rational reason for using these medications in the treatment of anxiety or depression. While they may occasionally have some benefit in these conditions, the risks of long-term harm are substantial, and may even occur with the first dose, no matter how small it may be. There are three main areas of danger: neuroleptic malignant syndrome, tardive dyskinesia, and agranulocytosis.

Neuroleptic Malignant Syndrome

Neuroleptic malignant syndrome (NMS) is a poorly understood, uncommon condition that can be fatal. It appears in patients who have been treated with antipsychotics, and seems to be independent of dosage and length of treatment. These patients present with symptoms of muscle rigidity, elevated temperature, sweating, blood pressure and pulse changes, as well as altered consciousness. It is treatable, but must be recognized quickly for treatment to succeed. The two essential symptoms are the muscle rigidity *and* elevated temperature. Treatment of NMS requires intensive care unit monitoring of vital signs, kidney function, etc.

Tardive Dyskinesia

Tardive dyskinesia is only one of a variety of muscle movement disorders caused by the antipsychotics. Other disorders include: sudden dystonia, (sudden abnormal muscle movements and spasms), akathisia (an extremely intense form of restlessness that causes people to actually want to "jump out of their skin"—in some patients this agitation can be mistaken for a worsening of the psychotic symptoms, leading to more medication, increased agitation, and even suicide. It is easily and quickly treatable within minutes, once recognized); and parkinsonism (minimal facial expressiveness, stiff walking movements, and characteristic movements of the hands). All of these movement disorders are treatable and reversible, *with the exception of tardive dyskinesia.*

Tardive dyskinesia was thought to occur only after prolonged treatment with antipsychotics, hence the descriptor tardive (late or tardy). Kinesia refers to the movement of the muscles, and the prefix dys means abnormal. Unfortunately, recent studies and case reports indicate that the onset of this often permanent condition does not seem to be related to time. In fact, tardive dyskinesia has been known, on rare occasions, to occur after the first dose of an antipsychotic medication.

Patients who are most at risk for tardive dyskinesia seem to include the elderly, women, people with depressive disorders, and those with previous brain damage. Frequently, the condition improves and is not permanent if the medication is discontinued, but this may take as long as one or two years. In a significant number of patients it is permanent. Recently, it has been suggested that high doses of vitamin E may reverse this disorder.

Tardive dyskinesia must be differentiated from the other movement disorders listed above, as the implications for treatment are different. The other disorders are usually easy to treat. It should be emphasized that tardive dyskinesia is not fatal, but is often permanent. Because of the possible permanence of this side effect, the major tranquilizers should only be used in schizophrenia, schizoaffective disorders (a combination of depressive and schizophrenic symptoms), Tourette's syndrome (muscle and vocal tic disorder), obsessive-compulsive disorder with tics which has responded poorly to standard medications, and, occasionally, organic brain syndromes of the elderly. Given the higher risk of tardive dyskinesia in populations with affective disorders, these medications should be avoided in their treatment. A sudden episode of mania can usually be treated and prevented very effectively without these medications.

Agranulocytosis

Agranulocytosis is mainly a concern with Clozaril (occurring in 1.3% of those treated), but may occur with Mellaril, Prolixin, Serentil, Thorazine, and Trilafon as well. It is an uncommon condition that can be caused by many medications used in general medicine. It occurs when the medication causes the body to stop producing a certain type of infection-fighting blood cell. It is potentially life-threatening unless detected early. For this reason, weekly monitoring of blood counts of patients using Clozaril (and less frequently, other medications) is necessary.

One might wonder why anyone would even consider the use of a medication like Clozaril. The answer lies in two facts: Clozaril is the first antipsychotic that does *not* cause tardive dyskinesia, and Clozaril has been statistically shown to be more effective than the standard antipsychotic medications, particularly in treatment-resistant schizophrenia and schizophrenia accompanied by the negative symptom domain (see Classification of Schizophrenia, chapter 3). It is therefore quite a breakthrough for treatment-resistant schizophrenic patients. Clozaril is the first of what will be a new group of antipsychotic medications that are more effective due to their selective action at the level of the limbic system (the mediator of emotional response). These new medications (Risperdal is another) have little effect on the part of the brain that controls muscle movement (the striatum), and therefore seem to lack the troublesome muscular side effects. Table 6.2 lists the antipsychotic medications, daily dosage range, degree of sedation, and other critical points of information.

How and Where Do the Major Tranquilizers Work?

These medications block the action of the chemical neurotransmitter dopamine, which inhibits nerve cell activity; these drugs seem to target certain areas of the brain that are under dopamine control. This initially results in increased rates of firing in certain areas of the brain; however, after long-term use, when the antipsychotic effect is clinically evident, these nerve pathways are almost completely inactive. It is commonly believed, but not yet proven, that this action is the reason for both the beneficial and adverse side effects of these

TABLE 6.2
Major Tranquilizers

BRAND NAME (GENERIC NAME)	DAILY DOSAGE	SEDATIVE EFFECTS	COMMENTS
Clozaril (clozapine)	300–900 mg	High	No tardive dyskinesia Risk of possibly fatal blood disorder requires close monitoring
Compazine (prochlorperazine)	5–10 mg 4 ×/day	High	Mainly used for nausea despite same risks as other drugs in this class
Haldol (haloperidol)	0.5–100 mg	Low	Also used in Tourette's syndrome (uncontrollable tics and vocal utterances)
Loxitane (loxapine)	5–250 mg	Moderate	
Mellaril (thioridazine)	10–800 mg	High	Some data indicate less likelihood to cause tardive dyskinesia
Moban (molindone)	5–200 mg	Low–moderate	The only antipsychotic that does not cause weight gain
Navane (thiothixene)	5–60 mg	Low	
Orap (pimozide)	1–10 mg	Low	Used in Tourette's syndrome
Prolixin (fluphenazine)	1–40 mg	Low	Can be administered on once-monthly basis
Risperdal (risperidone)	1–4 mg 2 ×/day	Moderate	More effective for negative symptoms; less extrapyramidal symptoms
Serentil (mesoridazine)	50–100 mg 3 ×/day	High	
Stelazine (trifluoperazine)	1–20 mg 1–2 ×/day	Low	
Thorazine (chlorpromazine)	25–800 mg/day	High	The first known antipsychotic
Trilafon (perphenazine)	2–32 mg 1–2 ×/day	Low	

medications. The specific areas of the brain whose nerve cells communicate via dopamine include:

- The area that connects the midbrain, limbic system (controlling emotion), and the frontal cortex (controlling executive activity, social awareness, reward and pleasure, and planning), called the mesolimbic, and mesocortical nerve pathways. The action of these medications on this nerve pathway probably accounts for the antipsychotic effects of these medications. These medications also affect the dopamine-containing nigrostriatal pathway, which accounts for the movement disorders associated with these drugs. Medications are currently being developed that may not affect this pathway (Clozaril is such a medication), eliminating many of the side effects caused by the action of these medications on the following areas.
- The striatum, which controls movement and muscle tone. Drug effects in this area are responsible for the side effects of muscle stiffness, movement disorders, as well as NMS (discussed above) caused by these medications.
- The hypothalamus and pituitary gland, which control hormonal regulation of appetite, milk production, sexual function, and temperature regulation. Medication action in this area is responsible for side effects such as breast enlargement, weight gain, and NMS.
- The reticular formation, which controls arousal. Medication action in this area accounts for the reduction in emotional reactivity to external stimuli, perhaps improved sensory filtering, as well as sedation.

THE ANTIDEPRESSANTS

The antidepressant medications are very useful in a broad range of disorders including depression, attention deficit disorder, panic disorder, generalized anxiety disorder, posttraumatic stress disorder, somatization disorder, ulcers, migraine headaches, and chronic pain syndromes. Because of this broad range of actions, the term antidepressants is a misnomer. The fact that these medications are effective in such a seemingly diverse group of disorders is an indicator that there may be common abnormalities underlying these disorders. The antidepressant medications may be grouped according to:

1. chemical nature (i.e., by the number of rings in their molecular structure such as tricyclics, heterocyclics, aminoketones)
2. mode of action (reuptake inhibitors, monoamine oxidase inhibitors, selective serotonin reuptake inhibitors)
3. side effects
4. the chronology of their development (i.e. first, second, third generation).

The grouping by side effects parallels the grouping by chronology of development, and is most practical for the nonpsychiatric mental health provider. Table 6.3 lists (alphabetically for easy reference) the antidepressants, daily dosage, side effects, and special uses/risks. The development of the antidepressant medications has occurred in three waves, or generations. In general, each succeeding generation has had fewer side effects and been more selective in chemical action, but has not improved in efficacy. No one antidepressant seems to be more effective than others for the treatment of depression. In individual patients it is common for one patient to respond to one specific agent and not another. This may be related to the probability that there are subtypes of depression, each affecting different neurotransmitters to different degrees (see below and table 6.4), as well as different stages of the neurotransmission and neuromodulation process.

The First Generation Antidepressants

The first generation antidepressants were discovered in the late 1950s and include:

- the tricyclics (so-called because they have three rings in their structure) and
- the MAO inhibitors.

TABLE 6.3
Antidepressants

BRAND NAME (GENERIC NAME)	DAILY DOSAGE	SIDE EFFECTS*	SPECIAL USES/ RISKS**
Anafranil (clomipramine)	25–75 mg 3 × /day with food	A, B, c	D, O, Bld; possibly P, M, C
Asendin (amoxapine)	25–600 mg/day	A, b, c	D; uniquely effective for psychotic depression
Desyrel (trazodone)	25–600 mg/day	a, b, c	D, Anx, SP, M, C
Effexor (venlafaxine)	25 mg–125 mg 3 × /day with food	N, T, h, i, a, b	D, possibly faster onset, treatment-resistant depression. May be useful in ADHD Active in serotonin and norepinephrine systems
Elavil (amitriptyline)	25–300 mg/day	A, B, C	D, U, M, C, Bld,
Ludiomil (maprotiline)	25–225 mg/day	a, b, c	D, must raise dose slowly
Luvox (fluvoxamine)	25–150 mg 2 × /day	a, b, h, n	O, probably P, C, D
Nardil (phenelzine)	15–105 mg/day	a, b, c	D, ADHD, P, SP, Anx, C (MAO inhibitor)
Norpramin (desipramine)	25–350 mg/day	A, b, c	D, ADHD, Bld
Pamelor (nortriptyline)	25–150 mg/day	A, b, c	D, Bld (therapeutic window level must be in specified range)
Parnate (tranylcypromine)	10–90 mg/day	a, c	D—energizing; dietary restrictions (MAO inhibitor)
Paxil (paroxetine)	5–20 mg/day	a, b, n	D; probably O, SP, SOM, C, M

TABLE 6.3
Continued

BRAND NAME (GENERIC NAME)	DAILY DOSAGE	SIDE EFFECTS*	SPECIAL USES/ RISKS**
Prozac (fluoxetine)	5–80 mg/day	b, n	D, O, P, M, SP
Serzone (nefazodone)	100–300 mg 2 ×/day	N, a, b, c	Soon to be approved; fewer sexual side effects; D, possibly Anx
Sinequan (doxepin)	25–300 mg/day	A, B, C	D, Anx, Bld, U, C, SOM
Surmontil (trimipramine)	75–150 mg/day	A, B, C	D, Anx
Tofranil (imipramine)	25–300 mg/day	A, B, C	D, ADHD, P, Anx, Bld; possibly useful in O, SP, SOM
Vivactil (protriptyline)	5–15 mg 3 ×/day	A, c	D—energizing; tolerated in patients with sleep apnea
Wellbutrin (bupropion)	75–450 mg/day in *divided* doses	a	D, ADHD, no weight gain; increased risk of seizures in certain populations
Zoloft	25–200 mg/day	b	D; possibly useful in O, Anx, C

*A,a = dry mouth, constipation, blurry vision; B,b = sedation; C,c = dizziness on standing; N,n = nausea; H,h = headache; I,i = insomnia; T,t = hypertension (upper case = significant effect; lower case = minor effect).
**ADHD = attention-deficit/hyperactivity disorder; Anx = anxiety; Bld = monitoring of the level of medication in the patient's blood is necessary; C = chronic pain; D = depression; M = migraine; O = obsessive-compulsive disorder; P = panic disorder; SOM = somatization disorder; SP = social phobia; U = ulcers.

The tricyclic medications have many side effects due to their wide-ranging biological actions and are almost impossible for some people to tolerate. This fact helped to spur the development of the second and third generation antidepressants. First generation medications are still very useful, despite the newer, well-tolerated medications (second and third generation) on the market.

TABLE 6.4
Behavioral Effects of the Neurotransmitters

SEROTONIN		NOREPINEPHRINE		DOPAMINE	
PRIMARY AREA OF EFFECT	SYMPTOMS OF DYSREG-ULATION	PRIMARY AREA OF EFFECT	SYMPTOMS OF DYSREG-ULATION	PRIMARY AREA OF EFFECT	SYMPTOMS OF DYSREG-ULATION
Sleep/arousal	Hypersom-nia, insomnia	Arousal	Altered dream stage of sleep	Mood	Dysphoria/mania
Sensation (pain, temper-ature, touch)	Altered (+/−) pain thresh-old, sexual sensation	Reward	Pleasure seek-ing, initiative, procrasti-nation	Affect (auto-matic facial expression)	Tearfulness, "flatness"
Activation/impulsivity	Altered (+/−) activation: + suicidality, compulsivity, aggression; − indecision	Survival (life/death) issues	Panic/fear, hypervigi-lance, excite-ment	Motor activity	Psychomotor slowness or agitation, in-voluntary motor move-ment
Anxiety	Obsessive-ness, anxiety, worry	Energy	Drive/initiative	Reward/pleasure/motivation	Initiative: ability to expect and experience pleasure
Appetite	Carbohydrate craving in-creases brain serotonin	Appetite	Decreased food intake	Appetite	Weight gain

The most commonly used MAO inhibitors include Nardil (phenelzine), and Parnate (tranylcypromine). These medications are quite effective in the treatment of depression, panic disorder, and various types of anxiety, but require strict adherence to a special diet in order to prevent the risk of sudden elevation of blood pressure (a hypertensive episode), which in rare cases may lead to stroke or even death. These two medications can only be used in responsible, compliant individuals who can closely follow such a diet as well as instructions about how to deal with a hypertensive crisis. In nearly every study comparing the efficacy of Nardil against other antidepressants, Nardil is equal to the other agents as an antidepressant and superior as an antianxiety agent. It is also a very effective anti-panic agent, which is useful in panic disorder and social phobia, as well as in hysteroid dysphoria (rejection-sensitive patients with hysterical, narcissistic, and borderline personality traits, chocolate cravings, and stimulant abuse).

Currently, new agents are being researched that can work as MAO inhibitors without the need for dietary restrictions. These agents work on a reversible inhibition of the same enzyme (as opposed to the current irreversible inhibition of the enzyme, which can only be undone slowly as the body manufactures new quantities of the enzyme). These new agents are called RIMAs (reversible inhibitors of monoamine-oxidase A) and include two agents in the experimental phase: brafaromine and moclobemide.

The tricyclic group includes two parent compounds: Elavil (amitriptyline, the first antidepressant) and Tofranil (imipramine). The remaining members of this group are either breakdown products of one of the parent compounds or have subtle changes in their chemical structure that confer different clinical properties. These other tricyclics include Asendin (amoxapine), Pamelor (nortriptyline, which is a breakdown product of Elavil), Norpramin (desipramine, the breakdown product of imipramine), Anafranil (clomipramine), Sinequan (doxepin), Surmontil (trimipramine), and Vivactil (protryptyline). See figure 6.1.

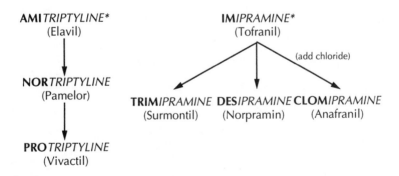

FIGURE 6.1. The relationship between some tricyclic antidepressants. An asterisk indicates the parent compound.

The Second Generation Antidepressants

The second generation of antidepressants include a group of chemically unrelated medications, which in general have fewer side effects than the tricyclics and were marketed in the early 1980s. Included in this group are Asendin (amoxapine), Ludiomil (maprotiline), and Desyrel (trazodone). Asendin seems to be particularly useful in psychotic depression as one of its breakdown products has antipsychotic effects. Ludiomil is very potent as a norepinephrine agent. Desyrel, often used as a sleep aid, can cause sustained and painful erection in males and therefore should be avoided in men. It is, however, useful in patients with epilepsy as it does not lower the seizure threshold.

The Third Generation Antidepressants

One of the distinguishing characteristics of the third generation antidepressants is the fact that they have few side effects. These compunds have brought about a revolution in psychopharmacology. It is now possible to treat the more subtle forms of depression, such as the chronically anxious, low-grade depressions, without significant side effects. The major decisions and life courses of these patients are altered on a subtle scale by their hyperresponsiveness to, and fears of, separation, avoidance of novelty and risk, chronic procrastination, and lack of initiative and assertiveness. These patients often are unable to tolerate the side effects of the first or second generation antidepressants. In these patients, treatment used to involve the use of MAO inhibitors (below), which are more dangerous to use but which are well-tolerated by this group.

The third generation antidepressants are also distinguished by their selectivity of action — they primarily affect only one neurotransmitter system (serotonin, norepinephrine, or dopamine). This specificity is making it possible to target one or two neurotransmitters selectively and it is therefore becoming possible to target specific symptoms in the depressive spectrum. Included in this group are four SSRIs (selective serotonin reuptake inhibitors): Prozac (fluoxetine), Zoloft (sertraline), Paxil (paroxetine), and Luvox (fluvoxamine). Serzone (nefazodone), Wellbutrin (buproprion) and Effexor (venlafaxine) are also third generation medications with reduced side effects. One of the most recently approved (in the United States) agents in the SSRI category is Luvox. Luvox is selectively active on the serotonin system and thus has side effects and efficacy similar to Prozac. It is indicated for obsessive-compulsive disorder and probably will be approved for depression and possibly for panic disorder. Another drug that has most recently been approved is Serzone (nefazodone). Serzone, a relative of Desyrel (above) is reported to have fewer sexual side effects than other third generation medications, and has different mechanisms of action than the SSRIs. It is too early to determine whether there will be significant clinical differences between some of the newer agents, such as Luvox and Serzone, and the earlier SSRIs, such as Prozac, Paxil, and Zoloft. Effexor is different from the SSRIs in that it has mild serotonin actions, norepinephrine actions, can cause elavated blood pressure, and is being tested as a possible treatment for ADHD.

The fact that these third generation medications are easily tolerated has expanded the scope of psychopharmacology, bringing into focus the nature of personality and its chemical, genetic, and environmental origins (chapter 2). This interaction between inborn biological response styles and environmental influences is being investigated by researchers.

Several questions have been raised by the third generation antidepressants, such as Prozac: Is it morally, socially, and ethically correct to alter the biological response style of a person? What are the personal and social consequences of such interventions when applied to a large segment of the population? Have we arrived at the brave new world where false happiness can be attained with a pill? What about creativity and art? Where would society be without such men as the biblical Job, and the modern-day Hertzl, Mozart, and Van Gogh? What if they took Prozac? These are complex questions, which are thoroughly addressed in other sources (e.g., Goodwin & Jamison, 1990). Experience has taught me that as long as we as individuals can make our choices, the risk to society (as opposed to the individual) is minimal. These dilemmas are nonexistent for some patients and central for others.

The recent controversy in the media regarding the safety of these medications (specifically Prozac) and whether they cause suicidal or homicidal behavior is not accurate. The fact is that any antidepressant, any psychiatric medication, as well as many nonpsychiatric medications, may cause psychosis or suicidal and homicidal behavior. Any antidepressant can make a patient worse, any antipsychotic may cause a patient to feel suicidal, and any minor tranquilizer can cause depression or agitation. The source of the problem is the sometimes poorly understood fact that these medications require careful evaluation of the patient before institution of the medication, close follow up, and good patient-physician communication.

In the United States, these medications are available only in the oral form. In Europe, some of these medications are available for intravenous use. Older preparations are still manufactured, which combine a tranquilizer of the minor or major type with an antidepressant. The use of these fixed dose combinations is generally discouraged, since the dosage cannot be individualized for each patient. These medications are not listed in table 6.3, but include Etrafon (Elavil and Trilafon), Limbitrol (Elavil and Librium), and Deprol (Miltown and benactyzine – a mild antidepressant not in general use).

How and Where Do the Antidepressants Work?

All of the antidepressant medications, with the exception of the MAO inhibitors, act by blocking the reuptake pump and are therefore often referred to as reuptake inhibitors. The reuptake pump removes excess neurotransmitter from the synapse by pumping it back into the nerve cell that had just released it. When this pump is blocked there is an immediate increase in the amount of neurotransmitter in the synapse. (This effect occurs within an hour or so after the first dose of an antidepressant.) Since there is more neurotransmitter in the synapse, more receptors are activated on the surface of the second nerve cell, which results in an increased firing rate. The second nerve cell recognizes this as too much stimulation, and after about 18-21 days the second nerve cell actually reduces the number of available receptors on its surface. This reduction in the number of available receptors is called down regulation. In effect, at this point the second nerve cell is less likely to react to stimulation. It is precisely at this point, when the number of available receptors has been reduced, that the antidepressant effects of the medication become clinically apparent. It is important to inform patients of this lag time, as it affects compliance. Since there is no immediate effect, patients can lose hope of responding to the medication or, once recovered, they can stop the medication without any immediate onset of depression, since the receptors would presumably take three weeks to return to the premedication state. Virtually all treatments of depression, medication, or electroconvulsive therapy (ECT) cause this down regulation of a particular type of receptor (the beta receptor). (Blood pressure medications actually can cause depression by increasing the activity of these receptors.)

The MAO inhibitor class of antidepressants also cause an increase in the amount of neurotransmitter in the synapse, but by a different mechanism. These drugs act by inhibiting the enzyme monoamine oxidase (MAO). After the neurotransmitter is released into the synapse, the excess is taken up into the first cell by the reuptake pump. Once inside the cell, MAO breaks down the neurotransmitter and either discards it or reuses its components. When this enzyme can no longer break down the neurotransmitters (due to the MAO inhibitor medication), the net effect is that the amount of neurotransmitter in the first cell is increased and more neurotransmitter is released into the synapse. As with the other antidepressants, this causes a down-regulation in the receptors within 18–21 days, which is usually when the first signs of clinical response appear.

At least three primary neurotransmitters are involved in the biology of depression, and there are numerous other chemical messengers that are involved as well; however, at this time we are only able to intervene pharmacologically with the function of norepinephrine, serotonin, and dopamine. In general, different areas of the brain may use only one of these three neurotransmitters to enable communication between nerve cells. This means that, in a simplified sense, if we know which functions of the brain are abnormal in depression (and by inference which parts of the brain are involved in those functions) and which neurotransmitter is used in that part of the brain, we should be able to look at the symptom picture of a patient, decide which brain areas are malfunctioning, and choose the antidepressant that most directly normalizes that particular neurotransmitter (see table 6.4) Simply put, we should be able to match the symptom profile to the appropriate drug. Because of the specificity of the third generation antidepressants, we are approaching that possibility. In table 6.4 the primary behavioral actions of the different neurotransmitters are outlined; these broad principles are routinely applied by the biological psychiatrist in addressing the different manifestations of neurotransmitter dysfunction—from depression to hypertension (see below). They are also used along with other factors in determining which of the numerous antidepressants to use in a given patient.

In reality, the situation is more complex because affecting one neurotransmitter will lead to secondary changes in other systems. It is not possible to change one neurotransmitter system without affecting others to a greater or lesser degree. As an example, when the serotonin balance is affected by a medication, there are often secondary effects on the norepinephrine system. Serotonin acts as a modulator of norepinephrine, functioning at different places in the brain. In fact, the effect that serotonin has on norepinephrine seems to depend on the initial state of the norepinephrine system. If the norepinephrine system is hyperactive, as in panic disorder, the serotonin influence would be to reduce activity of norepinephrine neurons. If, on the other hand, the norepinephrine system is underactive, as it may be in certain types of depression, it might have the opposite effect of increasing the norepinephrine activity! This interaction between serotonin and norepinephrine is one reason why some patients with high blood pressure (when caused by hyperarousal and anxiety) respond to serotoninergic medications with a normalization of blood pressure.

THE MOOD STABILIZERS

The mood stabilizers include a small group of chemically diverse medications that are useful primarily in the bipolar disorders, although they do have uses in other clinical situations (e.g., borderline personality, dissociative disorders, alcoholism). These medications tend to decrease mood cycling and mania as well as, to a lesser but significant degree, treat depression. The group includes lithium carbonate (Eskalith, Cibalith, Lithobid), carbamazepine (Tegretol), and valproic acid (Depakote). Klonopin, commonly used in the same disorders as the mood stabilizers, but not a mood stabilizer itself, is an antimanic, antipanic agent that is included in the minor tranquilizer class.

Lithium

Lithium is possibly the most thoroughly studied medication in all of medicine. Literally hundreds of new studies and reports of its effects are published each year. A clearinghouse for information on lithium has been established (The Lithium Information Center; Department of Psychiatry; University of Wisconsin; Madison, Wisconsin). Lithium is used in the treatment and prevention of mania, depression, alcoholism, and possibly cocaine abuse. It is often used to augment the effect of antidepressant medication when there has been a minimal or incomplete response. It has also been reported as useful in cluster headaches (a form of migraine), character disorders with unstable affect, aggressive male prisoners, late luteal phase dysphoric disorder (premenstrual syndrome), OCD (obsessive-compulsive disorders), and, of course, in its original use—in overactive thyroid conditions.

Risks and Side Effects of Lithium

Lithium is a natural element that in many ways is very similar to sodium (a component of table salt). In fact, the kidney, which is very sensitive to measuring the amount of sodium in the body, cannot distinguish between lithium and sodium. This is an important fact to remember since any condition that leads to an excessive loss of body salt (e.g., diarrhea, vomiting, excessive sweating) causes the kidney to react in such a way that it stops the loss of salt through the urine. If a patient is taking lithium, the kidney inadvertently stops the loss of lithium as well, and this can quickly lead to *lithium toxicity*—a potentially dangerous situation. Toxic effects of lithium include slurred speech, trouble with coordination and walking, and confusion. These are serious signs requiring immediate attention for a variety of reasons, including the possibility of permanent residual neurological changes, and alterations in heart function.

Lithium use has three primary risks: decreased thyroid function, altered kidney function, and a rare interaction with Haldol (a major tranquilizer). Because of these considerations, the use of lithium must be carefully monitored by periodic monitoring of the amount of lithium in the blood, kidney function, blood counts, thyroid function, and effects on the heart. More common side effects of lithium include upset stomach, diarrhea, tremor, excessive thirst, and increased urination. These side effects can often be avoided by increasing the dose gradually, taking the medication with meals, determining which preparation of lithium works best, and spacing dosage appropriately.

Tremor can be a serious concern for someone who works with their hands, but can often be treated by adjusting dosage or by the use of Inderal. A potentially troublesome effect for women is weight gain, which can be caused through three different mechanisms: a thyroid effect; a hormonal effect via the hypothalamus, appetite center, and serotonin; and a kidney effect. The cause of the weight gain can be determined by history and symptoms and can be treated appropriately. Nevertheless, this is a valid concern for many women.

The dosage of lithium varies from individual to individual, with most individuals requiring 300–2400 mg per day in divided doses. During a manic episode more lithium is required to obtain the same blood level than when that same patient is not manic. Thus the dosage is not as important as the amount of lithium in the blood. The amount of lithium in the blood must be maintained in a narrow range called the *therapeutic range* or *therapeutic window*. If the level of lithium is above the therapeutic window, toxic effects will occur. Side effects are more likely in the higher range of the therapeutic window, and lithium is not effective for manic depression when the level is below the therapeutic window.

How and Where Does Lithium Work?

Unfortunately, despite much investigation, we do not know how lithium works. In the body, lithium substitutes for sodium, calcium, potassium, and magnesium. It also interacts with the three main neurotransmitters studied in affective disorders: norepinephrine, dopamine, and serotonin. Finally, it seems to have an effect on the G proteins associated with the receptors on the surface of the nerve cells. On a nonmolecular level, lithium seems to normalize REM (rapid eye movement/dream) sleep abnormalities, which are present in the mood disorders. The most common measurement of these

REM abnormalities is called REM latency. REM latency is an excellent marker of the likelihood that a depressive disorder will respond preferentially to medication as opposed to psychotherapy. When a person goes into REM sleep too quickly after first falling asleep, they are said to have decreased REM latency. Lithium normalizes REM sleep, as do the antidepressants, moving dream sleep primarily to the second half of the night, where it belongs.

Carbamazepine

Carbamazepine (Tegretol) is a medication that has been used in the past primarily for certain seizure disorders. It has also been used for chronic pain syndromes and restless legs syndrome. Chemically it is similar to the tricyclic antidepressants. In the late 1970s researchers at the National Institute of Mental Health (Post, 1990) determined that Tegretol is effective in the treatment of manic depressive illness and possibly depression. This discovery was based on a theory that had been developed in the early 1900s by Kraepelin (1921), who suggested that the spectrum of manic depressive disorders (bipolar type I and II, as well as cyclothymia) shared many similar characteristics with the seizure disorders. Both disorders seem to have a periodic cycle. Initially, the disorder is quiet. This is followed by a prodrome (warning signs), followed by a severe stage, and finally a return over time to normal. This cycle is repeated and the more often it occurs, the more likely it is to recur spontaneously and without any stimulus. In fact, modern psychopharmacologists often view manic depressive disorders through this perspective.

In conjunction with this, a theory of kindling (see chapter 2) has been developed and applied to the mood disorders, specifically manic depression. While it is not absolutely certain that the kindling model is an accurate model of mood disorders, this discovery added a valuable new tool in the treatment of manic depression. Nevertheless, lithium remains the first-line treatment. Carbamazepine is reserved for those patients who are partially responsive or nonresponsive to lithium (as many as 40%), or those who cannot tolerate the side effects of lithium. Patients who are most likely to respond to carbamazepine are those who are less likely to respond to lithium: those with late-stage or severe bipolar disorder, a negative family history for bipolar disorder, and a clinical picture that contains mixed features of both mania (e.g., high energy) and depression (depressed, irritable mood).

Risks and Side Effects of Carbamazepine

Carbamazepine causes an increased frequency of abnormalities in the formation of blood cells. These disorders are called aplastic anemia and agranulocytosis, both having to do with a toxic effect of carbamazepine on the formation of different types of blood cells, and both disorders being potentially fatal. These risks require close monitoring of complete blood counts and iron before and during treatment. The occurrence of these disorders is rare, being anywhere from 16–80 cases per million people per year (5–8 times the normal frequency) for individuals who are taking carbamazepine. Patients should be alert for rash, fever, sore throat, or signs of easy bleeding and immediately report these to the physican, as discontinuation of the medication may be necessary.

Toxic effects of excessive doses of carbamazepine include muscular restlessness and twitching, tremor, trouble with balance, coordination, and walking, severe drowsiness, abnormal eye movements, and dizziness. These effects are aggravated by alcohol, and can also be caused when a large number of other drugs (such as erythromycin, an antibiotic; verapamil, a blood pressure medication; cimetidine, for stomach problems; fluoxetine, an antidepressant) are added or increased in dosage. There are many interactions between other medications and carbamazepine. These interactions must always be taken into account to avoid toxicity or a loss of effect of the carbamazepine due to a lowering of the blood level.

Common side effects during the early phases of therapy include dizziness, drowsiness, nausea, vomiting, and changes in thyroid function. Usually these effects are temporary, and certainly they can often be minimized by changing doses and timing of doses.

In order to avoid all of these risks and side effects and to maximize the best response, the physician must monitor the levels of carbamazepine in the blood, as well as the counts of certain blood cells, iron, and thyroid hormones. The average dosage of carbamazepine is 1000–1200 mg per day in divided doses of 250–500 mg each; however, it is the amount of medication in the blood that is the essential factor. Often, the side effects of carbamazepine lessen, and the dosage must be increased after the beginning of treatment, since the liver becomes adept at breaking down the carbamazepine for elimination from the body. When administered and monitored properly, carbamazepine is a very effective agent in the treatment of the above-mentioned disorders.

How And Where Does Carbamazepine Work?

Despite the analogy between seizures and bipolar disorders, it seems that different properties of the drug may account for its effectiveness in each of the disorders. Chemically, the carbamazepine molecule is very similar in structure to imipramine (Tofranil), one of the early antidepressant, antipanic medications, which is still in wide use today. But, carbamazepine has diverse effects on certain noradrenaline receptors, GABA receptors (receptors affected by the minor tranquilizers), and a wide variety of other molecules in the nervous system. Because of these diverse effects, it is not at all clear how it works—only that it does work.

Valproic Acid

Valproic acid (Depakote), like carbamazepine, is an antiseizure medication. It is being used more and more frequently in the United States in the treatment of bipolar disorders, (especially in rapidly cycling bipolars and those with mixed features). In fact, it has just become the first new drug approved for first-line treatment of bipolar disorder in 40 years. It is also used to treat schizoaffective disorder, panic disorder, some dissociative disorders, borderline personality disorder, and to assist in withdrawal from the minor tranquilizers, such as valium and xanax, among others.

Risks and Side Effects of Valproic Acid

Valproic acid has been in use for seizure disorders in Europe since the 1960s. As a result of this long history, certain risks have been found with the use of this medication. Liver failure, which can result in death, has been reported. Since this medication has usually been used with other antiseizure medications, it is difficult to determine the frequency with which this serious condition is caused by valproic acid itself. Nevertheless, this condition is rare. At particularly high risk for liver failure, however, are patients on multiple anticonvulsants (e.g., Tegretol or Klonopin [clonazepam]), those with inborn disorders of metabolism, organic brain disease, mental retardation in the presence of a severe seizure disorder, and children (particularly under age 2). As a person advances in age, he or she is significantly less likely to develop this problem.

Valproic acid can also cause decreased platelet counts, which result in abnormal bleeding and bruising. Because of these rare toxic effects, certain tests of liver function and platelets must be monitored both before and during treatment. Patients must report easy bruising, fatigue, muscle weakness, lethargy, swelling of the face, loss of appetite and vomiting to the physician. All of these problems usually occur in the first six months of treatment, if they occur, and thus monitoring should be more intense during that period.

Common side effects of valproic acid include nausea, vomiting, indigestion, diarrhea, tremor, sedation, temporary hair loss, depression, weakness, and abnormal menses.

The blood levels of valproic acid necessary for seizure control (the original use of this drug) may be different from the levels needed for the treatment of the various psychiatric conditions mentioned above. Sufficient research has not been conducted to address this question. Often, it takes several weeks to obtain the best regimen of valproic acid in an individual patient. Certain preparations are slowly released (e.g., sprinkle capsules for children) and better tolerated, but are only available in low strength, requiring that the patient take numerous pills. This can make compliance a problem; however, when the reason for the large number of pills is explained (to reduce side effects) patients do not seem to mind. The dosage range is wide, varying from 125 mg three times per day to as high as 750 mg three to four times per day. As with lithium and carbamazepine, the dose of medication is less important than the actual level of medication in the blood stream.

How and Where Does Valproic Acid Work?

As with lithium and carbamazepine, we do not know the exact mechanism of action of valproic acid in either seizures or bipolar disorders. There is much evidence that it affects the GABA nerve transmission in the brain, which seems to be calming and inhibitory. Increasing GABA activity seems to have antimanic, antipanic, antianxiety, and perhaps antidepressant effects. The GABA system seems to modify the activity level of the noradrenalin system as well, which has a role in bipolar disorders, depression, anxiety, and panic.

THE STIMULANTS

Stimulant medications (table 6.5) are used in the treatment of attention-deficit/hyperactivity disorder (ADHD), narcolepsy (a genetic

TABLE 6.5
Stimulants

BRAND NAME (GENERIC NAME)	DAILY DOSAGE	COMMENTS*
Cylert (pemoline)	18.75–112.5 mg/day	Less effective, less abuse potential, slow onset of action (3–4 weeks) Used for ADHD
Desoxyn (methamphetamine)	5–15 mg 1–2 × /day	High abuse potential Available as slow release (Gradumet tablets) Used for ADHD
Dexedrine (dextroamphetamine)	2.5–15 mg 2–4 × /day before meals	Peak effect at 2 hours Approved in children aged 3–6 High abuse potential Used in ADHD and narcolepsy
Dexedrine spansules**	5–60 mg/day	Slow release allows once daily dose High abuse potential
Ritalin (methylphenidate)	2.5–20 mg 2–4 × /day before meals	Peak effect at 2 hours Used for ADHD and narcolepsy
Ritalin-SR**	20 mg 1–2 × /day before meals	Slow release (SR) allows less frequent dosing May not work as well as Ritalin Used for ADHD and narcolepsy

*Avoid dosage late in day for all
**Slow release form

disorder characterized by sudden onset of dream sleep, loss of muscle control during daytime activities or with emotion, and associated with a sense of paralysis during dream sleep), at times in certain depressions in the elderly, and to treat the light-headedness side effect of Nardil (phenelzine). Included in this group of medications are Ritalin (methylphenidate), Dexedrine (dextroamphetamine), Desoxyn (methamphetamine), and Cylert (pemoline). Wellbutrin, and possibly Effexor, also seem to have stimulant properties, and are reviewed in the section on antidepressants.

The Use of the Stimulants

Stimulant medications are very useful in the treatment of narcolepsy. They enable the patient to engage in boring or repetitive tasks, such as driving, without falling asleep without warning or control. In the attentional disorders, however, there has been some controversy about the safety of these medications, specifically methylphenidate (Ritalin).

In general, medications must be used as one aspect of treatment in ADHD, along with family intervention, education about the disorder, behavioral interventions, and evaluation for learning and speech disorders and other conditions. The medications alone do not provide adequate or full treatment in this disorder.

Methylphenidate

Concerns and controversy about the use of methylphenidate (Ritalin) in children and adults have centered around the risk of addiction and impairment of growth. Long-term (four years) outcome studies have not born out the concern that children who use methylphenidate are more likely to develop drug or alcohol abuse (see Disorders of Attention, chapter 3). Similarly, long-term outcome studies have not shown any permanent reduction in weight or height. Short-term studies, which followed children for less than four years, have shown a lag in height and weight, which seems to be a temporary, initial effect of methylphenidate. If a child is in the 50th percentile in height and weight before starting methylphenidate, he will be in the same percentile range in four years, despite continuous medication use.

Risks and Side Effects of Methylphenidate

The most serious risk in the use of methylphenidate, (also dextroamphetamine and methamphetamine) is that about 1% of the children who receive methylphenidate develop tics and/or Tourette's syndrome. Tourette's syndrome is a genetic disorder that causes a person to experience involuntary muscle movements and tics, and involuntary verbal outbursts — usually profanities — which suddenly and briefly burst into the middle of normal speech. In the vast majority of children, these tics clear up with discontinuation of the medication. It is most likely that those who develop this side effect have a predisposition to the disorder. This predisposition can often be detected before using the medication by a careful personal and family history. In this case other medications can be used for treatment of ADHD. One might wonder then, why use methylphenidate at all? The answer seems to lie in its effectiveness, rapid onset of action, and the fact that most side effects are mild. Also, most studies being done in the treatment of ADHD use methylphenidate as the bench mark. An additional risk with methylphenidate is a very rare risk of seizures, particularly in those individuals with some history or vulnerability to seizures.

Common side effects of all of the stimulants include nervousness, insomnia, loss of appetite, irritability, headache, and stomach ache. These side effects can usually be managed by changes in dosage and timing of dosage.

Dextroamphetamine and Methamphetamine

Dextroamphetamine (Dexedrine) and methamphetamine (Desoxyn) are stimulant medications with a high abuse potential. They are often sold on the street as speed. Nevertheless, they have been shown to be effective in calming children and adults with ADHD and improving attention, performance, and conduct. Dextroamphetamine is approved for and useful in the treatment of narcolepsy as well. As with methylphenidate and the other stimulants, *dextroamphetamine and methamphetamine are only one part of a complete treatment approach to ADHD, including education, family intervention, and behavioral management, as well as evaluation for learning disabilities and other disorders.* Dextroamphetamine is the only stimulant medication approved for use in children between the ages of three to six years.

Risks and Side Effects of Dextroamphetamine and Methamphetamine

Common side effects of dextroamphetamine and methamphetamine include palpitations, increased blood pressure, rapid heart rate, overstimulation, insomnia, dry mouth, appetite loss, and weight loss. Psychosis may occur with hallucinations and mania. Dextroamphetamine may make tics and Tourette's syndrome worse (see methylphenidate, above).

Pemoline

Pemoline (Cylert) is a stimulant medication that is only useful in the treatment of ADHD, not narcolepsy. This medication is different than the three previously discussed medications in a number of ways. First, where the other stimulants work almost immediately (usually within 2–4 hours) pemoline has a gradual onset of effectiveness over the first 3–4 weeks. In part, due to this delayed effect, pemoline lacks the abuse potential of the other stimulants. In addition, pemoline is administered only once daily, where the other stimulants are usually administered 2–4 times per day. Unfortunately, studies seem to indicate that pemoline is less effective in the treatment of ADHD than the other stimulants, and as a result of this, and perhaps the risks listed below, its clinical use has been minimal.

Risks and Side Effects of Pemoline

Common side effects of pemoline include insomnia, which is usually temporary in nature, and appetite and weight loss in the early phases of treatment (3–6 months). Not uncommonly, mild liver disturbances occur which reverse upon discontinuation of the medication.

Risks associated with the use of pemoline include increased risk of seizures (see Methylphenidate, above), worsening of Tourette's syndrome, and, very rarely, liver damage possibly leading to death.

There have been isolated reports of aplastic anemia, a potentially fatal syndrome in which the body fails to make blood cells of various types. This leads to bleeding, fatigue, infections, and, if untreated, eventually death.

The Use of Stimulants in Addiction-Prone Individuals

Adults with histories of drug abuse can be treated cautiously with these stimulant medications if the evidence for ADHD is clear; however, pemoline, with its lack of abuse potential in adults, is a good first choice in this population. When other stimulants are used, these patients rarely increase the dose on their own, but they may develop marked tolerance, claiming loss of effect. This can be a sign of innappropriate diagnosis and psychological dependence. When this occurs, these patients may raise their dosage to a point where they develop psychosis. In addiction-prone patients, very careful evaluation for ADHD (including collateral history from family members, neuropsychological testing, and old report-cards — to help establish the onset in childhood), close monitoring of amounts prescribed, testing, and verification of the benefit of the medication from collateral sources are necessary. Evaluation of the patient via continuous performance tests (CPT) can be useful.

CPTs are computerized tests that measure impulsivity, inattention, and other variables. They are useful at times as one tool in the diagnosis and treatment of ADHD. If a patient with a history of drug abuse seems to have ADHD, a positive test result will confirm that and allow for an objective measure against which the proper dose can be chosen. Unfortunately, at this time a negative CPT does not mean that the patient doesn't have ADHD. The physician must then rely completely on historical data, collateral history, etc., for the diagnosis and dosage, which leaves more room for manipulation by the addictive personality.

How and Where Do the Stimulants Work?

Most of the available evidence supports the hypothesis that these stimulants act by stimulation of dopamine pathways in certain brain centers. Specifically, there seems to be two types of dopamine systems: Dopamine-1 (DA-1) and Dopamine-2 (DA-2). DA-1 seems to be inhibitory, while DA-2 is excitatory. It is suspected that the DA-2 system is responsible for ADHD. We suspect this because conditions that destroy dopamine nerves in the brains of rats cause a syndrome that is very similar to ADHD in humans. These rats show increased motor activity and a deficit of attention, manifested by overattention to irrelevant external stimuli, as well as nonresponsiveness to certain painful stimuli. This condition is reversed by methylphenidate. Just as with humans, these rats seem to outgrow these symptoms to some degree with age. Further support for the dopamine hypothesis comes from the fact that a certain type of encephalitis (swelling of the brain caused by a virus) causes ADHD in children, and Parkinson's disease in adults. Parkinson's disease is known to be caused by abnormal functioning of the dopamine system in a particular area of the brain.

ALPHA AGONISTS AND BETA BLOCKERS

This group of medications includes clonidine (Catapres) and propranolol (Inderal). Alpha agonists (agonist means to stimulate) and beta blockers are quite interesting in that they are used regularly in the traditional medical fields to lower blood pressure, although each one works by a different mechanism. Based on the understanding we are gaining of the receptors and neurotransmitters involved in anxiety states and mania, it has become clear that intervention with drugs such as these may have a role. The same mechanism that enables these medications to lower blood pressure is at least partially responsible for their therapeutic role in psychiatric disorders.

In general, these medications have not been approved by the FDA for psychiatric use, and in clinical practice these are not first-line medications for any psychiatric disorder, with the possible exception of propranolol for specific phobia.

Propranolol

Propranolol (Inderal) can be a good first choice when medication is needed for phobic situations, such as public speaking phobia, where elimination of a person's physical symptoms of the panic/anxiety might be useful on an occasional basis. In these situations this medication is used only as needed and is preferable to the minor tranquilizers because it does not cause sedation and is not associated with addiction or clouding of thinking. Propranolol blocks the physical symptoms of anxiety such as sweaty palms, tremor, palpitations (feeling one's heart pounding for no reason), and rapid heart rate. It has also been used to reduce the tremor caused by lithium, and in the treatment of migraine. The dosage range is usually low in psychiatric conditions, and may be anywhere from 10–160 mg once to twice per day. As a comparison, for high blood pressure the dose may be as high as 360–640 mg per day.

Risks and Side Effects of Propranolol

Common side effects of propranolol (Inderal) include dizziness, light-headedness, and nausea. Inderal should never be used in patients with a history of asthma, and all patients should be clear of any heart disease. Traditionally, it has been thought that propranolol may cause depression in as many as 50% of the people who take it. More recent reports do not find an association and, in fact, propranolol may be useful in seasonal depression.

How and Where Does Propranolol Work?

Propranolol works by blocking the beta adrenergic receptors in the body. The effect of this blockade is to reduce the adrenalin activity in the body, and since adrenalin activity is reduced, the physical effects of adrenalin (rapid heart rate, increased blood pressure, increased blood flow to the brain, hyperarousal, tremor, etc.) are negated.

Clonidine

Clonidine (Catapres) is not a first-line agent in psychiatric disorders, but is currently used in the treatment-resistant states of anxiety (such as panic and phobia), ADHD, and mania that have not responded to traditional medications. There is some evidence that tolerance to the antianxiety effects of clonidine can occur. It has been useful to help reduce anxiety and panic symptoms of nicotine, narcotic, methadone, and other types of drug withdrawal. It is very commonly used in the treatment of high blood pressure.

Risks and Side Effects of Clonidine

Clonidine *must* be tapered gradually when discontinued to avoid elevated blood pressure, agitation, headache, and rarely fatal hypertensive encephalopathy (abnormal brain function due to severely elevated blood pressure). Clonidine may increase the effect of alcohol or other sedatives.

Common side effects include dry mouth, sedation, nausea, dizziness, agitation, and vivid dreams. These side effects tend to diminish over the first several months of treatment. The dosage is 0.2–0.6 mg per day in divided doses, usually twice daily; higher doses are generally required when clonidine is used with tricyclic antidepressants.

How and Where Does Clonidine Work?

Clonidine is most interesting because of its mechanism of action. It acts to stimulate or activate the alpha-2 receptor of the noradrenalin nerves in the brain. These receptors are interesting because they are autoreceptors (self-stimulating nerve cell receptors). This means that when the nerve cell releases norepinephrine (NE) to stimulate a second nerve cell, some of the NE released actually inhibits the first cell from releasing more NE. Thus, stimulation of these alpha-2 receptors is like stepping on a brake — a built-in negative feedback system. Clonidine activates the brake, causing a dramatic decrease in the output of these NE cells. Not surprisingly, the cells that are responsible for the panic response to danger are cells of the NE system, and therefore clonidine blocks fear and panic responses in both humans and animals. The effectiveness of Clonidine in mania is much less clear, but if it is effective it is presumably through an inhibition of NE activity in the brain.

NOOTROPICS

The nootropics ("toward mind") are a group of primarily experimental compounds that are being designed to enhance memory. The goals of these drugs will be to accelerate the rate of learning and enhance memory retention.

The nootropics are often called "smart drugs," and are targeted to act on the mechanisms of memory that involve amino acid neurotransmitters, such as glutamate. Glutamate is a major excitatory neurotransmitter in the brain that acts by stimulation of the quick nerve response. The nootropics seem to act by decreasing the amount of stimulation necessary to produce the long-term memory. Currently, their effectiveness has only been demonstrated in rats, but FDA approval for clinical trials in humans with early Alzheimer's disease and mild dementia of other types is expected. The brand name of the most promising medication is *Ampalex.*

Also in the "memory enhancer" category is a medication called tacrine (Cognex). Tacrine has been approved for use in Alzheimer's disease and has been shown to cause improvement in memory and functioning in a substantial portion of patients or, in some cases, a slowing of deterioration. Those with early Alzheimer's disease are more likely to benefit. Unfortunately, a large number of patients are unable to tolerate the medication's side effects or toxic effects on the liver. Tacrine presumably works by acting on the cholinergic nerve cells—a different mechanism of action than the above-mentioned experimental drugs.

In addition to the above categories of "smart drugs," there are numerous other medications available in Europe and the United States that are being consumed by individuals who hope to enhance their memory. Unfortunately, there are no studies to support their clinical use for memory enhancement. The most commonly abused drugs from Europe are piracetam (Nootropil), aniracetam (Dragnon), and vincamine (Oxicebral). Piracetam is actually broken down by the body into a substance that impairs memory. American-made medications that have other legitimate uses, but are used by some to attempt to enhance memory, include ergoloid mesylate (Hydergine), selegiline (Eldepryl), and vasopressin (Diapid).

HORMONES AND PSYCHIATRY

The proper functioning of the human body depends on the assembly of groups of amino acids into proteins. The blueprint for this assembly is the DNA (genes) that is housed in the nucleus of the cell. Hormones, from the various glands in the body, attach themselves to the nucleus of the cell, sending a signal to the DNA, advising which types of proteins must be made. These proteins in turn are needed to make enzymes, which are necessary to make the neuro-transmitters. The proteins are also part of the structure of the receptors; it stands to reason, then, that abnormalities in the production of hormones will affect the function of the nervous system (in fact, every known hormonal disorder produces psychiatric symptoms). It also stands to reason that the use of hormones will be helpful in certain psychiatric conditions.

Thyroid Hormone

Thyroid hormone is used as an adjunct to other treatments in bipolar disorder in which there are rapid, frequent cycles between mania and depression, treatment-resistant depression, and postpartum depression. Also, since lithium can cause underfunctioning of the thyroid gland, thyroid supplementation is often needed to treat this side effect of lithium, which seems to occur more frequently in women. There is significant evidence that the thyroid system (also called the thyroid axis) does not respond normally in as many as 40% of patients with depression (i.e., it does not respond to stimulation with adequate output of thyroid hormone). There is no benefit to using thyroid hormone in the treatment of obesity.

Risks and Side Effects of Thyroid Hormone

Thyroid hormone replacement with either levothyroxine (Synthroid) or liothyronine (Cytomel) is generally safe. However, patients may be put at significant risk under a variety of conditions. If dosages are too high over a long period of time, osteoporosis (brittle bones) is more likely to occur in women. Thyroid hormone replacement in patients with any type of heart disease, high blood pressure, diabetes, or Addison's disease can cause an aggravation of the symptoms of these disorders, and may be contraindicated.

When patients are treated with thyroid replacement hormone it may be temporary (to ellicit an antidepressant response in a pharmacologically nonresponsive depression) or for the treatment of a concommitant thyroid disorder. In the latter case, patients must be thoroughly educated regarding side effects, delayed onset of action, and the need for life-long therapy. Too often patients discontinue thyroid hormone replacement on their own, risking potentially disruptive and even fatal consequences.

Side effects of these medications, when not related to the just-mentioned conditions, are rare, and can generally be attributed to excessive dosage. These signs and symptoms include weight loss, palpitations, nervousness, diarrhea, sweating, rapid heart rate, tremors, insomnia, heat intolerance, and menstrual irregularities. Mixing stimulants or appetite suppressants with thyroid supplementation can ellicit serious or even fatal reactions, and must be monitored if the mixture is therapeutically indicated (e.g., hypothyroidism and ADHD).

How and Where Does Thyroid Hormone Work?

There are three parts to the thyroid axis: the hypothalamus, the pituitary gland (both of these are in the brain), and the thyroid gland in the neck (see chapters 1 and 2). Depending on environmental and physical stress levels, as well as how much thyroid hormone is actually present in the blood, the hypothalamus starts the chain of events by releasing TRH (thyroid releasing hormone). TRH then stimulates the pituitary to produce TSH (thyroid stimulating hormone). TSH then travels through the blood to the thyroid gland in the neck, which releases the active thyroid hormone called thyroxine, levothyroxine, or T4. T4 is a thyroid hormone with four iodine molecules attached to it. T4 is converted in the body to T3 (called liothyronine) by removal of one iodine molecule. Both T4 and T3 are active thyroid hormones. These two hormones circulate throughout the body, entering all cells. In the brain, as well as other cells, thyroid hormone acts at the level of the cell nucleus, directing the activity and expression of genes. Antidepressant medication is often only partially effective in states of hypothyroidism, presumably because of impaired ability of the genes to respond to the increased signal density caused by the antidepressant.

There are a variety of abnormalities in the thyroid axis among depressed patients. When some depressed patients are given intravenous TRH (called the TRH stimulation test), as many as 40% of their pituitary glands produce an inadequate amount of TSH, despite normal amounts of thyroid hormone in the blood. (This result is not limited to depressive disorders, however; it is also common among alcoholics.) This inadequate response can be useful in predicting whether a patient will respond to lithium.

In depressed patients whose thyroid hormone levels are in the normal range, this same test may show an abnormally large response. This overresponse on the TRH stimulation test indicates that the patient is suffering from a low level of thyroid disease (called subclinical hypothyroidism), which is often not detected in normal screening. In fact, 12–20% of depressed patients, depending on the study, have been shown to have an underfunctioning thyroid gland.

Many studies (but not all) have shown that patients who have not responded to medication can be converted to responders by the addition of thyroid hormone supplements. Other studies show that the addition of thyroid hormone can actually accelerate the speed of the antidepressant response.

It is interesting that both depression and thyroid disease are more common in women than men, and studies indicate that the malfunction of the thyroid axis may be a part of the reason for this increased vulnerability to depressive disorders in women. Another reason may be the sex hormones—estrogen and progesterone, discussed next.

Sex Hormones

The evidence supporting the involvement of the sex hormones (progesterone, estrogen, and testosterone) in the psychiatric disorders is overwhelming. In women, vulnerability to affective disorders is twice that of men. Women are particularly vulnerable around puberty, premenstrually (the period of time *beginning* 15 days *after* the onset of menstruation), immediately after pregnancy, and around menopause. Many women who are treated with birth control pills, or progesterone alone, will respond with either a worsening or improvement of affective symptoms. It is very difficult to predict who will respond positively and who will respond negatively.

In England, Katrina Dalton (1984) has studied the correlation between the premenstrual phase and the onset of numerous disorders including seizures, criminal behaviors, and psychiatric disorders. The association she found was that "in women, about half of all such events as accidents, suicides, emergency hospital visits, and schoolgirls' punishments, occur during the paramenstrum" (the four days before menstruation and the first four days of menstruation).

Men with diminished testosterone (male sex hormone) levels, due to any number of causes, have increased vulnerability to depression. In men with low testosterone levels, testosterone supplements often alleviate mood disorders to some degree.

Despite the obvious association between psychiatric symptoms and sex hormones, the systematic, controlled study of their use in psychiatry, particularly in patients who are not responsive to traditional treatments, has not been done.

Risks and Side Effects of Sex Hormones

Progesterone may be associated with increased fats in the blood (hyperlipidemia) and should not be used in women who have had thrombophlebitis (blockage of blood vessels), a history of liver dysfunction, or suspected or known malignancy of breast or genital organs. The most common side effects are sedation and nausea.

Estrogen is associated with increased risk of endometrial cancer, and possibly breast cancer, in postmenopausal women. Higher doses are associated with cardiovascular problems, including blockages of blood vessels in the heart, lungs, or extremities. Estrogen is contraindicated in certain estrogen-dependent breast cancers. Estrogen is also associated with an increased risk of gallbladder disease. The most common side effects are abnormal menstruation, vaginal yeast infections, breast tenderness, nausea, bloating, weight changes, rashes, hair loss or growth, headache, migraine, depression, and rapid cycling of mood.

Testosterone has been associated with liver abnormalities, increased risk of prostatic hyperplasia (overgrowth of prostate cells), and prostate cancer, particularly in the elderly, in whom testosterone can also lead to congestive heart failure. Frequent side effects include increased baldness or hair growth, acne, breast enlargement, fluid retention, nausea, clotting abnormalities, headache, anxiety, depression, and increased cholesterol.

How and Where Do Sex Hormones Work?

Sex hormone levels, like thyroid hormone levels, are controlled by a three-part system involving the hypothalamus, pituitary gland, and gonads (ovaries and testicles). Sex hormones, also like thyroid hormone, work at the level of the cell nucleus where they regulate gene expression and, thus, the production of proteins. Sex hormones can cause changes in the activity levels of various brain regions, although they have numerous effects throughout the body as well.

Bibliography

CHAPTER 1

Damasio, A. R. (1994). *Descartes' error: Emotion, reason, and the human brain.* New York: Grosset/Putnam (pp. 94-95).

Engel, G. L. (1980). The clinical application of the biopsychosocial model. *American Journal of Psychiatry, 137,* 535-544.

Hendelman, W. J. (1994). *Student's atlas of neuroanatomy.* Philadelphia: Saunders.

Klein, D. F. (1993). False suffocation alarms, spontaneous panics, and related conditions: An integrative hypothesis. *Archives of General Psychiatry, 50,* 306-317.

Kluver, H., & Bucy, P. C. (1937). Psychic blindness and other symptoms following bilateral temporal lobe lobectomy in rhesus monkeys. *American Journal of Physiology, 119,* 352-353.

Koelle, G. B. (1975). Neurohumoral transmission and the autonomic nervous system. In L. S. Gooman & A. Gilman (Eds.), *The pharmacological basis of therapeutics* (5th ed., pp. 404-415). New York: Macmillan.

Luria, A. R. (1973). *The working brain: An introduction to neuropsychology.* New York: Basic.

Luria, A. R. (1980). *Higher cortical functions in man* (2nd ed.). New York: Basic.

MacLean, P. D. (1978). A mind of three minds: Educating the triune brain. In *Education and the brain* (p. 319). The National Society for the Study of Education, Chicago: University of Chicago Press.

Mapou, R. L, Spector, J., & Kay, G. G. (1995). In J. R. Rundell & M. G. Wise (Eds.), *Textbook of consultation-liason psychiatry.* Washington, DC: American Psychiatric Press.

Marin, R. S. (1991, Summer). Apathy: A neuropsychiatric syndrome. *Journal of Neuropsychiatry, 3*(3), 243-254.

CHAPTER 2

American Psychiatric Association. (1994). *Diagnostic and statistical manual of mental disorders* (4th ed.). Washington, DC: Author.

Ansseau, M., Troisfontaines, B., Papart, P., & von Frenckell, R. (1991). Compulsive personality as predictor of response to serotonergic antidepressants. *British Medical Journal, 303,* 760-761.

Ashton, H. (1992). *Brain function and psychotropic drugs.* New York: Oxford University Press.

Barbee, J. G. (1993). Memory, benzodiazepines, and anxiety: Integration of theoretical and clinical perspectives. *Jounal of Clinical Psychiatry, 54*(Suppl. 10), 86–97.

Bell, I. R., Amend, D., Kaszniak, A. W., Schwartz G. E., Peterson, J. M., William, A. S., Biederman, J., Rosenbaum, J. F., Hirschfeld, D. R., et al. (1990). Psychiatric correlates of behavioral inhibition in young children of parents with and without psychiatric disorders. *Archives of General Psychiatry, 47,* 21–26.

Bowen, M. (1978). *Family therapy in clinical practice.* New York: Aronson

Chuong, C. J., Coulam, C. B., Bergstralh, E. J., O'Fallon, W. M., & Steinmetz, G. I. (1988). Clinical trial of naltrexone in premenstrual tension. *Obstetrics & Gynecology, 72,* 332–336.

Clark, C. H., Hedaya, R. J., Rosenthal, N. E. (in press). Seasonal depression in patients with dissociative disorders. *Journal of Nervous and Mental Disease.*

Cloninger, R. C. (1987). A systematic method for clinical description and classification of personality variants. *Archives of General Psychiatry, 44,* 573–588.

Cloninger, R. C., Svrakic, D. M., & Przybeck, T. R. (1991). The tridimensional personality questionaire: US normative data. *Psychological Report, 69,* 1047–1057.

Cloninger, R. C., Svrakic D. M., & Przybeck, T. R. (1993). A psychobiological model of temperament and character. *Archives of General Psychiatry, 50,* 975–990.

Cotton, P. (1994). Medical news and perspectives: Biology enters repressed memory fray. *Journal of the American Medical Association, 272,* 1725–1726.

Crowe, R. R. (1995). Genetics. In F. E. Bloom & D. J. Kupfer (Eds.), *Psychopharmacology: The fourth generation of progress* (pp. 1821–1833). NewYork: Raven.

Dalton, K. (1984). *The premenstrual syndrome and progesterone therapy* (2nd ed.). Chicago: Year Book.

Depue, R. A., & Spoont, M. R. (1986). Conceptualizing a serotonin trait: A behavioral dimension of constraint. *Annals of the New York Academy of Science, 487,* 47–62.

Ehlers, C. L, Frank, E., Kupfer, D. J. (1988). Social zeitgebers and biological rhythms: A unified approach to understanding the etiology of depression. *Archives of General Psychiatry, 45,* 948–952.

Ellenberger, H. F. (1970). *The discovery of the unconscious: The history and evolution of dynamic psychiatry.* New York: Basic.

Faedda, G. L., Tondo, L., Teicher, M. H., Baldessarini, R. J., Gelbard, H. A., & Gianfranco, F. F. (1993). Seasonal mood disorders: Patterns of seasonal recurrence in mania and depression. *Archives of General Psychiatry, 50,* 17–23.

Glantz, S. A., Barnes, D. E., Bero, L., Hanauer, P., & Slade, J. (1995). Looking through a keyhole at the tobacco industry: The Brown and Williamson documents. *Journal of the American Medical Association, 274,* 219–224.

Goodwin, F. K., & Jamison, K. R. (1990). *Manic depressive illness.* New York: Oxford University Press.

Griffin, J. E. (1985). Dynamic tests of endocrine function. In J. D. Wilson & D. W. Foster (Eds.), *Textbook of endocrinology* (7th ed., pp. 147–154), Philadelphia: Saunders.

Jackson S. W. (1986). *Melancholia and depression from Hippocratic times to modern times.* New Haven: Yale University Press.

Joyce, P. R., Mudler, R. T., & Cloninger, R. C. (1994). Temperment predicts clomipramine and desipramine response in major depression. *Journal of Affective Disorders, 30,* 35–46.

Kagan, J. (1994). *Galen's prophesy: Temperament in human nature.* New York: Basic.

Kandel, E. R. (1989). Genes, nerve cells, and the remembrance of things past. *Journal of Neuropsychiatry, 1,* 103–125.

Kendler, K. S. (1983). Overview: A current perspective on twin studies of schizophrenia. *American Journal of Psychiatry, 140,* 1413–1425.

Kendler, K. S., Neale, M., Kessler, R., Heath, A. D., & Eaves, L. (1993). A twin study of recent life events and difficulties. *Archives of General Psychiatry, 50,* 789–796.

Kendler, K. S., Kessler, R.C., Walters, E. E., MacLean, C., Neale, M. C., Heath, A. C., Phil, D., & Eaves L. J. (1995a). Stressful life events, genetic liability, and onset of an episode of major depression in women. *American Journal of Psychiatry, 152*(6), 833–842.

Kendler, K. S., Mcguire, M., Gruenberg, A. M., & Walsh, D. (1995b). Schizotypal symptoms and signs in the Rosecommon family study: Their factor structure and familial relationship with psychotic and affective disorders. *Archives of General Psychiatry, 52,* 296–303.

Kendler, K. S., Walters, E. E., Neale, M. C., Kessler, R. C., Heath, A. C., & Eaves, L. J. (1995c). The structure of the genetic and environmental risk factors for six major psychiatric disorders in women. *Archives of General Psychiatry, 52,* 374–383.

Kerr, M. E., & Bowen, M. (1988). *Family evaluation: An approach based on Bowen theory.* New York: Norton.

Kety, S. S., Wender, P. H., Jacobsen, B., Ingraham, L. J., Jansson, L., Faber, B., & Kinney, D. K. (1994). Mental illness in the biological and adoptive relatives of schizophrenic adoptees: Replication of the Copenhagen study in the rest of Denmark. *Archives of General Psychiatry, 51,* 442–455.

Kupfer, D. J. (1992, October) Five-year outcome for maintenance therapies in recurrent depression. *Archives of General Psychiatry, 49,* 769–773.

McCarthy, G. (1995). Functional neuroimaging of memory. *The Neuroscientist, 1,* 155–163.

Mega, S. M., & Cummings, J. L. (1994). Frontal-subcortical circuits and neuropsychiatric disorders. *Journal of Neuropsychiatry and Clinical Neurosciences, 6,* 358–370.

Miller, J. W., & Selhub, J. (1995). Trait shyness in the elderly: Evidence for an association with Parkinson's disease in family members and biochemical correlates. *Journal of Geriatric Psychiatry and Neurology, 8,* 16–22.

Parry, B. L. (1995). Mood disorders linked to the reproductive cycle in women. In F. E. Bloom & D. J. Kupfer (Eds.), *Psychopharmacology: The fourth generation of progress* (pp. 1024–1042). New York: Raven.

Peselow, E. D., Fieve, R. R., & DiFiglia, C. (1992). Personality traits and response to desipramine. *Journal of Affective Disorders, 24,* 209–216.

Post, R. M. (1992). Transduction of psychosocial stress into the neurobiology of recurrent affective disorder. *American Journal of Psychiatry, 149,* 999–1010.

Rosenthal, N. E., Davenport, Y., Cowdry, R. W., Webster, M. H., & Goodwin, F. K. (1980). Monoamine metabolites in cerebrospinal fluid of depressive subgroups. *Psychiatry Research, 2,* 113–119.

Rosenthal, N. E., Sack, D. A., Skwerer, R. G., Jacobsen, F. M., & Wehr, T. A. (1988). Phototherapy for seasonal affective disorder. *Journal of Biological Rhythm, 3,* 101–120.

Siever, L. J., Klar, H., & Coccaro, E. (1985). Psychobiologic substrates of personality. In H. Klar & L. J. Siever (Eds.), *Biological response styles: Clinical implications* (pp. 38–66). Washington, DC: American Psychiatric Press.

Squire, L. R., Knowlton, B., & Musen, G. (1993). The structure and organization of memory. *Annual Review of Psychology, 44,* 453–495.

Squire, L. R., & Zola-Morgan, S. (1991). The medial temporal lobe memory system. *Science, 253,* 1380–1386.

Svrakic, D. M., Whitehead, C., Przybeck, T. R., & Cloninger R. C. (1993). Differential diagnosis of personality disorders by the seven-factor model of temperament and character. *Archives of General Psychiatry, 50,* 991–1000.

Wirz-Justice, A. (1995). Biological rhythms in mood disorders. In F. E. Bloom & D. J. Kupfer (Eds.), *Psychopharmacology: The fourth generation of progress.* New York: Raven.

Young, E. A., Haskett, R. F., Murphy-Weinberg, V., Watson, S. J., & Akil, H. (1991). Loss of glucocorticoid fast feedback in depression. *Archives of General Psychiatry, 48,* 693–698.

CHAPTER 3

Akbarian, S., Bunney, W. E., Potkin, S. G., Wigal, S. B., Hagman, J. O., Sandman, C.A., & Jones, E.G. (1993). Altered Distribution of nicotinamide-adenine dinucleotide phosphate-diaphorase cells in frontal lobe of schizophrenics implies disturbances of cortical development. *Archives of General Psychiatry, 50,* 169–177.

Akbarian, S., Kim, J. J., Potkin, S. G., Hagman, J. O., Tafazzoli, A., Bunney, W. E., & Jones, E.G. (1995). Gene expression for glutamic acid decarboxylase is reduced without loss of neurons in prefrontal cortex of schizophrenics. *Archives of General Psychiatry, 52,* 258–266.

Akiskal, H. S., Walker, P., & Puzantian, V. R. (1983). Bipolar outcome in the course of depressive illness: Phenomenologic, familial, and pharmacologic predictors. *Journal of Affective Disorders, 5*(2), 115-128.

Andreasen, N. C. (1994). Regional brain abnormalities in schizophrenia measured with magnetic resonance imaging. *Journal of the American Medical Association, 272*(22), 1763-1769.

Andreason, N. (1995). Posttraumatic stress disorder: Psychology, biology, and the Manichaen warfare between false dichotomies. *American Journal of Psychiatry, 152,* 963-965.

Andreasen, N., Nasrallah, H. A., & Dunn, V. (1986). Structural abnormalities in the frontal system in schizophrenia. *Archives of General Psychiatry, 43,* 136-144.

Anthenelli, R. M., Smith, T. L., Irwin, M. R., & Schuckit, M. A. (1994). A comparative study of criteria for subgrouping alcoholics: The primary/secondary diagnostic scheme versus variations of the type1/type2 criteria. *American Journal of Psychiatry, 151,* 1468-1474.

Asnis, M. G., Mcginn, L. K., & Sanderson, W. C. (1995). Atypical depression: Clinical aspects and noradrenergic function. *American Journal of Psychiatry, 152*(1), 31-36.

Barlow, D. H. (1988). Anxiety and its disorders: The nature and treatment of anxiety and panic. New York: Guilford.

Barr, C. E., Mednick, S. A., & Munk-Jorgensen, P. (1990). Exposure to influenza epidemics during gestation and adult schizophrenia: A 40-year study. *Archives of General Psychiatry, 47,* 869-874.

Baxter, L. R. (1995). Neuroimaging studies of human anxiety disorders: Cutting paths of knowledge through the field of neurotic phenomena. In F. E. Bloom & D. J. Kupfer (Eds.), *Psychopharmacology: The fourth generation of progress.* (pp. 1287-1299). New York: Raven.

Baxter, L. R., Schwartz, J. M., & Bergman, K. S. (1992). Caudate glucose metabolic rate changes with both drug and behavior therapy for obsessive-compulsive disorder. *Archives of General Psychiatry, 49,* 681-689.

Beck, A. T. (1967). *Depression.* New York: Hoeber.

Beck, A. T., Ward, G. H., & Mendelson, M. (1961). An inventory for measuring depression. *Archives of General Psychiatry, 4,* 561-571.

Berman, K. F., Torrey, E. F., Daniel, D. G., & Weinberger, D. R. (1992). Regional cerebral blood flow in monozygotic twins discordant and concordant for schizophrenia. *Archives of General Psychiatry, 49,* 927-934.

Bibring, E. (1953). The mechanism of depression. In P. Greenacre (Ed.), *Affective disorders.* New York: International Universities Press.

Biederman, J., Faraone, S. V., Keenan, K., & Tsuang, M. T. (1991). Evidence of familial association between attention deficit disorder and major affective disorders. *Archives of General Psychiatry, 48,* 633-642.

Biederman, J. et al. (1995). High risk for attention deficit hyperactivity disorder among children of parents with childhood onset of the disorder: A pilot study. *Archives of General Psychiatry, 152,* 431-435.

Black, D. W., Wesner, R., Bowers, W., & Gabel, J. (1993). A comparison of fluvoxamine, cognitive therapy, and placebo in the treatment of panic disorder. *Archives of General Psychiatry, 50,* 44-50.

Bleuler, E. (1950). *Dementia praecox and the group of schizophrenias.* New York: International Universities Press.

Bohman, M., Cloninger, C. R., Sigvardsson, S., & von Knorring, A. L. (1982). Predisposition to petty criminality in Swedish adoptees, I: Genetic and environmental heterogeneity. *Archives of General Psychiatry, 39,* 1233-1241.

Bohman, M., Cloninger, R., Sigvardsson, S., von Knorring, A.L. (1987). The genetics of alcoholisms and related disorders. *Journal of Psychiatric Research, 21,* 447-452.

Bracha, H. S., Torrey, E. F., Gottesman, I. I., Bigelow, L. B., & Cunniff, C. (1992). Second trimester markers of fetal size in schizophrenia: A study of monozygotic twins. *American Journal of Psychiatry, 149*(10), 1355-1361.

Braff, D. L., & Geyer, M. A. (1990). Sensorimotor gating and schizophrenia: Human and animal model studies. *Archives of General Psychiatry, 47,* 181-188.

Bremner, D. J., Randall, P., Scott, T. M., Broenen, R. A., & Seibyl, J. P. (1995). MRI-based measurement of hippocampal volume in patients with combat related posttraumatic stress disorder. *American Journal of Psychiatry, 152,* 973-981.

Breslau, N., Davis, G. C., & Andreski, P. (1995). Risk factors for PTSD-related traumatic events: A prospective analysis. *American Journal of Psychiatry, 152,* 529-535.

Breslau, N., Davis G. C., & Prabucki K. (1987). Searching for evidence on the validity of generalized anxiety disorder: Psychopathology in children of anxious mothers. *Psychiatry Research, 20,* 285-297.

Buckminister, S., Ugaglia, K., Jellinek, M. S., Steingard, R., Spencer, T., Norman, D., Kolodny, R., Kraus, I., Perrin, J., Keller, M.B., & Tsuang, M. T. (1992). Further evidence for family-genetic risk factors in attention deficit hyperactivity disorder: Patterns of co-morbidity in probands and relatives in psychiatrically and pediatrically referred samples. *Archives of General Psychiatry, 49,* 728-738.

Cadoret, R. J., Yates, W. R., Troughton, E., Woodworth, G., & Stewart, M.A. (1995). Adoption study demonstrating two genetic pathways to drug abuse. *Archives of General Psychiatry, 52,* 42-52.

Carpenter, W. T., Buchanan, R. W., Kirkpatrick, B., Tamminga, C., & Wood, F. (1993). Strong inference, theory testing and the neuroanatomy of schizophrenia. *Archives of General Psychiatry, 50,* 825-831.

Carrington, C. H. (1979). A comparison of cognitive and analytically oriented brief treatment approaches to depression in black women. *Dissertation Abstracts International, 40.* (University Microfilms No. 79-26513).

Carroll, K. M., Rounsaville, B. J., Nich, C., Lynn, G. T., Wirtz, P. W., Gawin, F. (1994). One-year follow-up of psychotherapy and pharmacotherapy for cocaine dependence: Delayed emergence psychotherapy effects. *Archives of General Psychiatry, 51,* 989-997.

Catts, S. V., Shelley, A. M., Ward, P. B., Liebert, B., McConaghy, N., Andrews, S., & Michie, P. T. (1995). Brain potential evidence for an auditory sensory memory deficit in schizophrenia. *American Journal of Psychiatry, 152,* 213-219.

Charney, D. S., Deutch, A. Y., Krystal, J. H., Southwick, S. M., & Davis, M. (1993). Psychobiologic mechanisms of posttraumatic stress disorder. *Archives of General Psychiatry, 50,* 294-305.

Chen, Y. W., & Dilsaver, S. C. (1995). Comorbidity of panic disorder in bipolar illness: Evidence from the epidemiologic catchement area survey. *American Journal of Psychiatry, 152,* 280-282.

Cloninger, C. R., Bohman, M., & Sigvardsson, S. (1981). Inheritance of alcohol abuse: Cross-fostering of adopted men. *Archives of General Psychiatry, 38,* 861-868.

Coffey, C. E., Wilkinson, W. E., Weiner, R. D. et al. (1993). Quantitative cerebral anatomy in depression. *Archives of General Psychiatry, 50,* 7-16.

Cohen, S. (1988). *The chemical brain: The neurochemistry of addictive disorders.* Minneapolis: CompCare.

Conrad, A. J., Abebe, T., Austin, R., Forsythe, S., & Scheibel, A. B. (1991). Hippocampal pyramidal cell disarray in schizophrenia as a bilateral phenomenon. *Archives of General Psychiatry, 48,* 413-417.

Copen, A. C. (1994). Depression as a lethal disease: Prevention strategies. *Journal of Clinical Psychiatry, 55*(Suppl. 4), 37-45.

Covi, L., & Lipman, R. S. (1987). Cognitive-behavioral group psychotherapy combined with imipramine in major depression: A pilot study. *Psychopharmacology Bulletin, 23,* 173-176.

Cowley, D. S., & Arana, G. W. (1990). The diagnostic utility of lactate sensitivity in panic disorder. *Archives of General Psychiatry, 47,* 277-284.

Crow, T. J. (1980). Molecular pathology of schizophrenia: More than one disease process. *British Medical Journal, 280,* 66-68.

Datlof, S., Coleman, P. D., Forbes, G. B., & Kreipe, R. E. (1986). Ventricular dilation on CAT scans of patients with anorexia nervosa. *American Journal of Psychiatry, 143,* 96-98.

Deakin, J. F. W., Slater, P., & Simpson, M. D. C. (1989). Frontal cortical and left temporal glutamatergic dysfunction in schizophrenia. *Journal of Neurochemistry, 52,* 1781-1786.

de Beurs, E., van Balkom, A. J. L. M., Lange, A., Koele, P., & van Dyck, R. (1995). Treatment of panic disorder with agoraphobia: Comparison of fluvoxamine, placebo, and psychological panic management combined with exposure and of exposure in vivo alone. *American Journal of Psychiatry, 152,* 683-691.

Deutsch, C. K., Matthysse, S., Swanson, J. M., & Farkas, L. G. (1990). Genetic latent structure analysis of dysmorphology in attention deficit disorder. *Journal of the American Academy of Child Psychiatry, 29,* 189–194.

DiMascio, A., Weissman, M. M., & Prusoff, B. A. (1979). Differential symptom reduction by drugs and psychotherapy in acute depression. *Archives of General Psychiatry, 36,* 1450–1456.

Dorovini-Zis, K., & Zis, A. P. (1987). Increased adrenal weight in victims of violent suicide. *American Journal of Psychiatry, 9,* 1214–1215.

Fairburn, C. G., Norman, P. A., Welch, S. L., Phil, D., O'Connor, M. E., Doll, H. A., & Peveler R. C. (1995). A prospective study of outcome in bulimia nervosa and long-term effects of three psychological treatments. *Archives of General Psychiatry, 52,* 304–312.

Faraone, S., Biederman, J., Chen, W. J., Krifcher, B., Keenan, K., Moore, C., Sprich, S., & Tsuang, M. T. (1992). Segregation analysis of attention deficit hyperactivity disorder. *Psychiatric Genetics, 2,* 257–275.

Fawcett, J. (1992). Suicide risk factors in depressive disorders and in panic disorder. *Journal of Clinical Psychiatry, 53*(March suppl.), 9–13.

Fesler, A. (1991). Valproate in combat-related posttraumatic stress disorder. *Journal of.Clinical Psychiatry, 52,* 361–364.

Foa, E. B., Riggs, D. S., & Gerhuny, B. S. (1995). Arousal, numbing, and intrusion: Symptom structure of PTSD following assault. *American Journal of Psychiatry, 152,* 16–120.

Freud, S. (1917). Mourning and melancholia. In J. Strachey (Ed. and Trans.), *The standard edition of the complete psychological works of Sigmund Freud* (Vol. XIV, pp. 239–258). New York: Norton, 1957.

Garfinkel, P. E., Lin, E., Goering, P., Spegg, C., Goldbloom, D. S., Kennedy, S., Kaplan, A. S., & Woodside, D. B. (1995). Bulimia nervosa in a Canadian community sample: Prevalence and comparison of subgroups. *American Journal of Psychiatry, 152,* 1052–1058.

Gerner, R. H., Post, R. M., & Bunney, W. E., Jr. (1976). A dopaminergic mechanism in mania. *American Journal of Psychiatry, 133,* 1177–1179.

Gershon, E. S., Hamovit, J., Guroff, J. J., Dibble, E., Leckman, J. F., Sceery, W., Targum, S. D., Nurmberger, J. I., Goldin, L. R., & Bunney, W. E. (1982). A family study of schizoaffective, bipolar I, bipolar II, unipolar and normal control probands. *Archives of General Psychiatry, 39,* 1157–1167.

Giedd, J., Castellanos, F. X., Casey, B. J., Kozuch, P., King, C. A., Hamburger, S. D., & Rapoport J. L. (1994). Quantitative morphology of the corpus collosum in attention deficit hyperactivity disorder. *American Journal of Psychiatry, 151,* 665–669.

Goddard, G. V., Dragunow, M., Maru, E. et al. (1986). Kindling and the forces that oppose it. In B. K. Doane, & K. F. Livingston (Eds.), *The limbic system: Functional organization and clinical disorders.* New York: Raven.

Golier, J. A., Marzuk, P. M., Leon, A. C., Weiner, C., & Tardiff, K. (1995). Low serum cholesterol level and attempted suicide. *American Journal of Psychiatry, 152*(3), 419–423.

Goodman, R., & Stevenson, J. (1989). A twin study of hyperactivity, II: The aetiological role of genes, family relationships, and perinatal adversity. *Journal of Child Psychology and Psychiatry, 30,* 691–709.

Goodwin, G. M., Fairburn, C. G., & Cowen, P. J. (1987). Dieting changes serotonergic function in women but not men: Implications for the eetiology of anorexia nervosa? *Psychological Medicine, 17,* 839–842.

Gorman, J. M., Liebowitz, M. R., Fyer, A. J., & Stein, J. (1989). A neuroanatomical hypothesis for panic disorder. *American Journal of Psychiatry, 146,* 148–161.

Greist, J. H., & March, J. (1995). Clinical advances in OCD. *Psychiatric Times, 12*(Suppl. 4), 38–41.

Gualtieri, C. T., & Hicks, R. E. (1991). Neuropharmacology of methylphenidate and a neural substrate for childhood hyperactivity. *Psychiatric Clinics of North America, 14,* 113–124.

Gwirstman, H. E., Kaye, W. H., & George, D. T. (1989). Central and peripheral ACTH and cortisol levels in anorexia nervosa and bulimia. *Archives of General Psychiatry, 46,* 61–69.

Hall, N. R., & Goldstein, A. L. (1981). Neurotransmitters and the immune system. In R. Adler (Ed.), *Psychoneuroimmunology.* New York: Academic.

Halmi, K. A. (1995). Basic biological overview of eating disorders. In F. E. Bloom & D. J. Kupfer (Eds.), *Psychopharmacology: The fourth generation of progress*. New York: Raven.

Halperin, J. M., Sharma, V., Siever, L. J., Schwartz, S. T., Matier, K., Wornell, G., & Newcorn, J. H. (1994). Serotinergic function in aggressive and nonaggressive boys with attention deficit hyperactivity disorder. *American Journal of Psychiatry, 151,* 243-248.

Hans, S. L., & Marcus, J. M. (1991). Neurobehavioral development of infants at risk for schizophrenia: A review. In E. Walker (Ed.), *Schizophrenia: A life-course developmental perspective* (pp. 33-57). Orlando, FL: Academic.

Hartmann, T. (1993). *Attention deficit disorder: A different perception*. Pennvalley, CA: Underwood-Miller.

Hauser, P., Zametkin, A. J., Martinez, P., Vitiello, B., Matochik, J. A., Mixson, A. J., & Weintraub, B. D. (1993). Attention deficit hyperactivity disorder in people with generalized resistance to thyroid hormone. *New England Journal of Medicine, 328,* 997-1001.

Hedaya, R. J. (1984). Pharmacokinetic factors in the clinical use of tryptophan. *Journal of Clinical Psychopharmacology, 4(6),* 347-348.

Helzer, J. E., Robins, L. N., & McEvoy, L. (1987). Posttraumatic stress disorder in the general population. *New England Journal of Medicine, 317,* 1630-1634.

Hemmingsen, R., Vorsrup, S., Clemmesen, L., Holm, S., & Tflet-Hansen, P. (1988). Cerebral blood flow during delerium tremens and related clinical states studied with Xenon-133 inhalation tomography. *American Journal of Psychiatry, 145,* 1384-1390.

Herceg-Baron, R. L., Prusoff, B. A., & Weissman, M. M. (1979). Pharmacotherapy and psychotherapy in acutely depressed patients: A study of attrition patterns in a clinical trial. *Comprehensive Psychiatry, 20,* 315-325.

Higuchi, S., Matsushita, S., Murayama, M., Takagi, S., & Hayashida, M. (1995). Alcohol and aldehyde dehydrogenase polymorphisms and the risk for alcoholism. *American Journal of Psychiatry, 152,* 1219-1221.

Hogarty, G. E. (1993). Prevention of relapse in chronic schizophrenic patients. *Journal of Clinical Psychiatry, 54*(Suppl. 3), 18-23.

Hogarty, G. E., Anderson, C. M., Reiss, D. J., Kornblith, S. J., Greenwald, D. P., Ulrich, R. F., & Carter, M. (1991). Family psychoeducation, social skills training, and maintenance chemotherapy in the aftercare treatment of schizophrenia, II: Two-year effects of a controlled study on relapse and adjustment. *Archives of General Psychiatry, 48,* 340-347.

Hollander, E. (1993). Obsessive compulsive spectrum disorders: An overview. *Psychiatric Annals, 23(7),* 355-358.

Hsiao, J. K., Colison, J., Bartko, J. J. et al. (1993). Monoamine neurotransmitter interactions in drug free and neuroleptic treated schizophrenics. *Archives of General Psychiatry, 5*(8), 606-614.

Hudson, J. I., & Pope, H. G. (1990). Affective spectrum disorder: Does antidepressant response identify a family of disorders with a common pathophysiology? *American Journal of Psychiatry, 5,* 552-564.

Hynd, G. W., Semrud-Clikeman, M., Lorys, A. R., Novery, E. S., & Eliopulos, D. (1991). Corpus collosum morphology in attention deficit-hyperactivity disorder (ADHD): Morphometric analysis of MRI. *Journal of Learning Disabilities, 24,* 141-146.

Imber-Mintz, L., Liberman, R. P., Miklowitz, D., et al. (1987). Expressed emotion: A clarion call for partnership. *Schizophrenia Bulletin, 13,* 227-235.

Insel, T. R. (1992). Toward a neuroanatomy of obsessive compulsive disorder. *Archives of General Psychiatry, 49,* 739-745.

Javitt, D. C., Doneshka, P., Grochowski, S., & Ritter, W. (1995). Impaired mismatch negativity generation reflects widespread dysfunction of working memory in schizophrenia. *Archives of General Psychiatry, 52,* 550-558.

Jensen, P. S., Sheruette, R. E., Xenakis, S. N., Richters, J. (1993). Anxiety and depressive disorders in attention deficit disorder with hyperactivity: New findings. *American Journal of Psychiatry, 150*(8), 1203-1209.

Judd, L. L., McAdams, L. A., Budnickm B., & Braff, D. L. (1992). Sensory gating deficits in schizophrenia: New results. *American Journal of Psychiatry, 149,* 488-493.

Kane, J. M. (1993). Academic highlights: Understanding and treating psychosis: Advances in research and therapy. *Journal of Clinical Psychiatry, 54,* 445-452.

Kaye, W. H., & Weltzin, T. E. (1991). Neurochemistry of bulimia nervosa. *Journal of Clinical Psychiatry, 52*(Suppl. 10), 21–28.

Kendler, K. S., & Diehl, S. R. (1993). The genetics of schizophrenia: A current genetic epidemiologic perspective. *Schizophrenia Bulletin, 19,* 261–285.

Kendler, K. S., Heath, A., & Martin, M. G. (1986). Symptoms of anxiety and depression in a volunteer twin population. *Archives of General Psychiatry, 43,* 213–221.

Kendler, K. S., Kessler, R. C., Neale, M. C., Heath, A. C., Phil, D., & Eaves, L. J. (1993). The prediction of major depression in women: Toward an integrated etiologic model. *American Journal of Psychiatry, 150*(8), 1139–1147.

Kendler, K. S., Mcguire, M., Gruenberg, A. M., & Walsh, D. (1994). Outcome and family study of the subtypes of schizophrenia in the west of Ireland. *American Journal of Psychiatry, 151,* 849–856.

Kendler, K. S., Mcguire, M., Gruenberg, A. M., & Walsh, D. (1995a). Schizotypal symptoms and signs in the Rosecommon family study: Their factor structure and familial relationship with psychotic and affective disorders. *Archives of General Psychiatry, 52,* 296–303.

Kendler, K. S., Walters, E. E., Neale, M. C., Kessler, R. C., Heath, A. C., & Eaves, L. J. (1995b). The structure of the genetic and environmental risk factors for six major psychiatric disorders in women. *Archives of General Psychiatry, 52,* 374–383.

Klein, D. F. (1993). False suffocation alarms, spontaneous panics, and related conditions: An integrative hypothesis. *Archives of General Psychiatry, 50,* 306–317.

Klerman, G. L., Lavori, P., Rice, J., Reich, T., Endicott, J., & Andreasen, N. (1985). Birth cohort trends in rates of major depressive disorders amoung relatives of patients with affective disorder. *Archives of General Psychiatry, 42,* 689–693.

Klerman, G. L., Weissman, M. M., Rounsaville, B. J., & Chevron, E. S. (1984). *Interpersonal psychotherapy of depression.* New York: Basic.

Kraepelin, E. (1919). Dementia praecox. (R. M. Barclay, Trans.). Edinburgh, Scotland: E. S. Livingstone.

Krieg, J. C., Pirke, K. M., Lauer, C., & Backmund, H. (1988). Endocrine, metabolic, and cranial computed tomographic findings in anorexia nervosa. *Biological Psychiatry, 23,* 377–387.

Krystal, J. H., Webb, E., Cooney, N., Kranzler, H. R., & Charney, D. S. (1994). Specificity of ethanollike effects elicited by serotonergic and noradrenergic mechanisms. *Archives of General Psychiatry, 51,* 898–911.

Kupfer, D. J., Frank, E., Jarrett, D. B., Reynolds, C. F., III, & Thase, M. E. (1988). Interrelationship of electroencephalographic sleep chronobiology and depression. In D. J. Kupfer, T. H. Monk, J. D. Barchas (Eds.), *Biological rhythms and mental disorders.* New York: Guilford.

Kupfer, D. J., Frank, E., Perel, J. M., Cornes, C., Mallinger, A. G., Thase, M. E., McEachran A. B., & Grochocinski, V. J. (1992). Five-year outcome for maintenance therapies in recurrent depression. *Archives of General Psychiatry, 49,* 769–773.

Kupfer, D. J., Frank, E., McEachran, A. B., & Grochocinski, V. J. (1990). Delta sleep ratio: A biological correlate of early recurrence in unipolar affective disorder. *Archives of General Psychiatry, 47,* 1100–1105.

Lauer, C. J., Wolfgang, S., Holsboer, F., & Krieg, J. C. (1995). In quest of identifying vulnerability markers for psychiatric disorders by all-night polysomnography. *Archives of General Psychiatry, 52,* 145–152.

Le Moal, M. (1995). Mesocorticolimbic dopaminergic neurons: Functional and regulatory roles. In F. E. Bloom & D. J. Kupfer (Eds.), *Psychopharmacology: The fourth generation of progress* (pp. 283–294). New York: Raven.

Leonard, H. L., Swedo, S. E., & Leane, M. C. (1991). A double blind desipramine substitution during long-term clomipramine treatment in children and adolescents with obsessive-compulsive disorder. *Archives of General Psychiatry, 48,* 922–927.

Liberman, R. P., & Corrigan, P. W. (1992). Is schizophrenia a neurological disorder? [Editorial]. *Journal of Neuropsychiatry, 4,* 119–124.

Liberthson, R., Sheehan, D. V., King, M. E., & Weyman, A. E. (1986). The prevalence of mitral valve prolapse in patients with panic disorders. *American Journal of Psychiatry, 143,* 511–515.

Lieberman, J. A. (1995). Signs and symptoms: What can they tell us about the clinical course and pathophysiologic processes of schizophrenia? [Commentary]. *Archives of General Psychiatry, 52,* 361–362.

Linnoila, M. (1994). *The pharmacotherapies of alcoholism* [Videotape]. (Available from Distinguished Professors of Pychiatry Series, 569 Applewood Drive, Dept. P., Ft. Washington, PA. 19034)

Lipska, B. K., & Weinberger, D. R. (1993). Delayed effects of neonatal hippocampal damage on haloperidol-induced catalepsy and apomorphine-induced stereotypic behaviors in the rat. *Developmental Brain Research, 75,* 213–222.

Litt, M. D., Babor, T. F., DelBoca, F. K., Kadden, R. M., & Cooney, N. L. (1992). Types of alcoholics, II: Application of an empirically derived typology to treatment matching. *Archives of General Psychiatry, 49,* 609–614.

Lydiard, R. B., Greenwald, S., Weissman, M. M., Johnson, J., Drossman, D. A., & Ballenger, J. C. (1994). Panic disorder and gastrointestinal symptoms: Findings from the NIMH epidemiologic catchment area project. *American Journal of Psychiatry, 151,* 64–70.

Marcus, J., Hans, S. L., Auerbach, J. G., & Auerbach, A. G. (1993). Children at risk for schizophrenia: The Jerusalem infant development study: Neurobehavioral deficits at school age. *Archives of General Psychiatry, 50,* 797–809.

Mathew, R. J., & Wilson, W. H. (1991). Substance abuse and cerebral blood flow. *American Journal of Psychiatry, 148,* 292–305.

McGlashan, T. H., & Fenton, W. S. (1992, January). The positive-negative distinction in schizophrenia: Review of natural history validators. *Archives of General Psychiatry, 49,* 63–72.

McGuffin, P., & Katz, R. (1989). The genetics of depression and manic depressive illness. *British Journal of Psychiatry, 155,* 294–304.

McNally, R. J., & Shin, L. M. (1995). Association of intelligence with severity of posttraumatic stress disorder symptoms in Vietnam combat veterans. *American Journal of Psychiatry, 152,* 936–938.

Mellman, T. A., Kulick-Bell, R., Ashlock, L. E., & Nolan, B. (1995). Sleep events among veterans with combat-related posttraumatic stress disorder. *American Journal of Psychiatry, 152,* 110–115.

Mendelwicz, J., & Rainer, J. (1977). Adoption study supporting genetic transmission in manic depressive illness. *Nature, 268,* 326–329.

Modell, J. G., & Mountz, J. M. (1995). Focal cerebral blood flow change during craving for alcohol measured by SPECT. *Journal of Neuropsychiatry, 7,* 15–22.

Nagy, L. M., Krystal, J. H., Woods, S. W., & Charney, D. S. (1989). Clinical and medication outcome after short-term alprazolam and behavioral group treatment in panic disorder: 2.5 year naturalistic follow-up study. *Archives of General Psychiatry, 46,* 993–999.

Nemiah, J. C. (1995). A few intrusive thoughts on posttraumatic stress disorder. *American Journal Psychiatry, 152,* 501–503.

Nestler, E. J. (1995). Molecular basis of addictive states. *The Neuroscientist, 1,* 212–220.

Nunes, E. V., McGrath, P. J., & Quitkin, F. M. (1995). Treating anxiety in patients with alcoholism. *Journal of Clinical Psychiatry, 56*(Suppl. 2), 3–9.

O'Brien, C., Eckardt, M. J., & Linnoila, M. (1995). Pharmacotherapy of alcoholism. In F. E. Bloom & D. J. Kupfer (Eds.), *Pharmacology: The fourth generation of progress.* New York: Raven.

O'Donnell, B. F., Faux, S. F., McCarley R. W., Kimble, M. O., Salisbury, D. F., Nestor, P. G., Kikinis, R., Jolesz, F. A., & Shenton, M. E. (1995). Increased rate of P300 latency prolongation with age in schizophrenia: Electrophysiological evidence for a neurodegenerative process. *Archives of General Psychiatry, 52,* 544–549.

Ornitz, E. M., & Pynoos, R. S. (1989). Startle modulation in children with posttraumatic stress disorder. *American Journal of Psychiatry, 146,* 866–870.

Pacholczyk, T., Blakely, R. D., & Amara, S. G. (1991). Expression cloning of a cocaine-and antidepressant-sensitive human noradrenaline transporter. *Nature, 350,* 350–354.

Pandy, G. N., Pandy, S. C., Dwivedi, Y., Sharma, R. P., Janicak, P. G., & Davis, J. M. (1995). Platelet serotonin-2A receptors: A potential biological marker for suicidal behavior. *American Journal of Psychiatry, 152*(6), 850–855.

Pauls, D. L., Alsobrook, J. P., Phil, M., Goodman, W., Rasmussen, S., & Leckman, J. F.

(1995). A family study of obsessive-compulsive disorder. *American Journal of Psychiatry, 152,* 76–84.

Pfefferbaum, A., Roth, W. T., & Ford, J. M. (1995). Event related potentials in the study of psychiatric disorders. *Archives of General Psychiatry, 52,* 559–563.

Plotnikoff, N., Murgo, A., Faith, R., & Wybran, J. (Eds.). (1991). *Stress and immunity.* Boca Raton, FL: CRC.

Post, R. M. (1992). Transduction of psychosocial stress into the neurobiology of recurrent affective disorder. *American Journal of Psychiatry, 149,* 999–1010.

Regier, D. A., Farmer, M. E., & Rae, D. (1990). Comorbidity of mental disorder with alcohol and other drug abuse: Results from the Epidemiologic Catchment Area (ECA) study. *Journal of the American Medical Association, 264,* 2511–2518.

Reich, T., Van Eerdewegh, P., Rice, J., Mullaney, J., Klerman, G. L., & Endicott, J. (1987). The family transmission of primary depressive disorder. *Journal of Psychiatric Research, 21,* 613–624.

Reynolds, G.P., Czudek, C., & Andrews, H. B. (1990). Deficit and hemispheric asymmetry of GABA uptake sites in the hippocampus in schizophrenia. *Biological Psychiatry, 27,* 1038–1044.

Ribeiro, S. C. M., Tandon, R., Grunhaus, L., & Greden, J. F. (1993). The DST as a predictor of outcome in depression: A meta-analysis. *American Journal of Psychiatry, 150*(11), 1618-1629.

Rickels, K., Schweizer, E., Weiss, S., & Zavodnick, S. (1993). Maintenance drug treatment for panic disorder. II. Short- and long-term outcome after drug taper. *Archives of General Psychiatry, 50,* 61–68.

Rogeness, G. A., Javors, M. A., & Pliska, S. R. (1992). Neurochemistry and child and adolescent psychiatry. *Journal of the American Academy of Child Adolescent Psychiatry, 31,* 765–781.

Root, M. P., Fallon, P., & Friedrich, W. N. (1986). *Bulimia: A systems approach to treatment.* New York: Norton.

Rosenthal, R. N. (1995, July/August). Comorbidity of psychiatric and substance use disorders. *Primary Psychiatry,* 42–45.

Rounsaville, B. J., Klerman, G. L., & Weissman, M. M. (1981). Do psychotherapy and pharmacotherapy for depression conflict? Evidence from a clinical trial. *Archives of General Psychiatry, 38,* 24–29.

Schwartz, S. R., & Africa, B. (1988). Schizophrenic disorders. In: H. H. Goldman (Ed.), *Review of general psychiatry.* Norwalk, CT: Appleton & Lange.

Seligman, M. E. P. (1975). *Helplessness: On depression, development, and death.* San Francisco, CA: Freeman.

Semrud-Clikeman, M., Filipek, P. A., & Biederman, J. (1994). Attention deficit hyperactivity disorder: Magnetic resonance imaging morphometric analysis of the corpus collosum. *Journal of the American Academy of Adolescent Psychiatry, 33,* 875–881.

Shaffer, D. (1994). Attention deficit hyperactivity disorder in adults [Editorial]. *American Journal of Psychiatry, 151,* 633–638.

Shaw, B. F. (1977). Comparison of cognitive therapy and behavior therapy in the treatment of depression. *Journal of Consulting Clinical Psychology, 45,* 543–551.

Shea, M. T., Elkin, I., Imber, S. D., Sotsky, S. M.,Watkins, J. T.,Collins, J. F., Pilkonis, P. A., Beckham, E., Glass, D. R., Dolan, R. T., & Parloff, M. B. (1992). Course of depressive symptoms over follow-up: Findings from the National Institute of Mental Health Treatment of Depression Collaborative Research Program. *Archives of General Psychiatry, 49,* 782–787.

Shear, K. M., Cooper, A. M., Klerman, G. L., Busch, F. N., & Shapiro, T. (1993). A psychodynamic model of panic disorder. *American Journal of Psychiatry, 150,* 859–866.

Siever, L. J., & Davis, K. L. (1985). Overview: Toward a dysregulation hypothesis of depression. *American Journal of Psychiatry, 142*(9), 1017–1028.

Silver, J. S., Shin, C., & McNamara, J. O. (1991). Antiepileptogenic effects of conventional anticonsultants in the kindling model of epilepsy. *Annals of Neurology, 5,* 356–363.

Smith, E. M., & North, C. S. (1993). Posttraumatic stress disorder in natural disasters and technological accidents: In J. P. Wilson & B. Raphael (Eds.), *International handbook of traumatic stress syndromes.* (pp. 405–419). New York: Plenum.

Sokoloff, P., Giros, B., Martres, M. P., Bouthenet, M. L., & Schwartz, J. C. (1990). Molecular cloning and characterization of a novel dopamine receptor (D3) as a target for neuroleptics. *Nature, 347,* 146–151.

Solomon, Z., Neria, Y., Ohry, A., Waysman, M., & Ginzburg, K. (1994). PTSD among Israeli former prisoners of war and soldiers with combat stress reaction: A longitudinal study. *American Journal of Psychiatry, 151,* 554–559.

Souetre, E., Salvah, E., Wehs, T., Sack, D., Krebs, B., & Darcourt, G. (1988). Twenty-four hour profiles of body temperature and plasma TSH in bipolar patients during depression and during remission and in normal control subjects. *American Journal of Psychiatry, 145*(9), 1133–1137.

Stein, L. I. (1993). A system approach to reducing relapse in schizophrenia. *Journal of Clinical Psychiatry, 54*(Suppl. 3), 7–12.

Steuer, J. L., Mintz, J., & Hammen, C. L. (1984). Cognitive-behavioral and psychodynamic group psychotherapy in treatment of geriatric depression. *Journal of Consulting Clinical Psychology, 52,* 180–189.

Suddath, R. L., Christison, G. W., Torrey, E. F. et al. (1990). Cerebral anatomical abnormalities in monozygotic twins discordant for schizophrenia. *New England Journal of Medicine, 322,* 541–545.

Sullivan, P. F. (1995). Mortality in anorexia nervosa. *American Journal of Psychiatry, 152,* 1073–1074.

Swedo, S. E., Rapoport, J. L., & Cheslow, D. L. (1989). High prevalence of obsessive-compulsive symptoms in patients with Sydenham's chorea. *American Journal of Psychiatry, 146,* 246–249.

Swerdlow, N. R., Braff, D. L., Taaid, N., & Geyer, M. A. (1994). Assessing the validity of an animal model of deficient sensorimotor gating in schizophrenic patients. *Archives of General Psychiatry, 51,* 139–154.

Thiel, A., Broocks, A., Ohlmeier, M., Jacoby, G. E., & Scubler, G. (1995). Obsessive-compulsive disorder amoung patients with anorexia nervosa and bulimia nervosa. *American Journal of Psychiatry, 152,* 72–75.

Tiihonen, J., Kuikka, J., Hakola, P., Paanila, J., & Airaksinen, J. (1994). Acute ethanol-induced changes in cerebral blood flow. *American Journal of Psychiatry, 151,* 1505–1508.

Torgersen, S. (1983). Genetic factors in anxiety disorder. *Archives of General Psychiatry, 40,* 1085–1089.

Torgersen, S. (1986). Childhood and family characteristics in panic and generalized anxiety disorders. *American Journal of Psychiatry, 143,* 630–632.

Tsai, G., Gastfriend, D. R., & Coyle, J. T. (1995). The glutamatergic basis of human alcoholism. *American Journal of Psychiatry, 152,* 332–340.

Voeller, K. K. S. (1991). What can models of attention, inattention and arousal tell us about attention-deficit hyperactivity disorder? *Journal of Neuropsychiatry, 3*(2), 209–215.

Volkow, N. D., Ding, Y. S., Fowler, J. S., Wang, G. J., Logan, J., Gatley, J. S., Dewey, S., Ashby, C., Lieberman, J., Hitzemann, R., & Wolf, A. P. (1995). Is methylphenidate like cocaine? Studies on their pharmacokinetics and distribution in the human brain. *Archives of General Psychiatry, 52,* 456–463.

Waddington, J. L., Torrey, E. F., Crow, T. J., & Hirsch, S. R. (1991, March). Schizophrenia, neurodevelopment, and disease. *Archives of General Psychiatry, 48,* 271–274

Walters, E. E., & Kendler, K. (1995). Anorexia nervosa and anorexia-like syndromes in a population based female twin sample. *American Journal of Psychiatry, 152,* 64–71.

Watson, R. R. (1992). *Drugs of abuse and neurobiology.* Boca Raton, FL: CRC.

Weinberger, D. R. (1994a, August). Biological basis of schizophrenia: Structural/functional considerations relevant to potential for antipsychotic drug response. *Journal of Clinical Psychiatry Monograph, 12*(2), 4–7.

Weinberger, D. R., Aloia, M. S., Goldberg, T. E., & Berman, K. F. (1994b). The frontal lobes and schizophrenia. *Journal of Neuropsychiatry and Clinical Neurosciences, 6,* 419–427.

Weinberger, D. R., Berman, K. F., Suddath, R., & Torrey, E. F. (1992). Evidence of dysfunctioin of a prefrontal-limbic network in schizophrenia: A magnetic resonance imaging and regional cerebral blood flow study of discordant monozygotic twins. *American Journal of Psychiatry, 149,* 890–897.

Weissman, M. M., Bland, R. C., Canino, G. J., Greenwald, S., Hwu, H. G., Lee, K. C., Newman, S. C., Oakley-Browne, M. A., Rubio-Stipec, M., Wickramaratne, P. J., Wittchen, H. U., & Yeh, E. K. (1994). The cross national epidemiology of obsessive compulsive disorder. *Journal of Clinical Psychiatry, 55*(Suppl. 3), 5–10.

Weissman, M. M., Prusoff, B. A., & DiMascio, A. (1979). The efficacy of drugs and psychotherapy in the treatment of acute depressive episodes. *American Journal of Psychiatry, 136,* 555–558.

Wender, P. H., Reimherr, F. W., & Wood, D. R. (1981). Attention deficit disorder ("minimal brain dysfunction") in adults: A replication study of diagnosis and drug treatment. *Archives of General Psychiatry, 38,* 449–456.

West, S. A., McElroy, S. L., Strakowski, S. M., Keck, P. E., McConville, B. J. (1995). Attention deficit hyperactivity disorder in adolescent mania. *American Journal of Psychiatry, 152*(2), 271–273.

Wexler, B. E. (1991). Failure at task-specific regional activation: New conceptualization of a disease entity. *Journal of Neuropsychiatry, 3,* 94–98.

Winokur, A., Maislin, G., Phillips, J. L., & Amsterdam, J. D. (1988). Insulin resistance after oral glucose tolerance testing in patients with major depression. *American Journal of Psychiatry, 3,* 325–330.

Withers, N. W., Pulvirenti, L., Koob, G. F., & Gillin, J. C. (1995). Cocaine abuse and dependence. *Journal of Clinical Psychopharmacology, 15,* 63–78.

Work Group On Eating Disorders (1993). Practice guideline for eating disorders. *American Journal of Psychiatry, 150*(2), 207–228.

Yehuda, R., Boisoneau, D., Lowy, M.T., & Giller, E. L. (1995). Dose-response changes in plasma cortisol and lymphocyte glucocorticoid receptors following dexamethasone administration in combat veterans with and without posttraumatic stress disorder. *Archives of General Psychiatry, 52,* 583–593.

Yehuda, R., Southwick, S. M., Krysta, J. H., Bremner, D., & Charney, D. S. (1993). Enhanced suppression of cortisol following dexamethasone administration in posttraumatic stress disorder. *American Journal of Psychiatry, 150,* 83–86.

Zametkin, A. J. (1995). Attention-deficit disorder: Born to be hyperactive? *JAMA, 273,* 1871–1874.

CHAPTER 4

Cutler, P. (1991). Iron overload in psychiatric illness [Letter to the editor]. *American Journal of Psychiatry, 148,* 147–148.

Drooker, M. A., & Byck, R. (1992, July). Physical disorders presenting as psychiatric illness: A new view. *The Psychiatric Times,* 19–24.

Fernandez, F., Levy, J. K., Lachar, B. L., & Small, G. W. (1995). The management of depression and anxiety in the elderly. *Journal of Clinical Psychiatry, 56*(Suppl. 2), 20–29.

Lindenbaum, J., Healton, E. B., Savage, D. G., Brust, J. C. M., & Garrett, T. J. (1988). Neuropsychiatric disorders caused by cobalamin deficiency in the absence of anemia or macrocytosis. *New England Journal of Medicine, 318,* 1720–1728.

Martin, M. J. (1983). A brief review of organic diseases masquerading as functional illness. *Hospital and Community Psychiatry, 34,* 328–332.

Tohen, M., Shulman, K. I., & Satlin, A. (1994). First-episode mania in late life. *American Journal of Psychiatry, 151,* 130–132.

Wise, M. G., & Griffiess, W. S. (1995). A combined treatment approach to anxiety in the medically ill. *Journal of Clinical Psychiatry, 56*(Suppl. 2), 14–19.

CHAPTER 5

Angst, J. (1988). *Suicides among depressive and bipolar patients.* Paper presented at the 141st annual meeting of the American Psychiatric Association, Los Angeles, CA.

Ansseau, M., & De Roeck, J. (1993). Trazodone in benzodiazepine dependence. *Journal of Clinical Psychiatry, 54,* 189–191.

Ashbrook, J. B. (1995). Psychopharmacology and pastoral counseling: Medication and meaning. *The Journal of Pastoral Care, 49,* 5–17.

Baldessarini, R. J., & Viguera, A. C. (1995). Neuroleptic withdrawal in schizophrenic patients. *Archives of General Psychiatry, 52,* 189–191.

Black, D. W., Winokur, G., & Nasrallah, A. (1987). Is death from natural causes still excessive in psychiatric patients? A follow-up of 1593 patients with major affective disorder. *Journal of Nervous and Mental Disease, 175,* 674–680.

Brandes, L. J., & Cheang, M. (1995). Letter regarding "Response to antidepessants and cancer: Cause for concern?" [Letter to the editor]. *Journal of Clinical Psychopharmacology, 15,* 84–85.

Dalton, K. (1984). *The premenstrual syndrome and progesterone therapy* (2nd ed.). Chicago: Year Book.

Do you put yourself at risk by doing medication backup? (1995, June 16). *Psychiatric News,* pp. 15, 20.

Fava, M., & Kaji, J. (1994). Continuation and maintenance treatments of major depressive disorder. *Psychiatric Annals, 24,* 281–290.

Fawcett, J. (1995). Compliance: Definitions and key issues. *Journal of Clinical Psychiatry, 56*(Suppl. 1), 4–8.

Frank, E., Kupfer, D. J., Perel, J. M., Cornes, C., Jarrett, D. B., & Mallinger, A. G. (1990). Three-year outcomes for maintenance therapies in recurrent depression. *Archives of General Psychiatry, 47,* 1093–1099.

Goodwin, F. K., & Jamison, K. R. (1990). *Manic depressive illness.* New York: Oxford University Press.

Greden, J. F. (1993). Antidepressant maintenance medications: When to discontinue and how to stop. *Journal of Clinical Psychiatry, 54*(Suppl. 8), 39–45.

Greden, J. F., & Tandon, R. (1995). Long-term treatment for lifetime disorders? *Archives of General Psychiatry, 52,* 197–199.

Greenblatt, D. J., & Shader, R. I. (1992). Mental Illness, psychopharmacotherapy, and automobile operation: What is the risk? [Editorial]. *Journal of Clinical Psychopharmacology, 12,* 382.

Hansten, P. D., & Horn, J. R. (1990). Drug interaction mechanisms and clinical characteristics. In *Drug interactions and updates.* Vancouver, WA: Applied Therapeutics.

Hedaya, R. J. (1984). Pharmacokinetic factors in the clinical use of tryptophan. *Journal of Clinical Psychopharmacology, 4*(6), 347–348.

Hirschfeld, R. M. A. (1994). Guidelines for the long-term treatment of depression. *Journal of Clinical Psychiatry, 55*(Suppl. 12), 61–69.

Hurowitz, G. I., & Liebowitz, M. (1993). Antidepressant-induced rapid cycling: Six case reprts. *Journal of Clinical Psychopharmacology, 13,* 52–56.

Jeste, D. V., Gilbert, P. L., McAdams, L. A., & Harris, M. J. (1995). Considering neuroleptic maintenance and taper on a continuum: Need for individual rather than dogmatic approach. *Archives of General Psychiatry, 52,* 209–212.

Kerr, M. E., & Bowen, M. (1988). *Family evaluation: An approach based on Bowen theory.* New York: Norton.

Kupfer, D. J., Frank, E., Perel, J. M., Cornes, C., Mallinger, A. G., Thase, M. E., McEachran, A. B., & Grochocinski, V. J. (1992). Five-year outcome for maintenance therapies in recurrent depression. *Archives of General Psychiatry, 49,* 769–773.

Leonard, H. L., Swedo, S. E., & Lenane, M. C. (1993). A 2- to 7-year follow-up study of 54 obsessive-compulsive children and adolescents. *Archives of General Psychiatry, 50,* 429–439.

Linnoila, M. (1992). Psychotropic medications and traffic safety. *Journal of Clinical Psychopharmacolgy, 12,* 384–385.

Maj, M., Veltro, F., Pirozzi, R., Lobrace, S., & Magliano, L. (1992). Pattern of recurrence of illness after recovery from an episode of major depression: A prospective study. *American Journal of Psychiatry, 149,* 795–800.

Matheson, I., Pande, H., & Alertsen, A. R. (1985). Respiratory depression caused by N-desmethyldoxepin in breast milk [Letter to the editor]. *Lancet, 2,* 1124.

Miller, G. M. (1995). Psychopharmacologic agents and cancer: A progress report [Editorial]. *Journal of Clinical Psychopharmacology, 15,* 160.

Miller, H. L., Pedro, D. L., Salomon, R. M., Licinio, J., Barr, L. C., & Carney, D. S. (1992). Acute tryptophan depletion: A method of studying antidepressant action. *Journal of Clinical Psychiatry, 53*(Suppl. 10), 28–35.

Miller, L. G. (1993). Antidepressants and cancer:cause for concern? [Editorial]. *Journal of Clinical Psychopharmacology, 13,* 1–2.

Nichol, M. B., Stimmel, G. L., & Lange, S. C. (1995). Factors predicting the use of multiple psychotropic medications. *Journal of Clinical Psychiatry, 56,* 60–66.

Parry, B. L. (1995). Mood disorders linked to the reproductive cycle in women. In F. E. Bloom & D. J. Kupfer (Eds.), *Psychopharmacology: The fourth generation of progress* (pp. 1024–1042). New York: Raven.

Pollack, M. H., & Otto, M. W. (1994). Long-term pharmacologic treatment of panic disorder. *Psychiatric Annals, 24,* 291–298.

Post, R. M. (1993). Issues in the long-term management of bipolar affective illness. *Psychiatric Annals, 23,* 86–93.

Racey, J. C. (1995, June). Integration of psychotherapy and pharmacotherapy. Part I: Applying theory to improve patient health. *Psychiatric Times,* 30–31.

Ratey, J. J. (Ed.). (1995). *Neuropsychiatry of personality disorders.* Cambridge, MA: Blackwell Science.

Rogers, W. H., Wells, K. B., Meredith, L. S., Sturm, R., Burnam, M. A. (1993). Outcomes for adult outpatients with depression under prepaid or fee-for-service financing. *Archives of General Psychiatry, 50*(7), 517–525.

Salzman, C., Wolfson, A. N., Schatzberg, A., Looper, J., Henke, R., & Albanese, M. (1995). Effect of fluoxetine on anger in symptomatic volunteers with borderline personality disorder. *Journal of Clinical Psychopharmacology, 15,* 23–29.

Schubiner, H., Tzelepis, A., Isaacson, H. J., Warbasse, L. H., Zacharek, M., & Musial, J. (1995). The dual diagnosis of attention deficit/hyperactivity disorder and substance abuse: Case reports and literature review. *Journal of Clinical Psychiatry, 56,* 146–150.

Schwartz, J. (1995, August 24). Pharmacies told to give patients full drug data. *The Washington Post,* p. A17.

Stokes, P. E. (1993). A primary care perspective on management of acute and long-term depression. *Journal of Clinical Psychiatry, 54*(Suppl. 8), 74–84.

Wisner, K. L., & Perel, J. M. (1988). Psychopharmacologic agents and electroconvulsive therapy during pregnancy and the puerperium. In R.L. Cohen (Ed.), *Psychiatric consultation in childbirth settings.* New York: Plenum.

Wisner, K. L., Perel, J. M., Foglia, J. P. (1995). Serum clomipramine and metabolite levels in four nursing mother-infant pairs. *Journal of Clinical Psychiatry, 56,* 17–20.

Wisner, K. L., Perel, J. M., & Wheeler, S. B. (1993). Tricyclic dose requirements across pregnancy. *American Journal of Psychiatry, 150,* 1541–1542.

CHAPTER 6

Dalton, K. (1984). *The premenstrual syndrome and progesterone therapy* (2nd ed.). Chicago: Year Book.

Goodwin, F. K., & Jamison, K. R. (1990). *Manic depressive illness.* New York: Oxford University Press.

Kraepelin, E. (1921). *Manic depressive insanity and paranoia* (R. M. Barclay, Trans., G. M. Robertson, Ed.). Edinburgh, Scotland: Livingstone.

Post, R. M. (1990). Alternatives to lithium for bipolar affective illness. In A. Tasman, S. M. Goldfinger, C. A. Kaufmann (Eds.), *Review of Psychiatry* (Vol. 9, pp. 170–202). Washington, DC: American Psychiatric Press.

Index

295